2012
YEAR BOOK OF
ONCOLOGY®

The 2012 Year Book Series

Year Book of Anesthesiology and Pain Management™: Drs Chestnut, Abram, Black, Gravlee, Lien, Mathru, and Roizen

Year Book of Cardiology®: Drs Gersh, Cheitlin, Elliott, Gold, Graham, and Thourani

Year Book of Critical Care Medicine®: Drs Dries, Zanotti-Cavazzoni, Latenser, Martinez, Rincon, and Zwank

Year Book of Dermatology and Dermatologic Surgery™: Dr Del Rosso

Year Book of Diagnostic Radiology®: Drs Elster, Abbara, Oestreich, Offiah, Rosado de Christenson, Stephens, and Strickland

Year Book of Emergency Medicine®: Drs Hamilton, Bruno, Handly, Minczak, Mullin, Quintana, and Ramoska

Year Book of Endocrinology®: Drs Schott, Apovian, Clarke, Eugster, Meikle, Oetgen, Ovalle, Schteingart, and Toth

Year Book of Hand and Upper Limb Surgery®: Drs Yao, Adams, Isaacs, Lee, and Rizzo

Year Book of Medicine®: Drs Barker, Garrick, Gersh, Khardori, LeRoith, Panush, Talley, and Thigpen

Year Book of Neonatal and Perinatal Medicine®: Drs Fanaroff, Benitz, Donn, Neu, Papile, and Van Marter

Year Book of Neurology and Neurosurgery®: Drs Klimo, Minagar, Gandhi, House, Kevill, Liu, Mazia, Panagariya, Ragel, Riesenburger, Robottom, Schwendimann, Shafazand, Uhm, and Yang

Year Book of Obstetrics, Gynecology, and Women's Health®: Drs Dungan and Shulman

Year Book of Oncology®: Drs Arceci, Bauer, Chiorean, Gordon, Lawton, Murphy, Thigpen, and Tsao

Year Book of Ophthalmology®: Drs Rapuano, Cohen, Flanders, Hammersmith, Milman, Myers, Nagra, Nelson, Penne, Pyfer, Sergott, Shields, Talekar, and Vander

Year Book of Orthopedics®: Drs Morrey, Huddleston, Rose, Swiontkowski, and Trigg

Year Book of Otolaryngology-Head and Neck Surgery®: Drs Sindwani, Balough, Franco, Gapany, and Mitchell

Year Book of Pathology and Laboratory Medicine®: Drs Raab and Bissell

Year Book of Pediatrics®: Dr Stockman

Year Book of Plastic and Aesthetic Surgery™: Drs Miller, Gosman, Gurtner, Gutowski, Ruberg, Salisbury, and Smith

Year Book of Psychiatry and Applied Mental Health®: Drs Talbott, Ballenger, Buckley, Frances, Krupnick, and Mack

Year Book of Pulmonary Disease®: Drs Barker, Jones, Maurer, Spradley, Tanoue, and Willsie

Year Book of Sports Medicine®: Drs Shephard, Cantu, Feldman, Galea, Jankowski, Janssen, Lebrun, and Nieman

Year Book of Surgery®: Drs Copeland, Behrns, Daly, Eberlein, Fahey, Huber, Klodell, Mozingo, and Pruett

Year Book of Urology®: Drs Andriole and Coplen

Year Book of Vascular Surgery®: Drs Moneta, Gillespie, Starnes, and Watkins

Year Book of Psychiatry and Applied Mental Health®: Drs Talbott, Ballenger, Buckley, Frances, Krupnick, and Mack

Year Book of Pulmonary Disease®: Drs Barker, Jones, Maurer, Spradley, Tanoue, and Willsie

Year Book of Sports Medicine®: Drs Shephard, Cantu, Feldman, Galea, Jankowski, Janssen, Lebrun, and Nieman

Year Book of Surgery®: Drs Copeland, Behrns, Daly, Eberlein, Fahey, Huber, Klodell, Mozingo, and Pruett

Year Book of Urology®: Drs Andriole and Coplen

Year Book of Vascular Surgery®: Drs Moneta, Gillespie, Starnes, and Watkins

2012 The Year Book of ONCOLOGY®

Editor-in-Chief

Robert J. Arceci, MD, PhD

King Fahd Professor of Pediatric Oncology, Johns Hopkins University, Johns Hopkins Hospital, Baltimore, Maryland

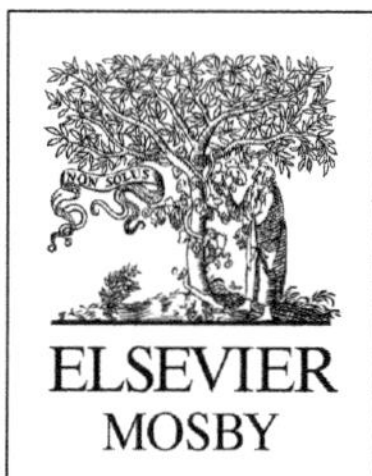

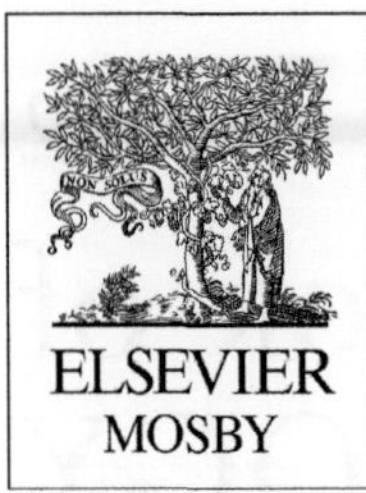

Vice President, Continuity: Kimberly Murphy
Editor: Yonah Korngold
Production Supervisor, Electronic Year Books: Donna M. Skelton
Electronic Article Manager: Emily Ogle
Illustrations and Permissions Coordinator: Dawn Vohsen

2012 EDITION

Composition by TNQ Books and Journals Pvt Ltd, India

Editorial Office:
Elsevier
Suite 1800
1600 John F. Kennedy Blvd.
Philadelphia, PA 19103-2899

International Standard Serial Number: 1040-1741
International Standard Book Number: 978-0-323-08885-5

Printed and bound by CPI Group (UK) Ltd, Croydon, CR0 4YY
Transferred to digital print 2012

Editorial Board

Contributors

Jeffrey M. Albert, MD

Department of Radiation Oncology, The University of Texas MD Anderson Cancer Center, Houston, Texas

Thomas A. Aloia, MD

Assistant Professor, Department of Surgical Oncology, The University of Texas MD Anderson Cancer Center, Houston, Texas

Matthew T. Ballo, MD

Professor, Department of Radiation Oncology, The University of Texas MD Anderson Cancer Center, Houston, Texas

John R. Benson, MA, DM (Oxon), MD (Cantab), FRCS

Consultant Surgeon, Cambridge Breast Unit, Addenbrooke's Hospital Cambridge, Fellow and Director of Clinical Studies, Selwyn College, Cambridge, Professor of Applied Surgical Sciences, Anglia Ruskin University, Cambridge, United Kingdom

Elizabeth S. Bloom, MD

Associate Professor of Radiation Oncology, Division of Radiation Oncology, The University of Texas MD Anderson Cancer Center, Radiation Treatment Center at Bellaire, Houston, Texas

Table of Contents

Editorial Board vii

Journals Represented xiii

1. Cancer Biology 1

2. Cancer Prevention 5

3. Cancer Therapies 7

4. Chemotherapy: Mechanisms and Side Effects 9

5. Breast Cancer 11

General Issues in Breast Cancer 11

Epidemiology 16

Prevention 18

Early Stage and Adjuvant Therapy 20

Breast Conserving Therapy 31

Diagnostic Imaging 34

Prognostic Factors 38

Radiation Therapy 42

Surgical Treatment 55

Tumor Biology 65

Axillary Management 66

Hormonal Therapy 68

Intraductal Cancer 71

Non-Invasive Cancer 72

Advanced 74

Miscellaneous 77

6. Genitourinary 81

Prostate 81

Testis 99

7. Gynecology 103

Ovarian 103

Cervix 122

Endometrial 127

Miscellaneous 132

8. Gastrointestinal 135
- Screening and Detection 135
- Esophagus, Stomach 136
- Pancreas 141
- Rectal Carcinoma 142
- Colorectal Cancer 145

9. Hematologic Malignancies 147
- Leukemia and Myelodysplastic Syndrome 147
- Lymphoma 167

10. Thoracic Cancer 169
- Biology 169
- Non–Small-Cell: Early Stage and Adjuvant Therapy 171
- First-Line Metastatic Non–Small-Cell Lung Cancer 178
- Second-Line Metastatic Non–Small-Cell Lung Cancer 187
- Small-Cell Lung Cancer 189
- Advanced Diseases 192
- Miscellaneous 196

11. Endocrine 199

12. Head and Neck 201

13. Pediatric Cancer 205
- Leukemia 205
- Neuro-Oncology 211
- Solid Tumors 215
- Miscellaneous 223

14. Melanoma 225

15. Sarcoma 227

16. Late Effects of Therapy 229

17. Novel Targets 237

18. Supportive Care 239

19. Miscellaneous 243

Article Index 245

Author Index 255

Journals Represented

Journals represented in this Year Book are listed below.

AJR American Journal of Roentgenology
American Journal of Clinical Nutrition
American Journal of Obstetrics and Gynecology
American Journal of Surgery
Annals of Internal Medicine
Annals of Surgical Oncology
Blood
Breast Journal
British Journal of Cancer
British Journal of Surgery
Cancer
European Journal of Surgical Oncology
Gynecologic Oncology
International Journal of Radiation Oncology Biology Physics
Journal of Clinical Oncology
Journal of the American College of Surgeons
Journal of the American Medical Association
Journal of the National Cancer Institute
Journal of Thoracic Oncology
Journal of Urology
Lancet
Nature
New England Journal of Medicine
Practical Radiation Oncology
Radiology
Radiotherapy & Oncology
Surgical Oncology

Standard Abbreviations

The following terms are abbreviated in this edition: acquired immunodeficiency syndrome (AIDS), cardiopulmonary resuscitation (CPR), central nervous system (CNS), cerebrospinal fluid (CSF), computed tomography (CT), deoxyribonucleic acid (DNA), electrocardiography (ECG), health maintenance organization (HMO), human immunodeficiency virus (HIV), intensive care unit (ICU), intramuscular (IM), intravenous (IV), magnetic resonance (MR) imaging (MRI), ribonucleic acid (RNA), ultrasound (US), and ultraviolet (UV).

Note

To facilitate the use of the YEAR BOOK OF ONCOLOGY as a reference tool, all illustrations and tables included in this publication are now identified as they appear in the original article. This change is meant to help the reader recognize that any illustration or table appearing in the YEAR BOOK OF ONCOLOGY may be only one of many in the original article. For this reason, figure and table numbers will often appear to be out of sequence within the YEAR BOOK OF ONCOLOGY.

1 Cancer Biology

Clinically Relevant Changes in Family History of Cancer Over Time

Ziogas A, Horick NK, Kinney AY, et al (Univ of California–Irvine; Massachusetts General Hosp Biostatistics Ctr, Boston; Huntsman Cancer Inst and Univ of Utah, Salt Lake City; et al)

JAMA 306:172-178, 2011

Context.—Knowledge of family cancer history is important for assessing cancer risk and guiding screening recommendations.

Objective.—To quantify how often throughout adulthood clinically significant changes occur in cancer family history that would result in recommendations for earlier or intense screening.

Design and Setting.—Descriptive study examining baseline and follow-up family history data from participants in the Cancer Genetics Network (CGN), a US national population-based cancer registry, between 1999 and 2009.

Participants.—Adults with a personal history, family history, or both of cancer enrolled in the CGN through population-based cancer registries. Retrospective colorectal, breast, and prostate cancer screening-specific analyses included 9861, 2547, and 1817 participants, respectively; prospective analyses included 1533, 617, and 163 participants, respectively. Median follow-up was 8 years (range, 0-11 years). Screening-specific analyses excluded participants with the cancer of interest.

Main Outcome Measures.—Percentage of individuals with clinically significant family histories and rate of change over 2 periods: (1) retrospectively, from birth until CGN enrollment and (2) prospectively, from enrollment to last follow-up.

Results.—Retrospective analysis revealed that the percentages of participants who met criteria for high-risk screening based on family history at ages 30 and 50 years, respectively, were as follows: for colorectal cancer, 2.1% (95% confidence interval [CI], 1.8%-2.4%) and 7.1% (95% CI, 6.5%-7.6%); for breast cancer, 7.2% (95% CI, 6.1%-8.4%) and 11.4% (95% CI, 10.0%-12.8%); and for prostate cancer, 0.9% (95% CI, 0.5%-1.4%) and 2.0% (95% CI, 1.4%-2.7%). In prospective analysis, the numbers of participants who newly met criteria for high-risk screening based on family history per 100 persons followed up for 20 years were 2 (95% CI, 0-7) for colorectal cancer, 6 (95% CI, 2-13) for breast cancer, and 8 (95% CI, 3-16) for prostate cancer. The rate of change in cancer family history was similar for colorectal and breast cancer between the 2 analyses.

Conclusion.—Clinically relevant family history of colorectal, breast, and prostate cancer that would result in recommendations for earlier or intense cancer screening increases between ages 30 and 50 years, although the absolute rate is low for prostate cancer.

▶ Documentation of family history of cancer is an important catalyst for primary care physicians to order screening tests. It is also critically important for the average person as they ponder which screening tests are worth having and therefore supporting financially. Certainly we as oncologists use family history of cancer routinely as we consider options for patients and as we give recommendations for screening of other (generally younger) family members.

The reality is, though, that family history changes over time; whereas a given person may have no first-degree relatives with cancer as a young adult, by the time they reach their 50s, this can change. Documenting this potential change in family history is the basis for the analysis of the Cancer Genetics Network.

The results of these data support the concern of a potential significant change in family history between the ages of 30 to 50 years. Given these results, it reinforces the point of updating family history with annual visits to primary care providers and oncologists. This updated information can help guide appropriate screening in these people.

C. Lawton, MD

Intratumor Heterogeneity and Branched Evolution Revealed by Multiregion Sequencing

Gerlinger M, Rowan AJ, Horswell S, et al (Cancer Res UK London Res Inst; et al)

N Engl J Med 366:883-892, 2012

Background.—Intratumor heterogeneity may foster tumor evolution and adaptation and hinder personalized-medicine strategies that depend on results from single tumor-biopsy samples.

Methods.—To examine intratumor heterogeneity, we performed exome sequencing, chromosome aberration analysis, and ploidy profiling on multiple spatially separated samples obtained from primary renal carcinomas and associated metastatic sites. We characterized the consequences of intratumor heterogeneity using immunohistochemical analysis, mutation functional analysis, and profiling of messenger RNA expression.

Results.—Phylogenetic reconstruction revealed branched evolutionary tumor growth, with 63 to 69% of all somatic mutations not detectable across every tumor region. Intratumor heterogeneity was observed for a mutation within an autoinhibitory domain of the mammalian target of rapamycin (mTOR) kinase, correlating with S6 and 4EBP phosphorylation in vivo and constitutive activation of mTOR kinase activity in vitro. Mutational intratumor heterogeneity was seen for multiple tumor-suppressor genes converging on loss of function; *SETD2, PTEN, and KDM5C* underwent multiple distinct and spatially separated inactivating mutations within a single tumor, suggesting convergent phenotypic evolution. Gene-expression signatures of good and poor prognosis were detected in different regions of the same tumor. Allelic composition and ploidy profiling analysis revealed extensive intratumor heterogeneity, with 26 of 30 tumor samples from four tumors harboring divergent allelic-imbalance profiles and with ploidy heterogeneity in two of four tumors.

Conclusions.—Intratumor heterogeneity can lead to underestimation of the tumor genomics landscape portrayed from single tumor-biopsy samples and may present major challenges to personalized-medicine and biomarker development. Intratumor heterogeneity, associated with heterogeneous protein function, may foster tumor adaptation and therapeutic failure through Darwinian selection. (Funded by the Medical Research Council and others.)

▶ The existence of de novo or acquired resistance to chemotherapeutic treatment for cancer remains the primary reason for disease progression and death. Most studies documenting such resistance signatures have been based on what one might best call *population* biology as a result of taking a tumor sample and assessing molecular changes that could be used to define pathways of resistance to chemotherapy. However, like most aspects of life, such a result is based on an oversimplification. As Einstein said, "Make it as simple as possible, but not too simple." Gerlinger et al now report on the regional molecular heterogeneity within primary renal cell cancer and metastases. The striking aspects of these data are that there exist quite profound regional differences within any tumor specimen, predicting that it will be particularly challenging to develop curative treatments. However, such studies have not addressed the issue of whether there exists a common (or possibly less heterogeneous) tumor-initiating population of cells that might be more effectively eradicated. After all, some patients with cancer are in fact cured. Future work will clearly need to find common molecular ground, or it shall be a long time before most patients with cancer can expect curative treatment.

R. J. Arceci, MD, PhD

2 Cancer Prevention

Effect of daily aspirin on risk of cancer metastasis: a study of incident cancers during randomised controlled trials

Rothwell PM, Wilson M, Price JF, et al (Univ of Oxford, UK; Univ of Edinburgh, UK; et al)

Lancet 379:1591-1601, 2012

Background.—Daily aspirin reduces the long-term incidence of some adenocarcinomas, but effects on mortality due to some cancers appear after only a few years, suggesting that it might also reduce growth or metastasis. We established the frequency of distant metastasis in patients who developed cancer during trials of daily aspirin versus control.

Methods.—Our analysis included all five large randomised trials of daily aspirin (≥75 mg daily) versus control for the prevention of vascular events in the UK. Electronic and paper records were reviewed for all patients with incident cancer. The effect of aspirin on risk of metastases at presentation or on subsequent follow-up (including post-trial follow-up of in-trial cancers) was stratified by tumour histology (adenocarcinoma *vs* other) and clinical characteristics.

Findings.—Of 17 285 trial participants, 987 had a new solid cancer diagnosed during mean in-trial follow-up of 6·5 years (SD 2·0). Allocation to aspirin reduced risk of cancer with distant metastasis (all cancers, hazard ratio [HR] 0·64, 95% CI 0·48–0·84, $p = 0{\cdot}001$; adenocarcinoma, HR 0·54, 95% CI 0·38–0·77, $p = 0{\cdot}0007$; other solid cancers, HR 0·82, 95% CI 0·53–1·28, $p = 0{\cdot}39$), due mainly to a reduction in proportion of adenocarcinomas that had metastatic versus local disease (odds ratio 0·52, 95% CI 0·35–0·75, $p = 0{\cdot}0006$). Aspirin reduced risk of adenocarcinoma with metastasis at initial diagnosis (HR 0·69, 95% CI 0·50–0·95, $p = 0{\cdot}02$) and risk of metastasis on subsequent follow-up in patients without metastasis initially (HR 0·45, 95% CI 0·28–0·72, $p = 0{\cdot}0009$), particularly in patients with colorectal cancer (HR 0·26, 95% CI 0·11–0·57, $p = 0{\cdot}0008$) and in patients who remained on trial treatment up to or after diagnosis (HR 0·31, 95% CI 0·15–0·62, $p = 0{\cdot}0009$). Allocation to aspirin reduced death due to cancer in patients who developed adenocarcinoma, particularly in those without metastasis at diagnosis (HR 0·50, 95% CI 0·34–0·74, $p = 0{\cdot}0006$). Consequently, aspirin reduced the overall risk of fatal adenocarcinoma in the trial populations (HR 0·65, 95% CI 0·53–0·82, $p = 0{\cdot}0002$), but not the risk of other fatal cancers (HR 1·06, 95% CI 0·84–1·32, $p = 0{\cdot}64$; difference, $p = 0{\cdot}003$). Effects were independent of age and sex, but absolute benefit was greatest in smokers.

A low-dose, slow-release formulation of aspirin designed to inhibit platelets but to have little systemic bioavailability was as effective as higher doses.

Interpretation.—That aspirin prevents distant metastasis could account for the early reduction in cancer deaths in trials of daily aspirin versus control. This finding suggests that aspirin might help in treatment of some cancers and provides proof of principle for pharmacological intervention specifically to prevent distant metastasis.

▶ This article looks at 5 randomized trials of aspirin versus no therapy to prevent vascular events in the United Kingdom. A total 17 285 individuals participated in these 5 studies. The objective of the study was to determine whether aspirin could reduce or prevent the diagnosis of cancers with metastases at initial diagnosis. Among the participants, 987 cancers were diagnosed. In the individuals on aspirin, the risk of a new solid cancer with metastases at diagnosis was reduced by 36% (hazard ratio [HR] = 0.64; *P* = .001). The likelihood of adenocarcinomas was impacted more (HR = 0.54; *P* = .0007) than other histologies. In particular, there was a major reduction in metastatic adenocarcinoma of the colon. In addition, the risk of fatal adenocarcinoma was reduced substantially (HR = 0.65; *P* = .0002). Low-dose, slow release formulations were as effective as higher doses of aspirin. These data suggest that the beneficial effects of daily aspirin extend beyond vascular disease and include a reduction in the likelihood of developing metastatic adenocarcinomas particularly of the colon. Aspirin, anyone?

J. T. Thigpen, MD

3 Cancer Therapies

American society for radiation oncology (ASTRO) and american college of radiology (ACR) practice guideline for the performance of high-dose-rate brachytherapy

Erickson BA, Demanes DJ, Ibbott GS, et al (Med College of Wisconsin, Milwaukee; Univ of California, Los Angeles; MD Anderson Cancer Ctr, Houston, TX; et al)

Int J Radiat Oncol Biol Phys 79:641-649, 2011

High-Dose-Rate (HDR) brachytherapy is a safe and efficacious treatment option for patients with a variety of different malignancies. Careful adherence to established standards has been shown to improve the likelihood of procedural success and reduce the incidence of treatment-related morbidity. A collaborative effort of the American College of Radiology (ACR) and American Society for Therapeutic Radiation Oncology (ASTRO) has produced a practice guideline for HDR brachytherapy.

The guideline defines the qualifications and responsibilities of all the involved personnel, including the radiation oncologist, physicist and dosimetrists. Review of the leading indications for HDR brachytherapy in the management of gynecologic, thoracic, gastrointestinal, breast, urologic, head and neck, and soft tissue tumors is presented. Logistics with respect to the brachytherapy implant procedures and attention to radiation safety procedures and documentation are presented. Adherence to these practice guidelines can be part of ensuring quality and safety in a successful HDR brachytherapy program.

► Brachytherapy is a form of radiation therapy that has been used for over a century. The number of tumor types for which brachytherapy has been used is large, and equally large is the number of ways in which brachytherapy has been applied to these varied malignancies.

Most of the brachytherapy that has been performed over the last century would be considered low dose rate. This article is a discussion of appropriate guidelines for high-dose-rate (HDR) brachytherapy, (HDR being defined as > 20 cGy/minute to a point or volume).

The take-home message from this article is 2-fold. First, HDR brachytherapy is excellent treatment for a wide variety of malignancies if done correctly. Second, to perform HDR brachytherapy well, there must be a well-informed team of physicians, physicists, dosimetrists, radiation therapists, and nurses who work in concert to bring about the best results for the patient.

C. Lawton, MD

4 Chemotherapy: Mechanisms and Side Effects

Appropriate Chemotherapy Dosing for Obese Adult Patients With Cancer: American Society of Clinical Oncology Clinical Practice Guideline

Griggs JJ, Mangu PB, Anderson H, et al (Univ of Michigan, Ann Arbor; American Society of Clinical Oncology, Alexandria, VA; Breast Cancer Coalition of Rochester, NY; et al)

J Clin Oncol 30:1553-1561, 2012

Purpose.—To provide recommendations for appropriate cytotoxic chemotherapy dosing for obese adult patients with cancer.

Methods.—The American Society of Clinical Oncology convened a Panel of experts in medical and gynecologic oncology, clinical pharmacology, pharmacokinetics and pharmacogenetics, and biostatistics and a patient representative. MEDLINE searches identified studies published in English between 1996 and 2010, and a systematic review of the literature was conducted. A majority of studies involved breast, ovarian, colon, and lung cancers. This guideline does not address dosing for novel targeted agents.

Results.—Practice pattern studies demonstrate that up to 40% of obese patients receive limited chemotherapy doses that are not based on actual body weight. Concerns about toxicity or overdosing in obese patients with cancer, based on the use of actual body weight, are unfounded.

Recommendations.—The Panel recommends that full weight–based cytotoxic chemotherapy doses be used to treat obese patients with cancer, particularly when the goal of treatment is cure. There is no evidence that short- or long-term toxicity is increased among obese patients receiving full weight–based doses. Most data indicate that myelosuppression is the same or less pronounced among the obese than the non-obese who are administered full weight-based doses. Clinicians should respond to all treatment-related toxicities in obese patients in the same ways they do for non-obese patients. The use of fixed-dose chemotherapy is rarely justified, but the Panel does recommend fixed dosing for a few select agents. The

Panel recommends further research into the role of pharmacokinetics and pharmacogenetics to guide appropriate dosing of obese patients with cancer.

▶ This article reports the results of the deliberations of an American Society of Clinical Oncology expert panel on the questions surrounding appropriate dosing for the obese patients. Traditionally, these patients have had doses of chemotherapeutic agents capped usually at a body surface area of either 2 or 2.2 m^2. The panel concluded that obese patients should be treated with full doses based on either weight or body surface area as calculated by standard formulae. These recommendations seem relatively straightforward but deserve a cautionary note. As noted in the panel's report, the conclusions are based on a very limited number of randomized clinical trials, and it seems unlikely that there will be more data forthcoming addressing these questions. Most oncologists recognize the importance of maintaining relative dose intensity at least up to a point, but if the recommendations are to be followed, the patient should be informed of the potential risk of being overdosed. Furthermore, the oncologist must be prepared to deal with anticipated toxicity and to adjust doses as needed based on observed toxicity.

J. T. Thigpen, MD

5 Breast Cancer

General Issues in Breast Cancer

Characteristics and Outcomes of Breast Cancer in Women With and Without a History of Radiation for Hodgkin's Lymphoma: A Multi-Institutional, Matched Cohort Study

Elkin EB, Klem ML, Gonzales AM, et al (Memorial Sloan Kettering Cancer Ctr, NY; Exempla St Joseph Hosp, Denver, CO; et al)

J Clin Oncol 29:2466-2473, 2011

Purpose.—To compare characteristics and outcomes of breast cancer in women with and without a history of radiation therapy (RT) for Hodgkin's lymphoma (HL).

Patients and Methods.—Women with breast cancer diagnosed from 1980 to 2006 after RT for HL were identified from eight North American hospitals and were matched three-to-one with patients with sporadic breast cancer by age, race, and year of breast cancer diagnosis. Information on patient, tumor and treatment characteristics, and clinical outcomes was abstracted from medical records.

Results.—A total of 253 patients with breast cancer with a history of RT for HL were matched with 741 patients with sporadic breast cancer. Median time from HL to breast cancer diagnosis was 18 years. Median age at breast cancer diagnosis was 42 years. Breast cancer after RT for HL was more likely to be detected by screening, was more likely to be diagnosed at an earlier stage, and was more likely to be bilateral at diagnosis. HL survivors had an increased risk of metachronous contralateral breast cancer (adjusted hazard ratio [HR], 4.3; 95% CI, 1.7 to 11.0) and death as a result of any cause (adjusted HR, 1.9; 95% CI, 1.1 to 3.3). Breast cancer–specific mortality was also elevated, but this difference was not statistically significant (adjusted HR, 1.6; 95% CI, 0.7 to 3.4).

Conclusion. In women with a history of RT for HL, breast cancer is diagnosed at an earlier stage, but these women are at greater risk for bilateral disease and are more likely to die as a result of causes other than breast cancer. Our findings support close follow-up for contralateral tumors in these patients and ongoing primary care to manage comorbid conditions.

▶ To understand the implications of the data presented by Elkin and colleagues, we need to understand the background.

On the one hand, a high cure rate after combined chemotherapy and RT in patients with HL is a great achievement. On the other hand, the chemoradiation regimen applied in this setting in the early days from 1950 until the beginning of the 1990s was costly. Patients who survived for decades eventually suffered from secondary side effects, including cardiac toxic effects and second malignancies, and the latter became the leading cause of death in long-term HL survivors.[1,2]

The realization that the treatment of HL caused such toxic effects led to several randomized trials that shifted the practice of both medical and radiation oncologists. The toxic chemotherapy regimen of mechlorethamine, vincristine, procarbazine, and prednisone was replaced by doxorubicin, bleomycin, vinblastine, and dacarbazine[3,4]; eventually, the number of cycles of doxorubicin, bleomycin, vinblastine, and dacarbazine was reduced, and the number of cycles is now determined according to risk groups. Radiation dose, field, and dose per fraction were also reduced as a result of the many randomized trials that showed the same survival outcome with a less toxic approach.[5,6]

The outcomes of breast cancer in women with and without a history of RT for HL presented here provide extremely important and long-awaited data that confirm several points.

1. The treatment of HL, especially in the early days, increased the risk of breast cancer related specifically to the RT fields; the following are the characteristics of these patients: (1) higher risk for both synchronous and metachronous bilateral breast cancer; (2) younger age at diagnosis; (3) lower disease stage at diagnosis (stage 0 and 1); (4) less likely to have axillary lymph node involvement; (5) less likely to have a family history of breast cancer; and (6) therapeutic options were limited due to previous RT.
2. Although malignancies in this population are more likely to be early-stage disease and screen detected, these patients still have the same risk of locoregional failure, distant failure, and death as their counterparts with sporadic breast cancer.
3. Other competing risks lead to poorer outcomes for these patients in addition to the second malignancy, in this case breast cancer. These risks are related to possible genetic predisposition and the HL treatment received, including chemotherapy.

Considering these factors, it is important to recognize the risk of second malignancy when treating this group of highly curable patients and to use the therapy that is appropriate for the risk group as defined by recently published data. It is also important that oncologists follow long-term survivors closely and conduct adequate screening tests for secondary malignancies and cardiac toxic effects.

One drawback of the study is that the authors did not report on the actual locations of the cancers in relation to the radiation field, which means that we cannot assume that all breast cancers in patients with HL are secondary to RT.

Although the results of this study are valuable, the take-home message from these data is not relevant to patients currently being treated for HL in view of the dramatic improvements in the field of RT:

1. Radiation oncologists now use computed tomography for treatment planning, which implies a 3-dimensional view of the patient as opposed to the 2-dimensional x-rays used in the patients analyzed in this study.
2. The recent advances in therapy delivery using computer planning systems have become the standard of care. Most radiation oncologists use intensity-modulated radiation therapy, which can deliver the therapeutic dose to the target while delivering only a small fraction of that dose to the surrounding normal tissue; with this technique, the normal tissue receives only a small fraction of the daily dose, which is much safer.
3. Because of increased awareness of the risks associated with RT, radiation oncologists make every effort to avoid delivering any radiation to the breasts. For example, we recently published a paper showing how using an inclined board can in all cases further avoid the breasts while delivering radiation to the mediastinum in young women with HL.[7]

B. S. Dabaja, MD

References

1. Aleman BM, van den Belt-Dusebout AW, Klokman WJ, Van't Veer MB, Bartelink H, van Leeuwen FE. Long-term cause-specific mortality of patients treated for Hodgkin's disease. *J Clin Oncol.* 2003;21:3431-3439.
2. Hancock SL, Tucker MA, Hoppe RT. Breast cancer after treatment of Hodgkin's disease. *J Natl Cancer Inst.* 1993;85:25-31.
3. Bonadonna G, Bonfante V, Viviani S, Di Russo A, Villani F, Valagussa P. ABVD plus subtotal nodal versus involved-field radiotherapy in early-stage Hodgkin's disease: long-term results. *J Clin Oncol.* 2004;22:2835-2841.
4. Canellos GP, Anderson JR, Propert KJ, et al. Chemotherapy of advanced Hodgkin's disease with MOPP, ABVD, or MOPP alternating with ABVD. *N Engl J Med.* 1992;327:1478-1484.
5. Engert A, Plütschow A, Eich HT, et al. Reduced treatment intensity in patients with early-stage Hodgkin's lymphoma. *N Engl J Med.* 2010;363:640-652.
6. Eich HT, Diehl V, Görgen H, et al. Intensified chemotherapy and dose-reduced involved-field radiotherapy in patients with early unfavorable Hodgkin's lymphoma: final analysis of the German Hodgkin Study Group HD11 trial. *J Clin Oncol.* 2010; 28:4199-4206.
7. Dabaja BS, Rebueno NC, Mazloom A, et al. Radiation for Hodgkin's lymphoma in young female patients: a new technique to avoid the breasts and decrease the dose to the heart. *Int J Radiat Oncol Biol Phys.* 2011;79:503-507.

Quality-of-Life Measurement in Randomized Clinical Trials in Breast Cancer: An Updated Systematic Review (2001–2009)

Lemieux J, Goodwin PJ, Bordeleau LJ, et al (Service d'hémato-oncologie du CHA and Centre des Maladies du Sein Deschênes-Fabia du CHA, Quebec, Canada; Univ of Toronto, Ontario, Canada; McMaster Univ and Juravinski Cancer Centre, Hamilton, Ontario, Canada; et al)

J Natl Cancer Inst 103:178-231, 2011

Background.—Quality-of-life (QOL) measurement is often incorporated into randomized clinical trials in breast cancer. The objectives of this systematic review were to assess the incremental effect of QOL measurement in addition to traditional endpoints (such as disease-free survival or toxic effects) on clinical decision making and to describe the extent of QOL reporting in randomized clinical trials of breast cancer.

Methods.—We conducted a search of MEDLINE for English-language articles published between May–June 2001 and October 2009 that reported: 1) a randomized clinical trial of breast cancer treatment (excluding prevention trials), including surgery, chemotherapy, hormone therapy, symptom control, follow-up, and psychosocial intervention; 2) the use of a patient self-report measure that examined general QOL, cancer-specific or breast cancer-specific QOL or psychosocial variables; and 3) documentation of QOL outcomes. All selected trials were evaluated by two reviewers, and data were extracted using a standardized form for each variable. Data are presented in descriptive table formats.

Results.—A total of 190 randomized clinical trials were included in this review. The two most commonly used questionnaires were the European Organization for Research and Treatment of Cancer QOL Questionnaire and the Functional Assessment of Cancer Therapy/Functional Assessment of Chronic Illness Therapy. More than 80% of the included trials reported the name(s) of the instrument(s), trial and QOL sample sizes, the timing of QOL assessment, and the statistical method. Statistical power for QOL was reported in 19.4% of the biomedical intervention trials and in 29.9% of the nonbiomedical intervention trials. The percentage of trials in which QOL findings influenced clinical decision making increased from 15.2% in the previous review to 30.1% in this updated review for trials of biomedical interventions but decreased from 95.0% to 63.2% for trials of nonbiomedical interventions. Discordance between reviewers ranged from 1.1% for description of the statistical method (yes vs no) to 19.9% for the sample size for QOL.

Conclusion.—Reporting of QOL methodology could be improved.

▶ In this systematic review, Lemieux and colleagues addressed the measurement of QOL in biomedical and nonbiomedical clinical trials. Overall, this study adequately summarizes the literature and adds to the growing body of evidence supporting the measurement of QOL in clinical trials. On the basis of this article, it appears that QOL may not be an appropriate outcome in many biomedical interventions. The inability of studies to detect significant differences between treatment arms could be due to methodological flaws such as limited sample size or the instrument's inability to capture "specific" deficits. Psychosocial and behavioral interventions appear to have fewer methodological concerns in clinical trial research, but additional improvements can be made. In the next few paragraphs, we describe 2 specific examples of measurement concerns in QOL research and future directions.

Universal measurement concerns

Let's say, for example, that we are interested in comparing the effects of 2 different breast surgical approaches. In view of the fact that breast cancer surgery often limits upper body mobility, commonly used QOL instruments may not be sensitive enough to capture "specific" upper body deficits that may occur as a result of breast cancer surgery. In addition, there may be symptom-related issues (ie, nausea and constipation/diarrhea) that are not detected because a symptom inventory was not included or composite and subscale measures were not sensitive enough to detect item-level variability. Strategies for addressing these limitations may include (1) incorporating mixed-method approaches (ie, both quantitative and qualitative); (2) considering supplemental instruments; and (3) identifying specific items that need further exploration. Moreover, studies involving patients with breast cancer may benefit from the Late-Life Function and Disability Instrument (LLFDI).[1,2] The LLFDI may be relevant to investigators involved in breast cancer clinical trials because it has demonstrated concurrent and predictive validity with objective measures of performance and contains a subscale for upper extremity function.[3]

Future directions

More research is needed that evaluates the psychometric properties of QOL instruments. Although previous studies have established the validity of these instruments, they may not be stable in the population in which they are being administered. Aspects of the measurement characteristics, including the construct validity and measurement equivalence/invariance, should be established prior to examining mean differences between groups or across time.[4,5] Comparisons that are most relevant and may confound study results include comparisons between (1) race/ethnicity, (2) socioeconomic status, and (3) disease (eg, stage of diagnosis, years from diagnosis, and age at diagnosis) groups. Once the structural aspects of validity are established, between- or within-group comparisons can be made.

In summary, the measurement of QOL in biomedical and nonbiomedical interventions is promising; however, future studies should consider conducting a power analysis prior to recruitment and establishing the validity of these instruments prior to assessing differences between groups or across time. As researchers become more innovative and the complexity of experimental designs increases, universal outcomes such as QOL instruments will be able to reliably quantify intervention efficacy and effectiveness.[6]

R. J. Paxton, PhD
L. A. Jones, PhD

References

1. Haley SM, Jette AM, Coster WJ, et al. Late life function and disability instrument: II. Development and evaluation of the function component. *J Gerontol A Biol Sci Med Sci.* 2002;57:M217-M222.
2. Jette AM, Haley SM, Coster WJ, et al. Late life function and disability instrument: I. Development and evaluation of the disability component. *J Gerontol A Biol Sci Med Sci.* 2002;57:M209-M216.
3. Sayers SP, Jette AM, Haley SM, Heeren TC, Guralnik JM, Fielding RA. Validation of the late-life function and disability instrument. *J Am Geriatr Soc.* 2004;52:1554-1559.
4. Stommel M, Wang S, Given CW, Given B. Confirmatory factor analysis (CFA) as a method to assess measurement equivalence. *Res Nurs Health.* 1992;15:399-405.

5. Drasgow F, Kanfer R. Equivalence of psychological measurement in heterogeneous populations. *J Appl Psychol.* 1985;70:662-680.
6. Prochaska JJ, Spring B, Nigg CR. Multiple health behavior change research: an introduction and overview. *Prev Med.* 2008;46:181-188.

Epidemiology

Dietary fiber intake and risk of breast cancer: a meta-analysis of prospective cohort studies

Dong J-Y, He K, Wang P, et al (Soochow Univ, Suzhou, China; Univ of North Carolina at Chapel Hill; Peking Univ, Beijing, China)
Am J Clin Nutr 94:900-905, 2011

Background.—Observational and preclinical studies suggest that dietary fiber intake may reduce the risk of breast cancer, but the results are inconclusive.

Objective.—We aimed to examine the association between dietary fiber intake and risk of breast cancer by conducting a meta-analysis of prospective cohort studies.

Design.—Relevant studies were identified by a PubMed database search through January 2011. Reference lists from retrieved articles were also reviewed. We included prospective cohort studies that reported RRs with 95% CIs for the association between dietary fiber intake and breast cancer risk. Both fixed- and random-effects models were used to calculate the summary risk estimates.

Results.—We identified 10 prospective cohort studies of dietary fiber intake and risk of breast cancer involving 16,848 cases and 712,195 participants. The combined RR of breast cancer for the highest compared with the lowest dietary fiber intake was 0.89 (95% CI: 0.83, 0.96), and little evidence of heterogeneity was observed. The association between dietary fiber intake and risk of breast cancer did not significantly differ by geographic region, length of follow-up, or menopausal status of the participants. Omission of any single study had little effect on the combined risk estimate. Dose-response analysis showed that every 10-g/d increment in dietary fiber intake was associated with a significant 7% reduction in breast cancer risk. Little evidence of publication bias was found.

Conclusion.—This meta-analysis provides evidence of a significant inverse dose-response association between dietary fiber intake and breast cancer risk.

▶ Dietary fiber is found in fruits, vegetables, and whole grains. Most Americans get less than half the recommended amount of fiber each day. Adequate dietary fiber intake is important for normal bowel function in humans. There is evidence that people who eat higher amounts of dietary fiber had a lower risk of heart disease.[1] Dietary fiber may also lessen the risk of type 2 diabetes.[2] However, the link between low consumption of dietary fiber and increased breast cancer risk has been inconsistent, probably because of methodologic study design issues. In the current analysis of data from 10 large prospective cohort studies that followed over 700 000 women and identified 16 848 breast cancer cases, Dong and colleagues reported that women who consumed the highest level of dietary fiber had a significant 11% (relative risk, 0.89; 95% confidence interval, 0.83-0.96) reduction in breast cancer risk compared with women who consumed the lowest level of dietary fiber, irrespective of menopausal status. The article also estimated that, in general, if a woman increases her dietary fiber intake by 10 g per day, her risk of breast cancer would be reduced by approximately 7%. The inclusion criteria for selecting studies for this meta-analysis, as well as the data extraction, were well planned, and the results do not seem to be spurious. The findings could have the substantial public health effect of reducing the breast cancer burden by increasing dietary fiber intake.

The strength of Dong and colleagues' study lies in the statistical power derived from the large size of the cohort (n = 712 195) and the large number of breast cancer cases (n = 16 848). In cancer epidemiology, prospective cohort studies are considered superior study designs because subjects are enrolled prior to the onset of the disease and followed over time. However, like other study designs, including randomized controlled trials, prospective cohort studies have limitations. In Dong and colleagues' article, it is not clear whether dietary fiber intake was measured throughout the course of the cohort follow-up. Due to funding issues, most prospective studies collect dietary data at baseline only and follow up the cohort for cancer occurrence. It is quite possible that during the follow-up period, dietary behavior could change. Thus, multiple dietary assessments would be preferable and would make the results more credible. In addition, it is highly probable that women who consume high amounts of fiber have healthier lifestyles overall that would protect against breast cancer, such as either not drinking or consuming small amounts of alcohol, eating healthier diets, and exercising more. Also, the study focused on total dietary fiber intake. It would have been more beneficial for women to know which foods contributed the most to total fiber intake and reduced breast cancer risk. The identification of potentially beneficial foods would offer a modifiable way to prevent a portion of breast cancers. For example, refined foods are generally low in fiber and some nutrients such as minerals. Whether refined foods should be avoided to protect against breast cancer could have been addressed in the analysis if such dietary assessments were done.

Despite the limitations of Dong and colleagues' study, it adds to the epidemiologic evidence that high dietary fiber intake reduces breast cancer risk for both pre- and postmenopausal women. Future prospective epidemiologic studies investigating the links between dietary fiber consumption and breast cancer will have to address outstanding issues such as whether the association is affected by the hormone receptor status of breast tumors, obesity, race/ethnicity, and genetic/epigenetic factors. Furthermore, an emerging paradigm in cancer research is that early-life exposures, including diet, influence the subsequent development of breast cancer. For example, higher soy consumption during the adolescent years has been associated with a lower risk of breast cancer later in life.[3,4] Soybeans are a good source of dietary fiber. Consumption of dietary fiber during childhood and adolescence may reduce risk during critical windows of susceptibility for breast cancer development; therefore, opportunities to unravel the links between early dietary exposures and breast cancer should be addressed in future studies.

An important criterion that must be accounted for in weighing the evidence of the apparent protective association between high intake of dietary fiber and breast cancer risk is the biologic plausibility. What is the mechanism by which dietary fiber protects against breast cancer? Since exposure to endogenous and exogenous estrogens are important risk factors for breast cancer, clear evidence that dietary fiber intake decreases concentrations of serum hormones associated with breast cancer would suggest a mechanism by which dietary fiber decreases breast cancer risk. A review published in 2007 reported that several low-fat, high-fiber dietary interventions reduced serum estradiol concentrations in girls and pre- and postmenopausal women.[5] And as indicated by Dong and colleagues, dietary fiber may affect the gut microbiome by suppressing bacterial β-glucuronidase activity, which inhibits estrogen reabsorption in the colon and increases estrogen excretion in the feces, thereby decreasing estrogen concentrations in the serum.

Overall, this meta-analysis of prospective cohort studies provides good evidence that increasing dietary fiber intake among all women could translate into a substantial benefit in our efforts to prevent breast cancer. Increasing dietary fiber intake starting from childhood and continuing across the life course needs to be addressed.

S. Mahabir, PhD, MPH

References

1. Park Y, Subar AF, Hollenbeck A, Schatzkin A. Dietary fiber intake and mortality in the NIH-AARP diet and health study. *Arch Intern Med.* 2011;171:1061-1068.
2. de Munter JS, Hu FB, Spiegelman D, Franz M, van Dam RM. Whole grain, bran, and germ intake and risk of type 2 diabetes: a prospective cohort study and systematic review. *PLoS Med.* 2007;8:e261.
3. Lee SA, Shu XO, Li H, et al. Adolescent and adult soy food intake and breast cancer risk: results from the Shanghai Women's Health Study. *Am J Clin Nutr.* 2009;89:1920-1926.
4. Korde LA, Wu AH, Fears T, et al. Childhood soy intake and breast cancer risk in Asian American women. *Cancer Epidemiol Biomarkers Prev.* 2009;18:1050-1059.
5. Forman MR. Changes in dietary fat and fiber and serum hormone concentrations: nutritional strategies for breast cancer prevention over the life course. *J Nutr.* 2007;137:170S-174S.

Prevention

Tumor-Infiltrating CD8$^+$ Lymphocytes Predict Clinical Outcome in Breast Cancer

Mahmoud SMA, Paish EC, Powe DG, et al (Univ of Nottingham, UK; Nottingham Univ Hosps Natl Health Service Trust, Nottingham, UK; Mansoura Univ, Egypt)
J Clin Oncol 29:1949-1955, 2011

Breast carcinomas are often infiltrated by inflammatory cells, particularly macrophages and T lymphocytes, but the significance of these cells remains unclear. One possible role of these inflammatory cells is that they represent a cell-mediated immune response against the carcinoma. $CD8^+$ lymphocytes are a known crucial component of cell-mediated immunity. The purpose of this study was to explore the prognostic value of tumor-infiltrating $CD8^+$ cytotoxic lymphocytes in breast cancer. Tumor-infiltrating $CD8^+$ lymphocytes were assessed by immunohistochemical staining of tissue microarray cores from 1,334 unselected breast tumors from patients with long-term follow-up. The number of $CD8^+$ T cells was counted in tumor nests (intratumoral), in stroma adjacent to tumor cells, and in stroma distant to tumor cells, and their relationship with clinical outcome was determined. The total number of $CD8^+$ cells was positively correlated with tumor grade ($r_s = 0.20$; $P < .001$) and inversely correlated with patient's age at diagnosis, estrogen receptor—alpha (ER-α), and progesterone receptor (PgR) expression (Mann-Whitney *U* test, $P < .001$). The total patient cohort was randomly divided into two separate training and validation sets before performing univariate survival analysis. Total number and distant stromal $CD8^+$ lymphocytes were associated with better patient survival ($P = .041$ and $P < .001$, respectively) in the training set. In multivariate analysis, total $CD8^+$ T-cell count was an independent prognostic factor in both training and validation sets. These results suggest that tumor-infiltrating $CD8^+$ T lymphocytes have antitumor activity as judged by their favorable effect on patients' survival and could potentially be exploited in the treatment of breast cancer.

► Breast cancer remains a serious life-threatening malignancy for tens of thousands of US women annually. While screening mammograms and self—breast examinations are helpful in identifying the disease early, they are just the beginning of the story of a disease that varies from a slow-growing non—life-threatening problem to a very aggressive often fatal disease process. Therefore, the ability to identify factors that help oncologists and patients understand the gravity of the disease is critically important.

Many factors, such as hormone receptor status, have already been identified to help define aggressive tumors. Work continues to further outline favorable or unfavorable tumor characteristics. These authors have evaluated the role of tumor infiltration by $CD8^+$ lymphocytes. $CD8^+$ lymphocytes are associated with cell-mediated immunity, and its presence potentially predicts a favorable outcome.

The analysis presented here suggests that $CD8^+$ T-cell count in a breast cancer tumor is an independent prognostic variable and should be investigated further to define its potential role in breast cancer outcomes.

C. Lawton, MD

Early Stage and Adjuvant Therapy

Adjuvant Therapy in Stage I Carcinoma of the Breast: The Influence of Multigene Analyses and Molecular Phenotyping

Schwartz GF, Bartelink H, Burstein HJ, et al (Jefferson Med College, Philadelphia, PA; The Netherlands Cancer Inst, Amsterdam; Harvard Med School, Boston, MA; et al)

Breast J 18:303-311, 2012

A consensus conference was held in order to provide guidelines for the use of adjuvant therapy in patients with Stage I carcinoma of the breast, using traditional information, such as tumor size, microscopic character, Nottingham index, patient age and co-morbidities, but also incorporating steroid hormone and Her-2-neu data as well as other immunohistochemical markers. The role of the genetic analysis of breast cancer and proprietary gene prognostic signatures was discussed, along with the molecular profiling of breast cancers into several groups that may predict prognosis. These molecular data are not currently sufficiently mature to make them part of decision making algorithms of recommendations for the treatment of individual patients.

▶ This article summarizes the deliberations of a consensus conference on the use of molecular profiling as a basis for determining adjuvant treatment. The panel focused primarily on stage I cancers but also discussed briefly some node-positive patients. There are several noteworthy recommendations. First, the panel concluded that current molecular profiling (OncotypeDx and Mammaprint) should not be used as a substitute for clinical judgment in determining adjuvant therapy for stage I breast cancers. Second, they felt that assigning breast cancer type (basal, luminal A, luminal B) on the basis of molecular profiling was not sufficiently consistent among the various tests that it should be routinely done as a basis for clinical decision making. Third, they recommended that molecular profiling, if ordered, should be ordered from 1 source per patient because the various tests can give discordant answers and lead to confusion. Fourth, they felt that molecular profiling, at its current state, should be adjunct to other factors in clinical decision making. Finally, they recommended that molecular profiling not be used in node-positive patients because this is already a major adverse prognostic factor. The panel also encouraged further clinical studies to validate the clinical utility of these tests. The article is worth reading in detail if one plans to use these tests in the clinical management of patients.

J. T. Thigpen, MD

Association of Occult Metastases in Sentinel Lymph Nodes and Bone Marrow With Survival Among Women With Early-Stage Invasive Breast Cancer

Giuliano AE, Hawes D, Ballman KV, et al (John Wayne Cancer Inst at Saint John's Health Ctr, Santa Monica; Univ of Southern California Norris Comprehensive Cancer Ctr, Los Angeles; Mayo Clinic, Rochester, MN; et al)

JAMA 306:385-393, 2011

Context.—Immunochemical staining of sentinel lymph nodes (SLNs) and bone marrow identifies breast cancer metastases not seen with routine pathological or clinical examination.

Objective.—To determine the association between survival and metastases detected by immunochemical staining of SLNs and bone marrow specimens from patients with early-stage breast cancer.

Design, Setting, and Patients.—From May 1999 to May 2003, 126 sites in the American College of Surgeons Oncology Group Z0010 trial enrolled women with clinical T1 to T2N0M0 invasive breast carcinoma in a prospective observational study.

Interventions.—All 5210 patients underwent breast-conserving surgery and SLN dissection. Bone marrow aspiration at the time of operation was initially optional and subsequently mandatory (March 2001). Sentinel lymph node specimens (hematoxylineosin negative) and bone marrow specimens were sent to a central laboratory for immunochemical staining; treating clinicians were blinded to results.

Main Outcome Measures.—Overall survival (primary end point) and disease-free survival (a secondary end point).

Results.—Of 5119 SLN specimens (98.3%), 3904 (76.3%) were tumor-negative by hematoxylin-eosin staining. Of 3326 SLN specimens examined by immunohistochemistry, 349 (10.5%) were positive for tumor. Of 3413 bone marrow specimens examined by immunocytochemistry, 104 (3.0%) were positive for tumors. At a median follow-up of 6.3 years (through April 2010), 435 patients had died and 376 had disease recurrence. Immunohistochemical evidence of SLN metastases was not significantly associated with overall survival (5-year rates: 95.7%; 95% confidence interval [CI], 95.0%-96.5% for immunohistochemical negative and 95.1%; 95% CI, 92.7%-97.5% for immunohistochemical positive disease; $P = .64$; unadjusted hazard ratio [HR], 0.90; 95% CI, 0.59-1.39; $P = .64$). Bone marrow metastases were associated with decreased overall survival (unadjusted HR for mortality, 1.94; 95% CI, 1.02-3.67; $P = .04$), but neither immunohistochemical evidence of tumor in SLNs (adjusted HR, 0.88; 95% CI, 0.45-1.71; $P = .70$) nor immunocytochemical evidence of tumor in bone marrow (adjusted HR, 1.83; 95% CI, 0.79-4.26; $P = .15$) was statistically significant on multivariable analysis.

Conclusion.—Among women receiving breast-conserving therapy and SLN dissection, immunohistochemical evidence of SLN metastasis was not associated with overall survival over a median of 6.3 years, whereas occult bone marrow metastasis, although rare, was associated with decreased survival.

Trial Registration.—clinicaltrials.gov Identifier: NCT00003854.

▶ It has long been speculated that breast cancer is a systemic disease at diagnosis and that circulating breast cancer cells can set up housekeeping even years after the diagnosis and local treatment. It has also been proven that many cancers such as breast and prostate can result in cells that can be found in the blood stream. Yet most never do cause life-threatening problems.

How to comprehend the fact that circulating cancer cells can exist yet most cause no problems is a challenge that these authors have pondered. Specifically, they have evaluated the survival effect of circulating cancer cells that have produced occult metastasis in sentinel lymph nodes and the occult metastasis in the bone marrow of patients with early-stage invasive breast cancer (clinical T1 and T2N0M0 tumors).

It is encouraging to learn that in this large data set, with fairly long follow-up (median 6.3 years), women with occult metastasis in the sentinel lymph nodes did not succumb to their disease more often than those without occult sentinel lymph node metastasis. The fact that occult bone marrow metastasis was associated with decreased overall survival remains concerning and supports the use of aggressive systemic therapy in these patients.

C. Lawton, MD

Bevacizumab Added to Neoadjuvant Chemotherapy for Breast Cancer

Bear HD, Tang G, Rastogi P, et al (Natl Surgical Adjuvant Breast and Bowel Project (NSABP), Pittsburgh, PA)

N Engl J Med 366:310-320, 2012

Background.—Bevacizumab and the antimetabolites capecitabine and gemcitabine have been shown to improve outcomes when added to taxanes in patients with metastatic breast cancer. The primary aims of this trial were to determine whether the addition of capecitabine or gemcitabine to neoadjuvant chemotherapy with docetaxel, followed by doxorubicin plus cyclophosphamide, would increase the rates of pathological complete response in the breast in women with operable, human epidermal growth factor receptor 2 (HER2)–negative breast cancer and whether adding bevacizumab to these chemotherapy regimens would increase the rates of pathological complete response.

Methods.—We randomly assigned 1206 patients to receive neoadjuvant therapy consisting of docetaxel (100 mg per square meter of body-surface area on day 1), docetaxel (75 mg per square meter on day 1) plus capecitabine (825 mg per square meter twice a day on days 1 to 14), or docetaxel (75 mg per square meter on day 1) plus gemcitabine (1000 mg per square meter on days 1 and 8) for four cycles, with all regimens followed by treatment with doxorubicin–cyclophosphamide for four cycles. Patients were also randomly assigned to receive or not to receive bevacizumab (15 mg per kilogram of body weight) for the first six cycles of chemotherapy.

Results.—The addition of capecitabine or gemcitabine to docetaxel therapy, as compared with docetaxel therapy alone, did not significantly increase the rate of pathological complete response (29.7% and 31.8%, respectively, vs. 32.7%; $P = 0.69$). Both capecitabine and gemcitabine were associated with increased toxic effects — specifically, the hand–foot syndrome, mucositis, and neutropenia. The addition of bevacizumab significantly increased the rate of pathological complete response (28.2% without bevacizumab vs. 34.5% with bevacizumab, $P = 0.02$). The effect of bevacizumab on the rate of pathological complete response was not the same in the hormone-receptor–positive and hormone-receptor–negative subgroups. The addition of bevacizumab increased the rates of hypertension, left ventricular systolic dysfunction, the hand–foot syndrome, and mucositis.

Conclusions.—The addition of bevacizumab to neoadjuvant chemotherapy significantly increased the rate of pathological complete response, which was the primary end point of this study. (Funded by the National Cancer Institute and others; ClinicalTrials.gov number, NCT00408408.)

▶ This trial studied neoadjuvant systemic therapy in patients with operable HER2− breast cancer. Patients received either docetaxel, docetaxel plus capecitabine, or docetaxel plus gemcitabine with each regimen followed by doxorubicin/cyclophosphamide. No differences among the chemotherapeutic regimens were observed. All patients were also randomly assigned to receive either bevacizumab or no targeted therapy. The addition of bevacizumab was associated with a statistically significantly increased pathologic complete response rate (34.5% vs 28.2%, $P = .02$), which was the primary endpoint of the trial. Pathologic complete response to neoadjuvant systemic therapy is associated with an improved survival. These results suggest that bevacizumab is an active agent in breast carcinoma associated with significant patient benefit. This increase in the pathological complete response rate was bought at the expense of a small increase in the incidence of hypertension, hand-foot syndrome, left ventricular systolic dysfunction, and mucositis. Across a number of randomized phase III trials, bevacizumab has demonstrated a consistent if modest clinical benefit for patients receiving it in conjunction with chemotherapy.

J. T. Thigpen, MD

Comparisons between different polychemotherapy regimens for early breast cancer: meta-analyses of long-term outcome among 100 000 women in 123 randomised trials

Early Breast Cancer Trialists' Collaborative Group (EBCTCG) (Clinical Trial Service Unit (CTSU), Oxford, UK)

Lancet 379:432-444, 2012

Background.—Moderate differences in efficacy between adjuvant chemotherapy regimens for breast cancer are plausible, and could affect treatment choices. We sought any such differences.

Methods.—We undertook individual-patient-data meta-analyses of the randomised trials comparing: any taxane-plus-anthracycline-based regimen versus the same, or more, non-taxane chemotherapy (n = 44 000); one anthracycline-based regimen versus another (n = 7000) or versus cyclophosphamide, methotrexate, and fluorouracil (CMF; n=18 000); and polychemotherapy versus no chemotherapy (n = 32 000). The scheduled dosages of these three drugs and of the anthracyclines doxorubicin (A) and epirubicin (E) were used to define standard CMF, standard 4AC, and CAF and CEF. Log-rank breast cancer mortality rate ratios (RRs) are reported.

Findings.—In trials adding four separate cycles of a taxane to a fixed anthracycline-based control regimen, extending treatment duration, breast cancer mortality was reduced (RR 0·86, SE 0·04, two-sided significance [2p] = 0·0005). In trials with four such extra cycles of a taxane counterbalanced in controls by extra cycles of other cytotoxic drugs, roughly doubling non-taxane dosage, there was no significant difference (RR 0·94, SE 0·06, 2p = 0·33). Trials with CMF-treated controls showed that standard 4AC and standard CMF were equivalent (RR 0·98, SE 0·05, 2p = 0·67), but that anthracycline-based regimens with substantially higher cumulative dosage than standard 4AC (eg, CAF or CEF) were superior to standard CMF (RR 0·78, SE 0·06, 2p = 0·0004). Trials versus no chemotherapy also suggested greater mortality reductions with CAF (RR 0·64, SE 0·09, 2p < 0·0001) than with standard 4AC (RR 0·78, SE 0·09, 2p = 0·01) or standard CMF (RR 0·76, SE 0·05, 2p < 0·0001). In all meta-analyses involving taxane-based or anthracycline-based regimens, proportional risk reductions were little affected by age, nodal status, tumour diameter or differentiation (moderate or poor; few were well differentiated), oestrogen receptor status, or tamoxifen use. Hence, largely independently of age (up to at least 70 years) or the tumour characteristics currently available to us for the patients selected to be in these trials, some taxane-plus-anthracycline-based or higher-cumulative-dosage anthracycline-based regimens (not requiring stem cells) reduced breast cancer mortality by, on average, about one-third. 10-year overall mortality differences paralleled breast cancer mortality differences, despite taxane, anthracycline, and other toxicities.

Interpretation.—10-year gains from a one-third breast cancer mortality reduction depend on absolute risks without chemotherapy (which, for oestrogen-receptor-positive disease, are the risks remaining with appropriate endocrine therapy). Low absolute risk implies low absolute benefit, but information was lacking about tumour gene expression markers or quantitative immunohistochemistry that might help to predict risk, chemosensitivity, or both.

▶ It should always be remembered that meta-analyses do not represent the highest form of evidence, although we are often impressed by the massive numbers. This meta-analysis does provide some interesting information concerning adjuvant therapy for early stage breast cancer. It confirms an observation in an earlier meta-analysis that cyclophosphamide, methotrexate, and fluorouracil (CMF) and anthracycline (AC) yield essentially the same efficacy and that CAF appears to have a slight advantage over either CMF or AC. A regimen containing a taxane and an AC appears to offer some advantage. Unfortunately, data regarding gene expression markers were insufficient to allow these markers to be factored into the equation. Two thoughts represent a reasonable bottom line: First, current approaches to adjuvant therapy for breast cancer clearly reduce mortality. What we lack is solid information about the very best approach to use in each individual situation. Second, we need improved information about the assessment of risk so we can properly evaluate whether benefit outweighs risk in a given situation. These needs should be met as our knowledge of the biology of the disease continues to grow.

J. T. Thigpen, MD

Disease-Related Outcomes With Long-Term Follow-Up: An Updated Analysis of the Intergroup Exemestane Study

Bliss JM, Kilburn LS, Coleman RE, et al (The Inst of Cancer Res, Sutton, Surrey, UK; Weston Park Hosp, Sheffield, UK; et al)

J Clin Oncol 30:709-717, 2012

Purpose.—Intergroup Exemestane Study (IES), an investigator-led study in 4,724 postmenopausal patients with early-stage breast cancer has demonstrated clinically important benefits from switching adjuvant endocrine therapy after 2 to 3 years of tamoxifen to exemestane. Now, with longer follow-up, a large number of non—breast cancer—related events have been reported. Exploratory analyses describe breast cancer—free survival (BCFS) and explore incidence and patterns of the different competing events.

Patients and Methods.—Patients who were disease-free after 2 to 3 years of adjuvant tamoxifen were randomly assigned to continue tamoxifen or switch to exemestane to complete 5 years of adjuvant endocrine therapy. At this planned analysis, the median follow-up was 91 months. Principal analysis focuses on 4,052 patients with estrogen receptor (ER)—positive and 547 with ER-unknown tumors.

Results.—In all, 930 BCFS events have been reported (exemestane, 423; tamoxifen, 507), giving an unadjusted hazard ratio (HR) of 0.81 (95% CI, 0.71 to 0.92; $P = .001$) in favor of exemestane in the ER-positive/ER unknown group. Analysis partitioned at 2.5 years after random assignment showed that the on-treatment benefit of switching to exemestane (HR, 0.60; 95% CI, 0.48 to 0.75; $P < .001$) was not lost post-treatment, but that there was no additional gain once treatment had ceased (HR, 0.94; 95% CI, 0.80 to 1.10; $P = .60$). Improvement in overall survival was demonstrated, with 352 deaths in the exemestane group versus 405 deaths in the tamoxifen group (HR, 0.86; 95% CI, 0.75 to 0.99; $P = .04$). Of these, 222 were reported as intercurrent deaths (exemestane, 107; tamoxifen, 115).

Conclusion.—The protective effect of switching to exemestane compared with continuing on tamoxifen on risk of relapse or death was maintained for at least 5 years post-treatment and was associated with a continuing beneficial impact on overall survival.

▶ Studies have shown that in the postmenopausal population, switching adjuvant endocrine therapy after a defined period of time from tamoxifen to an aromatase inhibitor in the early stages of breast cancer provides benefits in terms of disease-free survival. This article provides a longer-term follow-up of 1 of these trials. Patients with early-stage breast cancer were randomized after 2.5 years of tamoxifen adjuvant therapy to either continue tamoxifen for 2.5 more years or switch to exemestane for 2.5 years. With a median follow-up of 91 months, this report shows clear superiority for switching in regard to both disease-free and overall survival. This clearly shows the value of the aromatase inhibitor but does not clearly establish that both agents are necessary to achieve optimal results. It should also be noted that the study shows that the effect of the adjuvant therapy continues beyond cessation of the treatment and is associated with no difference in long-term side effects. In short, in postmenopausal patients, aromatase inhibitors should be a part of adjuvant therapy in those who have estrogen-receptor–positive cancers.

J. T. Thigpen, MD

Preoperative Chemotherapy Plus Trastuzumab, Lapatinib, or Both in Human Epidermal Growth Factor Receptor 2–Positive Operable Breast Cancer: Results of the Randomized Phase II CHER-LOB Study

Guarneri V, Frassoldati A, Bottini A, et al (Modena Univ Hosp, Italy; AO Istituti Ospitalieri di Cremona, Italy; et al)
J Clin Oncol 30:1989-1995, 2012

Purpose.—This is a noncomparative, randomized, phase II trial of preoperative taxane-anthracycline in combination with trastuzumab, lapatinib, or combined trastuzumab plus lapatinib in patients with human epidermal growth factor receptor 2 (HER2) –positive, stage II to IIIA operable breast cancer. The primary aim was to estimate the percentage of pathologic complete response (pCR; no invasive tumor in breast and axillary nodes).

Patients and Methods.—In the three arms, chemotherapy consisted of weekly paclitaxel (80 mg/m^2) for 12 weeks followed by fluorouracil, epirubicin, and cyclophosphamide for four courses every 3 weeks. The patients randomly assigned to arm A received a 4-mg loading dose of trastuzumab followed by 2 mg weekly; in arm B patients received lapatinib 1,500 mg orally (PO) daily; and in arm C, patients received trastuzumab and lapatinib 1,000 mg PO daily.

Results.—A total of 121 patients were randomly assigned. Diarrhea and dermatologic and hepatic toxicities were observed more frequently in patients receiving lapatinib. No episodes of congestive heart failure were observed. The rates of breast-conserving surgery were 66.7%, 57.9%, and 68.9% in arms A, B and C, respectively. The pCR rates were 25% (90%

CI, 13.1% to 36.9%) in arm A, 26.3% (90% CI, 14.5% to 38.1%) in arm B, and 46.7% (90% CI, 34.4% to 58.9%) in arm C (exploratory $P = .019$).

Conclusion.—The primary end point of the study was met, with a relative increase of 80% in the pCR rate achieved with chemotherapy plus trastuzumab and lapatinib compared with chemotherapy plus either trastuzumab or lapatinib. These data add further evidence supporting the superiority of a dual-HER2 inhibition for the treatment of HER2-positive breast cancer.

► Trastuzumab and lapatinib represent 2 different ways of attacking tumor cells that overexpress *HER2*-neu. Trastuzumab is a monoclonal antibody directed at the cell membrane receptor for human epidermal growth factor-2, whereas lapatinib is a small-molecule tyrosine kinase inhibitor that works at an intracellular location to inhibit dimerization within the epidermal growth factor receptor family and thus signaling within the cell. Both should be complementary to each other; hence, there has been interest in combining the 2 agents.

This trial was undertaken to determine whether there was sufficient promise of at least an additive effect to warrant evaluating the combination of both agents with chemotherapy in *HER2* positive breast cancer. A total of 121 patients with *HER2* positive locally advanced breast cancer were randomized to chemotherapy plus either trastuzumab, lapatinib, or both in this randomized phase II study. A statistically significant improvement in pathologic complete response was seen with the combination of the 2 agents than was the case with either alone. This supports a phase III trial to determine whether this approach should become the new standard of care for these cancers.

J. T. Thigpen, MD

Effect of Obesity on Prognosis After Early-Stage Breast Cancer

Ewertz M, Jensen M-B, Gunnarsdóttir KÁ, et al (Univ of Southern Denmark, Odense, Denmark; Aarhus Univ Hosp, Denmark; Vejle Hosp, Denmark; et al)

J Clin Oncol 29:25-31, 2011

Purpose.—This study was performed to characterize the impact of obesity on the risk of breast cancer recurrence and death as a result of breast cancer or other causes in relation to adjuvant treatment.

Patients and Methods.—Information on body mass index (BMI) at diagnosis was available for 18,967 (35%) of 53,816 women treated for early-stage breast cancer in Denmark between 1977 and 2006 with complete follow-up for first events (locoregional recurrences and distant metastases) up to 10 years and for death up to 30 years. Information was available on prognostic factors and adjuvant treatment for all patients. Univariate analyses were used to compare the associations of known prognostic factors and risks of recurrence or death according to BMI categories. Cox proportional hazards regression models were used to assess the influence of BMI after adjusting for other factors.

Results.—Patients with a BMI of 30 kg/m^2 or more were older and had more advanced disease at diagnosis compared with patients with a BMI below 25 kg/m^2 ($P < .001$). When data were adjusted for disease characteristics, the risk of developing distant metastases after 10 years was significantly increased by 46%, and the risk of dying as a result of breast cancer after 30 years was significantly increased by 38% for patients with a BMI of 30 kg/m^2 or more. BMI had no influence on the risk of locoregional recurrences. Both chemotherapy and endocrine therapy seemed to be less effective after 10 or more years for patients with BMIs greater than 30 kg/m^2.

Conclusion.—Obesity is an independent prognostic factor for developing distant metastases and for death as a result of breast cancer; the effects of adjuvant therapy seem to be lost more rapidly in patients with breast cancer and obesity.

▶ Obesity for men and women is a huge health concern in the United States. Increased risk of heart disease, diabetes, and cancer all relate to our obesity epidemic. The extra fat that exists in obese patients is known to increase estrogen levels and is thought to play a role in the incidence of both breast and prostate cancer in our country.

What has not been well studied is the role of obesity and overall outcome of patients with breast cancer. It has been shown that obesity can negatively affect outcomes in breast cancer patients, but exactly why has not been well elucidated.

These data confirm the finding of an association between obesity and an increased risk of breast cancer deaths in patients with early stage breast cancer. The interesting fact that the breast cancer deaths are related to an increase in distant metastasis and not related to an increase in local regional recurrences should be an aid to oncologists. It should prompt us to work on more effective systemic agents for this population of breast cancer patients.

C. Lawton, MD

Effect of Occult Metastases on Survival in Node-Negative Breast Cancer

Weaver DL, Ashikaga T, Krag DN, et al (Univ of Vermont College of Medicine and Vermont Cancer Ctr, Burlington; et al)

N Engl J Med 364:412-421, 2011

Background.—Retrospective and observational analyses suggest that occult lymph-node metastases are an important prognostic factor for disease recurrence or survival among patients with breast cancer. Prospective data on clinical outcomes from randomized trials according to sentinel-node involvement have been lacking.

Methods.—We randomly assigned women with breast cancer to sentinel-lymph-node biopsy plus axillary dissection or sentinel-lymph-node biopsy alone. Paraffin-embedded tissue blocks of sentinel lymph nodes obtained from patients with pathologically negative sentinel lymph nodes were centrally evaluated for occult metastases deeper in the blocks. Both routine staining and immunohistochemical staining for cytokeratin were used at two widely spaced additional tissue levels. Treating physicians were unaware of the findings, which were not used for clinical treatment decisions. The initial evaluation at participating sites was designed to detect all macrometastases larger than 2 mm in the greatest dimension.

Results.—Occult metastases were detected in 15.9% (95% confidence interval [CI], 14.7 to 17.1) of 3887 patients. Log-rank tests indicated a significant difference between patients in whom occult metastases were detected and those in whom no occult metastases were detected with respect to overall survival ($P = 0.03$), disease-free survival ($P = 0.02$), and distant-disease–free interval ($P = 0.04$). The corresponding adjusted hazard ratios for death, any outcome event, and distant disease were 1.40 (95% CI, 1.05 to 1.86), 1.31 (95% CI, 1.07 to 1.60), and 1.30 (95% CI, 1.02 to 1.66), respectively. Five-year Kaplan-Meier estimates of overall survival among patients in whom occult metastases were detected and those without detectable metastases were 94.6% and 95.8%, respectively.

Conclusions.—Occult metastases were an independent prognostic variable in patients with sentinel nodes that were negative on initial examination; however, the magnitude of the difference in outcome at 5 years was small (1.2 percentage points). These data do not indicate a clinical benefit of additional evaluation, including immunohistochemical analysis, of initially negative sentinel nodes in patients with breast cancer. (Funded by the National Cancer Institute; ClinicalTrials.gov number, NCT00003830.)

▶ Breast cancer continues to affect tens of thousands of women annually and results in over 35 000 deaths per year in the United States alone. Many female patients feel completely overwhelmed with the diagnosis. So we as treating oncologists need to continue to develop prognostic factors to help quantitate the diagnosis and its possible effects on a given patient's life.

It is well understood that tumor size and number of positive axillary lymph nodes predict for breast cancer outcomes in terms of local control, distant metastasis, and overall survival. One question that has been debated is whether occult nodal metastasis (lymph nodes that are pathologically negative, but with further analysis via deeper cuts in the tissue blocks and immunohistochemical analysis show evidence of tumor) is another independent predictor of breast cancer outcomes. These authors have done excellent work in evaluating patients with occult lymph node metastases on their sentinel lymph nodes and found occult metastasis to be an independent prognostic variable.

Although this is an important finding, the other aspect of this information is equally, if not more, important, that being the magnitude of the effect, which is only a 1.2% difference in overall survival at 5 years. Thus the clinical benefit is likely too small to warrant this additional evaluation in breast cancer patients with negative sentinel lymph nodes.

C. Lawton, MD

Lapatinib with trastuzumab for HER2-positive early breast cancer (NeoALTTO): a randomised, open-label, multicentre, phase 3 trial

Baselga J, on behalf of the NeoALTTO Study Team (Massachusetts General Hosp Cancer Ctr, Boston; et al)

Lancet 379:633-640, 2012

Background.—The anti-HER2 monoclonal antibody trastuzumab and the tyrosine kinase inhibitor lapatinib have complementary mechanisms of action and synergistic antitumour activity in models of HER2-overexpressing breast cancer. We argue that the two anti-HER2 agents given together would be better than single-agent therapy.

Methods.—In this parallel groups, randomised, open-label, phase 3 study undertaken between Jan 5, 2008, and May 27, 2010, women from 23 countries with HER2-positive primary breast cancer with tumours greater than 2 cm in diameter were randomly assigned to oral lapatinib (1500 mg), intravenous trastuzumab (loading dose 4 mg/Kg, subsequent doses 2 mg/kg), or lapatinib (1000 mg) plus trastuzumab. Treatment allocation was by stratified, permuted blocks randomisation, with four stratification factors. Anti-HER2 therapy alone was given for the first 6 weeks; weekly paclitaxel (80 mg/m^2) was then added to the regimen for a further 12 weeks, before definitive surgery was undertaken. After surgery, patients received adjuvant chemotherapy followed by the same targeted therapy as in the neoadjuvant phase to 52 weeks. The primary endpoint was the rate of pathological complete response (pCR), analysed by intention to treat. This trial is registered with ClinicalTrials.gov, NCT00553358.

Findings.—154 patients received lapatinib, 149 trastuzumab, and 152 the combination. pCR rate was significantly higher in the group given lapatinib and trastuzumab (78 of 152 patients [51·3%; 95% CI 43·1–59·5]) than in the group given trastuzumab alone (44 of 149 patients [29·5%; 22·4–37·5]; difference 21·1%, 9·1–34·2, $p = 0·0001$). We recorded no significant difference in pCR between the lapatinib (38 of 154 patients [24·7%, 18·1–32·3]) and the trastuzumab (difference −4·8%, −17·6 to 8·2, $p = 0·34$) groups. No major cardiac dysfunctions occurred. Frequency of grade 3 diarrhoea was higher with lapatinib (36 patients [23·4%]) and lapatinib plus trastuzumab (32 [21·1%]) than with trastuzumab (three [2·0%]). Similarly, grade 3 liver-enzyme alterations were more frequent with lapatinib (27 [17·5%]) and lapatinib plus trastuzumab (15 [9·9%]) than with trastuzumab (11 [7·4%]).

Interpretation.—Dual inhibition of HER2 might be a valid approach to treatment of HER2-positive breast cancer in the neoadjuvant setting.

▶ Trastuzumab and lapatinib are 2 breast cancer agents directed at tumor that overexpresses HER2-neu. Their mechanisms of action are very different and, at least theoretically, complementary to one another. Trastuzumab is a monoclonal antibody directed against the receptor at the surface of the cell membrane. Lapatinib is a small-molecule tyrosine kinase inhibitor that acts inside the cell to prevent dimerization and subsequent signaling. This trial sought to evaluate the combination of the 2 in HER2+ breast carcinoma. A total of 455 patients with larger (>2 cm) tumors were randomized to either trastuzumab, lapatinib, or the combination of the 2. The primary endpoint of the trial was pathologic complete response rate. The combination demonstrated a striking advantage (51.3% vs 29.5% vs 24.7% for the combination, trastuzumab, and lapatinib, respectively). In the neoadjuvant setting, the combination of trastuzumab and lapatinib appears to have a significant advantage over either agent alone.

J. T. Thigpen, MD

Breast Conserving Therapy

Ductal Carcinoma In Situ Treated With Breast-Conserving Surgery and Accelerated Partial Breast Irradiation: Comparison of the Mammosite Registry Trial With Intergroup Study E5194

Goyal S, Vicini F, Beitsch PD, et al (Cancer Inst of New Jersey and UMDNJ/ Robert Wood Johnson Med School, New Brunswick; William Beaumont Hosp, Royal Oak, MI; Dallas Breast Ctr, TX; et al)

Cancer 117:1149-1155, 2011

Background.—The purpose of this study was to determine the ipsilateral breast tumor recurrence (IBTR) in ductal carcinoma in situ (DCIS) patients treated in the American Society of Breast Surgeons MammoSite Breast Brachytherapy Registry Trial who met the criteria for E5194 treated with local excision and adjuvant accelerated partial breast irradiation (APBI).

Methods.—A total of 194 patients with DCIS were treated between 2002 and 2004 in the Mammosite registry trial; of these, 70 patients met the enrollment criteria for E5194: 1) low to intermediate grade (LIG)—pathological size >0.3 but <2.5 cm and margins ≥3 mm (n = 41) or 2) high grade (HG)—pathological size <1 cm and margins ≥3 mm (n = 29). All patients were treated with lumpectomy followed by adjuvant APBI using MammoSite. Median follow-up was 52.7 months (range, 0-88.4). SAS (version 8.2) was used for statistical analysis.

Results.—In the LIG cohort, the 5-year IBTR was 0%, compared with 6.1% at 5 years in E5194. In the HG cohort, the 5-year IBTR was 5.3%, compared with 15.3% at 5 years in E5194. The overall 5-year IBTR was 2%, and there were no cases of elsewhere or regional failures in the entire cohort. The 5-year contralateral breast event rate was 0% and 5.6% in LIG and HG patients, respectively (compared with 3.5% and 4.2%, respectively, in E5194).

Conclusions.—This study found that patients who met the criteria of E5194 treated with APBI had extremely low rates of recurrence (0% vs 6.1% in the LIG cohort and 5.3% vs 15.3% in the HG cohort).

► The role of accelerated partial breast irradiation (APBI) as treatment for early-stage breast cancer is being evaluated in multiple trials. There are several ways to deliver APBI following lumpectomy, including interstitial implants, external beam radiation, and the MammoSite breast brachytherapy catheter. The results for well-selected patients with early-stage breast cancer look promising, although longer follow-up is needed on most of the trials reported to date.

This article is a report of patients with ductal carcinoma in situ (DCIS) entered on the American Society of Breast Surgeons MammoSite Breast Brachytherapy Registry Trial. It is unique in that APBI has not been extensively studied in patients with DCIS, and this protocol had very strict criteria for enrollment resulting in enrollment of more favorable patients (eg, those with a solitary lesion, older than 45 years of age, pure DCIS, clear margins, node-negative disease, etc). The use of MammoSite APBI resulted in very low rates of in-breast recurrence. At 5 years, the in-breast recurrence event rate was 0% for the low- and intermediate-grade patients and 5.6% in the high-grade patients.

Just which DCIS patients need radiotherapy (RT) after lumpectomy is still not clear and needs further research. But of those who do, APBI should be considered in further trials as a method of RT delivery.

C. Lawton, MD

Comparison of treatment outcome between breast-conservation surgery with radiation and total mastectomy without radiation in patients with one to three positive axillary lymph nodes

Kim SI, Park S, Park HS, et al (Yonsei Univ College of Medicine, Seoul, Korea)
Int J Radiat Oncol Biol Phys 80:1446-1452, 2011

Purpose.—To test the difference in treatment outcome between breast-conservation surgery with radiation and total mastectomy without radiation, to evaluate the benefits of adjuvant radiotherapy in patients with one to three positive axillary lymph nodes.

Methods and Materials.—Using the Severance Hospital Breast Cancer Registry, we divided the study population of T1, T2 and one to three axillary node–positive patients into two groups: breast–conservation surgery with radiation (BCS/RT) and total mastectomy without radiation (TM/no-RT). Data related to locoregional recurrence, distant recurrence, and death were collected, and survival rates were calculated.

Results.—The study population consisted of 125 patients treated with BCS/RT and 365 patients treated with TM/no-RT. With a median follow-up of 68.4 months, the 10-year locoregional recurrence–free survival rate with BCS/RT and TM/no-RT was 90.5% and 79.2%, respectively ($p = 0.056$). The 10-year distant recurrence-free survival rate was 78.8% for patients treated with BCS/RT vs. 68.0% for those treated with TM/no-RT ($p = 0.012$). The 10-years overall survival rate for patients treated with BCT/RT and TM/no-RT was 87.5% and 73.9%, respectively ($p = 0.035$). After multivariate analysis, patients treated with BCT/RT had better distant recurrence-free survival (hazard ratio [HR], 0.527; 95% confidence interval [CI], 0.297–0.934; $p = 0.028$), with improving locoregional recurrence-free survival (HR, 0.491; 95% CI, 0.231–1.041; $p = 0.064$) and overall survival trend (HR, 0.544; 95% CI, 0.277–1.067; $p = 0.076$).

Conclusions.—This study provides additional evidence that adjuvant radiation substantially reduces local recurrence, distant recurrence, and mortality for patients with one to three involved nodes.

▶ In this retrospective analysis, Kim and colleagues compared breast conservation treatment, including BCS/RT, with total mastectomy without radiation in patients with T1 to T2 breast cancer with 1 to 3 positive nodes. Patients in the BCS/RT group had fewer locoregional (LR) recurrences, fewer distant metastases, and better overall survival rates. Retrospective analyses have well-recognized shortcomings, and some of the authors' results were of borderline statistical significance. Nevertheless, their findings are consistent with a growing number of studies that have shown improved breast cancer outcomes with RT.

In a recent study of women with T1 to T2 N0 triple-negative breast cancer, Abdulkarim and colleagues[1] showed that those who underwent mastectomy had more LR relapses than those who underwent breast conservation treatment, including radiation therapy (RT). As in the present study, patients with 1 to 3 positive nodes did not receive supraclavicular RT. The low axilla is included in the breast tangential fields, however. Interestingly, the American College of Surgeons Oncology Group Z0011 study,[2] in which all patients received whole-breast RT (no supraclavicular RT), showed equivalent outcomes between patients who underwent completion axillary dissection for positive sentinel nodes and those who did not. A long time ago, the Danish Breast Cancer Cooperative Group showed a survival advantage of postmastectomy RT.[3] These patients received comprehensive nodal irradiation. Preliminary results of the National Cancer Institute of Canada Clinical Trials Group MA.20 study[4] showed improved LR relapse-free survival, distant disease-free survival, and disease-free survival when regional nodal irradiation was added to whole-breast irradiation.

The present study and this existing body of evidence provide empirical data that more extensive surgery (whether mastectomy or axillary dissection) does not improve outcomes. Irradiation, and in some cases irradiation of a wider field, however, does. Moreover, the improvement not only is limited to local control but also includes survival end points. How can this be explained? The view that cancer is a primarily systemic disease enjoys considerable currency. Are positive lymph nodes and adverse primary tumor characteristics the only markers of aggressive disease that are likely to manifest systemically regardless of LR treatment, or are they themselves the source of distant disease? The success of an LR treatment such as RT flies in the face of received wisdom by arguing the latter. The philosopher of science Karl Popper argued for a scientific method based on empirical falsification, meaning that observations are used to disprove theories.[5] As we learn more about what does and does not work in the treatment of cancer, we will come to a better understanding of the disease itself.

R. Gopal, MD, PhD

References

1. Abdulkarim BS, Cuartero J, Hanson J, Deschênes J, Lesniak D, Sabri S. Increased risk of locoregional recurrence for women with T1–2N0 triple-negative breast cancer treated with modified radical mastectomy without adjuvant radiation therapy compared with breast-conserving therapy. *J Clin Oncol.* 2011;29:2852-2858.

2. Giuliano AE, Hunt KK, Ballman KV, et al. Axillary dissection vs no axillary dissection in women with invasive breast cancer and sentinel node metastasis: a randomized clinical trial. *JAMA*. 2011;305:569-575.
3. Overgaard M, Hansen PS, Overgaard J, et al. Postoperative radiotherapy in high-risk premenopausal women with breast cancer who receive adjuvant chemotherapy. Danish Breast Cancer Cooperative Group 82b Trial. *N Engl J Med.* 1997;337:956-962.
4. Whelan TJ, Olivotto I, Ackerman I, et al. NCIC-CTG MA.20: an intergroup trial of regional nodal irradiation in early breast cancer (abstract LBA1003). *J Clin Oncol.* 2011:29.
5. Popper K. *The Logic of Scientific Discovery.* New York, NY: Basic Books; 1959.

Diagnostic Imaging

Breast Imaging Training and Attitudes: Update Survey of Senior Radiology Residents

Bassett LW, Bent C, Sayre JW, et al (David Geffen School of Medicine at UCLA)
AJR Am J Roentgenol 197:263-269, 2011

Objective.—The purpose of this study was to investigate the training and attitudes of senior residents regarding breast imaging.

Materials and Methods.—In 2008 a follow-up survey was completed by a chief or senior resident at 201 radiology training programs in North America. Questions included organization of breast imaging rotation, resident responsibilities, clinical practice protocols at the institution, resident impressions regarding breast imaging, and resident interest in performing breast imaging after residency. Results were compared with those of a survey completed in 2000.

Results.—Of 201 training programs, 200 (99.5%) had dedicated breast imaging rotations; 190 (95%), 12 weeks or longer; and 39 (19%), 16 weeks or longer. Residents regularly performed real-time ultrasound imaging in 138 programs (69%), needle localization in 159 (79%), ultrasound-guided biopsy in 154 (77%), and stereotactically guided biopsy in 145 programs (72%). One hundred sixty-two residents (81%) reported that interpreting mammograms was more stressful than interpretation of other imaging studies; 143 (71%) believed that only breast imaging subspecialists should interpret mammograms; and 104 (52%) would not consider pursuing a breast imaging fellowship. As in 2000, the most common reasons cited for not considering a fellowship were lack of interest in the field, fear of lawsuits, and the stressful nature of the job.

Conclusion.—Residency programs have devoted more time to breast imaging and made improvements in their curricula, but current residents report decreased opportunities to perform some studies and procedures. Although most residents would not consider a fellowship and did not want to interpret mammograms in future practice, the percentage of residents who would not consider breast imaging as a subspecialty has decreased since 2000. An accurate picture of current breast imaging curricula and

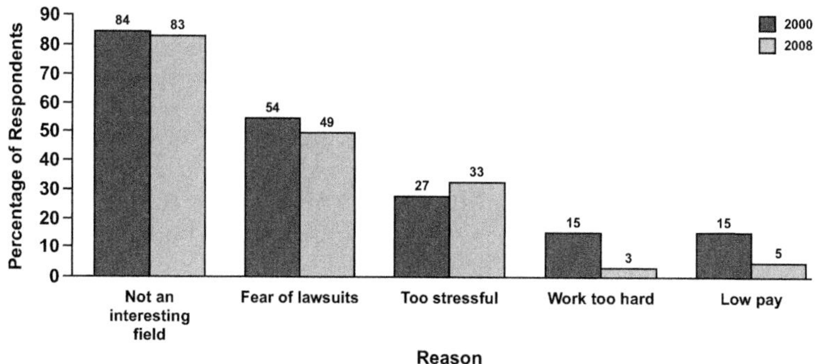

FIGURE 1.—Graph shows most common reasons selected by residents who would not consider doing breast imaging fellowship if offered. Residents could select as many reasons as they thought applied to them. *Y*-axis shows percentage of all residents who would not consider breast imaging fellowship. (Reprinted with permission from the American Journal of Roentgenology, Bassett LW, Bent C, Sayre JW, et al. Breast Imaging Training and Attitudes: Update Survey of Senior Radiology Residents. *AJR Am J Roentgenol.* 2011;197:263-269.)

variations among residency programs is necessary to identify and correct systemic problems and to improve the training of future breast imagers (Fig 1).

▶ Based on a national survey conducted in 2008, this article provides an update on the attitudes of radiology residents toward breast imaging. It is a sequel to an article that presented similar data from a survey conducted in 2000.[1] According to the study results, improvements have been made in many aspects of breast imaging training during residency. A dedicated breast imaging rotation with at least 12 weeks of clinical exposure has become the norm across the country.

However, some areas of concern still exist. Because the majority of mammograms in the United States are read by general radiologists, breast imaging training during residency must provide a high-quality experience.[2] Compared to the earlier survey, this study revealed that a smaller proportion of residents routinely perform real-time breast ultrasonography as part of their training. In 2000, 64% of residents reported that they "always" or "frequently" performed real-time breast ultrasonography. In 2008, this number had decreased to 44%. Proficiency in scanning the breast requires practice. Even in settings in which a technologist performs the scans or ultrasonography is automated, the radiologist must have a clear understanding of breast ultrasonographic anatomy and the ability to personally evaluate or re-scan problem cases. Furthermore, in 13% of programs, the breast imaging faculty did not interpret the breast ultrasonography findings. Correlating breast ultrasonography findings with mammography findings is an essential part of breast imaging care and an important part of the breast imaging training curriculum.[3]

Another potential area for concern is the volume of cases during residency. Although the mean volume reported was 119 cases per week, the range was between 10 and 500 cases per week. The authors do not report how many programs had lower volumes of cases. Although no existing data indicate how many mammograms a resident should see to become "competent," a volume of only 10 cases per week raises concerns.

This article also underscores the point that breast imaging is not the specialty of choice for many residents, primarily because of factors that are unique to the field and hard to change, such as high malpractice risk, high stress, and contact with anxious patients. However, at least 1 other factor can be changed. The authors make an excellent point that residents do not always get experience in breast imaging before they need to make important decisions about fellowship choices. Hopefully, the new Society of Chairs of Academic Radiology Departments (SCARD) recommendations regarding the timeline for fellowship interviews and selection will give residents a chance to experience breast imaging before they need to make these decisions. This SCARD resolution recommends that the fellowship application process begin in the spring of the third year of residency, which will give residents more clinical exposure before deciding on a career path.

D. M. Farria, MD, MPH

References

1. Bassett LW, Monsees BS, Smith RA, et al. Survey of radiology residents: breast imaging training and attitudes. *Radiology.* 2003;227:862-869.
2. Lewis RS, Sunshine JH, Bhargavan M. A portrait of breast imaging specialists and of the interpretation of mammography in the United States. *AJR Am J Roentgenol.* 2006;187:W456-W468.
3. Sickles EA, Philpotts LE, Parkinson BT, et al. American College of Radiology/Society of Breast Imaging curriculum for resident and fellow education in breast imaging. *J Am Coll Radiol.* 2006;3:879-884.

Screening Breast MR Imaging in Women with a History of Chest Irradiation

Sung JS, Lee CH, Morris EA, et al (Memorial Sloan-Kettering Cancer Ctr, NY)

Radiology 259:65-71, 2011

Purpose.—To assess the utility of screening magnetic resonance (MR) imaging in detecting otherwise occult breast cancers in women with a history of radiation therapy to the chest.

Materials and Methods.—This HIPAA-compliant study was approved by the authors' institutional review board. The need for informed consent was waived. Retrospective review of the radiology department database identified 247 screening breast MR imaging examinations performed between January 1999 and December 2008 in 91 women with a history of chest irradiation. Findings and recommendations for each breast MR study and on the most recent mammogram were reviewed. The number of cancers diagnosed, their method of detection, and tumor characteristics were examined. The exact 95% binomial proportion confidence intervals were calculated by using methods described by Clopper and Pearson.

Results.—Biopsy was recommended for 32 suspicious lesions on 27 (11%) of 247 MR imaging studies in 21 women. Seven cancers were identified in 30 lesions sampled (23%). Biopsy was recommended in five additional patients on the basis of mammographic findings, and malignancy was detected in three. Ten cancers were detected during the study period: four detected with MR imaging alone, three with MR imaging and mammography, and three with mammography alone. The four cancers detected with MR imaging alone were invasive carcinomas. Two of three cancers detected with mammography alone were ductal carcinoma in situ (DCIS), and the third was DCIS with microinvasion.

Conclusion.—MR imaging is a useful adjunct modality to screen high-risk women with a history of chest irradiation, resulting in a 4.4% (95% confidence interval: 1.2%, 10.9%) incremental cancer detection rate; the sensitivity for detecting breast cancers by using a combination of MR imaging and mammography was higher than that for either modality alone.

▶ Women who undergo chest irradiation as a component of cancer treatment have an increased risk of subsequent breast cancer.[1,2] The magnitude of the risk increases with higher radiation doses and larger radiation fields, both of which increase the amount of radiation delivered to the breast tissue. Patient age at the time of chest irradiation also influences the risk, with the highest risk seen in women who undergo radiation therapy at a young age (35 years or younger). Young women are thought to have a more pronounced risk of radiation-induced breast cancer because proliferating and developing breast tissue is more sensitive to the tumorigenic effects of radiation therapy.

For women who have undergone chest radiation therapy, the National Comprehensive Cancer Network (NCCN) guidelines recommend annual mammography starting 8-10 years after the completion of radiation therapy but not before 25 years of age.[3] The sensitivity of annual screening mammography may be limited in survivors who have a higher risk of breast cancer and who are often screened at a younger age than are those in the general population, when the breast tissue has greater density. Therefore, both the NCCN and American Cancer Society guidelines also recommend annual breast MR imaging for women who underwent radiation therapy to the chest between age 10 and 30 years.[3,4] However, these recommendations for MR imaging are based on expert opinion extrapolated from the benefit seen in women at high risk of breast cancer because of a family history of breast cancer or genetic mutations. Data that demonstrate a benefit of breast MR imaging in women who have undergone chest radiation therapy are lacking.

This study by Sung and colleagues provides some of the first evidence of a benefit of screening breast MR imaging in cancer survivors who underwent chest radiation therapy. In this retrospective review of 91 women who underwent screening via breast MR imaging after prior chest radiation therapy, 10 cancers were diagnosed. Four cancers were diagnosed via MR imaging alone; 3 were diagnosed via MR imaging and mammography; and 3 were diagnosed via mammography alone. The sensitivity for cancer detection in this high-risk population was higher when MR imaging and mammography were combined than when either modality was used alone. These results support existing recommendations for screening women who have a history of prior chest radiation therapy with annual breast MR imaging in conjunction with annual mammography.

Although guidelines recommend screening mammography and breast MR imaging for women who received chest radiation therapy between age 10 and 30 years, studies indicate that breast cancer screening is underutilized in high-risk populations. A study of women who underwent chest irradiation at a young age showed that nearly half of the women younger than 40 years had never undergone mammography.[5] Similarly, in a study of women for whom radiologists specifically recommended MR imaging screening in the mammography report because of a 20% or greater risk of breast cancer on the basis of a family history of breast cancer, only 14% of the at-risk women returned for the recommended screening breast MR imaging.[6] This underutilization of breast cancer screening tests highlights the need to educate both cancer survivors and clinicians on the importance of mammography and MR imaging screening in women who have undergone chest radiation therapy.

K. E. Hoffman, MD, MHSc, MPH
G. J. Whitman, MD

References

1. Ng AK, LaCasce A, Travis LB. Long-term complications of lymphoma and its treatment. *J Clin Oncol.* 2011;29:1885-1892.
2. Ng AK, Travis LB. Radiation therapy and breast cancer risk. *J Natl Compr Canc Netw.* 2009;7:1121-1128.
3. NCCN Clinical Practice Guidelines in Oncology. Breast Cancer Screening and Diagnosis. Version 1.2011. http://www.nccn.org/professionals/physician_gls/pdf/breast-screening.pdf. Accessed March 16, 2012.
4. Saslow D, Boetes C, Burke W, et al; American Cancer Society Breast Cancer Advisory Group. American Cancer Society guidelines for breast screening with MRI as an adjunct to mammography. *CA Cancer J Clin.* 2007;57:75-89.
5. Oeffinger KC, Ford JS, Moskowitz CS, et al. Breast cancer surveillance practices among women previously treated with chest radiation for a childhood cancer. *JAMA.* 2009;301:404-414.
6. Brinton JT, Barke LD, Freivogel ME, Jackson S, O'Donnell CI, Glueck DH. Breast cancer risk assessment in 64,659 women at a single high-volume mammography clinic. *Acad Radiol.* 2012;19:95-99.

Prognostic Factors

Effect of HER2 status on risk of recurrence in women with small, node-negative breast tumours

Tanaka K, Kawaguchi H, Nakamura Y, et al (Natl Kyushu Cancer Centre, Minami-ku, Fukuoka, Japan)
Br J Surg 98:1561-1565, 2011

Background.—Adjuvant trastuzumab for small, node-negative, human epidermal growth factor receptor 2 (HER2)-positive breast cancer remains controversial. The purpose of this study was to investigate the risk of recurrence in women with pathological tumour node (pTN) T1 N0 tumours.

Methods.—Patients with pT1 N0 breast cancer diagnosed at the National Kyushu Cancer Centre between 2001 and 2007 were reviewed. Patients were categorized according to HER2 status.

Results.—Four hundred and fifty-four patients who had pT1 N0 tumours, and had not received adjuvant trastuzumab, were identified. The HER2-negative and -positive groups comprised 376 and 78 patients (17·2 per cent) respectively. At a median follow-up of 46·3 months, there were 18 recurrences. The 5-year relapse-free survival (RFS) rates were 97·2 and 88 per cent in the HER2-negative and -positive groups respectively ($P < 0{\cdot}001$). Multivariable analysis identified HER2-positive tumour as an independent predictor of RFS in patients with pT1 N0 tumours (hazard ratio 6·65, 95 per cent confidence interval 2·53 to 17·49; $P < 0{\cdot}001$).

Conclusion.—Women with pT1 N0 HER2-positive breast cancer have a high risk of recurrence.

▶ In this article, Tanaka and colleagues provide a retrospective review of the data on relapse-free survival for a group of patients assessed as having pathologic T1 N0 HER2-positive breast cancers. The data were derived from a breast cancer database and were collected prior to the onset of the use of adjuvant trastuzumab therapy in Japan.

The study provides detailed analyses of patient and tumor characteristics. Using univariate and multivariable analyses, the authors demonstrated that HER2-positive status in tumors resulted in an increased risk of relapse (local, regional, and distant metastases were included as relapse endpoints).

The authors noted that the HER2-positive tumors were more likely to be histologic grade 3 and more likely to have lymphatic invasion within the breast. Multivariable analysis confirmed lymphatic invasion and HER2 status as significant risk factors for breast cancer recurrence. This was noted even though a greater proportion of patients with HER2-positive disease had been treated with chemotherapy.

The results of this manuscript are consistent with those of other retrospective analyses, including studies from Finland, Korea, and the United States that also reported an association between HER2-positive status and poor prognosis and increased risk of relapse of the primary breast cancer.

I concur with the authors' conclusions that HER2-positive breast cancers, even those conventionally considered to be "low risk" such as pathologic T1 N0 stage disease, can no longer be included in a low-risk category. Estimates of recurrence risk range up to 30%,[1] and confirmation of substantial risk reduction with the use of adjuvant systemic therapy, such as chemotherapy plus trastuzumab, awaits confirmatory clinical trials. If the risk reduction benefit of adjuvant therapy for these tumors is proportional to that for more advanced disease, substantial clinical benefit may accrue as a result of systemic therapy with chemotherapy and trastuzumab. In the interim, it is prudent to discuss with individual patients the potential risks and harms of cancer recurrence in relation to the risks, harms, and potential benefits of systemic adjuvant therapy.

In the absence of comorbidities or advanced age, systemic therapy should be considered an option for those with pathologic T1 N0 HER2-positive breast carcinomas.

R. Theriault, DO, MBA

Reference

1. Theriault RL, Litton JK, Mittendorf EA, et al. Age and survival estimates in patients who have node-negative T1ab breast cancer by breast cancer subtype. *Clin Breast Cancer.* 2011;11:325-331.

Factors influencing survival in patients with breast cancer and single or solitary brain metastasis

Niwińska A, Pogoda K, Murawska M, et al (The Maria Skłodowska-Curie Memorial Cancer Centre and Inst of Oncology, Warsaw, Poland; Erasmus Med Ctr, Rotterdam, Netherlands; et al)

Eur J Surg Oncol 37:635-642, 2011

Aim.—To perform a comprehensive analysis of patients with breast cancer and solitary or single brain metastasis and to analyze factors influencing survival from brain metastasis.

Methods.—One hundred consecutive patients with single or solitary brain metastasis were treated in one institution in the years 2003–2009. Brain lesions were diagnosed by magnetic resonance imaging (MRI). A total of 57% of patients underwent resection of brain metastasis, 95% of patients received whole-brain radiation therapy (WBRT) and 67% were treated systemically after WBRT.

Results.—Median survival from the detection of brain metastasis was 13 months and 28% of patients survived for 2 years. In 29 patients with solitary brain metastasis, median survival was 20 months (2–80 months) and in 71 patients with single brain metastasis it was 11 months (1–79 months) $p = 0.01$. Median survival from brain metastasis in patients with Recursive Partitioning Analysis Radiation Therapy Oncology Group (RPA RTOG) prognostic class I, II and III was 22 months (4–80 months), 13 months (2–79 months) and 6 months (0.4–28 months), respectively, $p < 0.0001$. Median survival from brain metastasis in triple-negative, HER2, luminal B and luminal A subtypes was 11 months, 13 months, 16 months and 15 months, respectively ($p = 0.60$). Multivariate analysis revealed that RPA RTOG prognostic class I, neurosurgery and systemic therapy after WBRT were factors that correlated with survival.

Conclusions.—In patients with one metastatic lesion in the brain, affiliation to RPA RTOG prognostic class I and intensive local and systemic treatment had a strong correlation with survival. There was no significant correlation between biological subtype of cancer and survival.

▶ Compared with many malignancies that metastasize to the brain, breast cancer is more sensitive to radiation and systemic therapies. Despite this, the median survival after diagnosis of a brain metastasis from breast cancer is only 12 months.[1] Therefore, identifying patient, tumor, and treatment factors that correlate with improved survival will be critical for improving outcomes in this group of patients.

This article by Niwińska and colleagues illustrates the contributions of both local and systemic control to the survival of patients with breast cancer that metastasizes to the brain. The importance of local control is supported by the improved survival of patients who underwent neurosurgery. This may reflect selection bias, but it is consistent with randomized data from Patchell and colleagues that showed that surgery adds a survival benefit for patients with single brain metastases.[2] More recent randomized data from the RTOG also support the importance of local control, with the finding that the addition of stereotactic radiosurgery (SRS) to WBRT provides a survival benefit in patients with single brain metastases.[3] The decision regarding which local therapy to use, SRS or surgery, depends on patient and tumor characteristics and is made with multidisciplinary input at my institution.

The role of systemic disease control in survival is also supported by Niwińska and colleagues' study. The finding that patients with solitary brain metastases had a median survival of 20 months compared with 11 months for patients with single brain metastases supports the hypothesis that metastatic disease outside the brain contributes significantly to decreased survival. Perhaps most intriguing, patients with solitary brain metastases who received systemic therapy had a median survival of 34 months compared with 8 months for those who did not. Similar results were seen for patients with single brain metastases, with median survivals of 13 months versus 4 months for patients who did or did not receive systemic therapy. The authors posit 2 possible explanations for this: control of extracranial occult micrometastases and disruption of the blood-brain barrier by WBRT resulting in increased permeability of systemic agents into the brain. Support for the former comes from a recent study showing that patients whose breast tumors had human epidermal growth factor receptor 2 (HER2)/neu amplification and who received trastuzumab after developing central nervous system metastases had longer survival than patients who did not receive the targeted therapy.[4] The latter hypothesis suggests intriguing possibilities for treating brain metastases with combination therapy and is under active investigation by several ongoing clinical trials testing concurrent systemic therapy with cranial irradiation.[5]

This study upheld the utility of the RPA RTOG classification as a prognostic tool.[6] Patients in RPA class I, II, and III had median survival durations of 22 months, 13 months, and 6 months, respectively. Given that only 12% of the patients included in the development of the RPA classification model had breast cancer, it is worthwhile to ask how well this classification applies to breast cancer patients. To address this question, a revised, disease-specific classification model has recently been developed based on updated RTOG data.[1] After analysis of several factors, only Karnofsky performance status (KPS) remained a discriminator of prognosis in the breast cancer–specific model. Using this model, a breast cancer patient with a brain metastasis and a KPS of 70 has a median survival of 6.1 months, and a similar patient with a KPS of 100 has a median survival of 18.7 months. Therefore, KPS continues to be a powerful predictor of outcome for these patients.

In addition to clinical characteristics, there is increasing interest in using hormone receptor and HER2/neu status as prognostic markers in the metastatic setting. This study by Niwińska and colleagues did not find survival differences after the diagnosis of brain metastasis between luminal A, luminal B, HER2/neu amplified, or triple-negative subtypes. This may be the result of the relatively small numbers of patients in each subgroup or the availability of effective systemic therapies. Triple-negative breast cancer remains a notable challenge in this setting, and more research into novel therapies is sorely needed.

In summary, this study provided a detailed view of prognostic factors for breast cancer patients with solitary or single brain metastases. Known clinical factors, including RPA classification, were again identified as important discriminators of survival. Future work will be needed to establish the influence of biological subtype on outcomes for breast cancer patients with brain metastases.

S. L. McGovern, MD, PhD

References

1. Sperduto PW, Chao ST, Sneed PK, et al. Diagnosis-specific prognostic factors, indexes, and treatment outcomes for patients with newly diagnosed brain metastases: a multi-institutional analysis of 4,259 patients. *Int J Radiat Oncol Biol Phys.* 2010;77:655-661.
2. Patchell RA, Tibbs PA, Walsh JW, et al. A randomized trial of surgery in the treatment of single metastases to the brain. *N Engl J Med.* 1990;322:494-500.
3. Andrews DW, Scott CB, Sperduto PW, et al. Whole brain radiation therapy with or without stereotactic radiosurgery boost for patients with one to three brain metastases: phase III results of the RTOG 9508 randomised trial. *Lancet.* 2004;363: 1665-1672.
4. Brufsky AM, Mayer M, Rugo HS, et al. Central nervous system metastases in patients with HER2-positive metastatic breast cancer: incidence, treatment, and survival in patients from registHER. *Clin Cancer Res.* 2011;17:4834-4843.
5. Lapatinib in combination with radiation therapy in patients with brain metastases from HER2-positive breast cancer. http://clinicaltrials.gov/ct2/show/NCT00470847. Accessed November 30, 2011.
6. Gaspar L, Scott C, Rotman M, et al. Recursive partitioning analysis (RPA) of prognostic factors in three Radiation Therapy Oncology Group (RTOG) brain metastases trials. *Int J Radiat Oncol Biol Phys.* 1997;37:745-751.

Radiation Therapy

Accelerated partial breast irradiation with interstitial implants: risk factors associated with increased local recurrence

Ott OJ, Hildebrandt G, Pötter R, et al (Univ Hosp Erlangen, Germany; Univ Hosp Leipzig, Germany; Univ Hosp AKH Vienna, Austria; et al)

Int J Radiat Oncol Biol Phys 80:1458-1463, 2011

Purpose.—To analyze patient, disease, and treatment-related factors regarding their impact on local control after interstitial multicatheter accelerated partial breast irradiation (APBI).

Methods and Materials.—Between November 2000 and April 2005, 274 patients with early breast cancer were recruited for the German–Austrian APBI Phase II trial (ClinicalTrials.gov identifier: NCT00392184). In all, 64% (175/274) of the patients received pulsed-dose-rate (PDR) brachytherapy and 36% (99/274) received high-dose-rate (HDR) brachytherapy. Prescribed reference dose for HDR brachytherapy was 32 Gy in eight fractions of 4 Gy, twice daily. Prescribed reference dose in PDR brachytherapy was 49.8 Gy in 83 consecutive fractions of 0.6 Gy each hour. Total treatment time was 3 to 4 days.

Results.—The median follow-up time was 64 months (range, 9–110). The actuarial 5-year local recurrence free survival rate (5-year LRFS) was 97.7%. Comparing patients with an age <50 years (49/274) vs. ≥50 years (225/274), the 5-year LRFS resulted in 92.5% and 98.9% (exact $p = 0.030$; 99% confidence interval, 0.029–0.032), respectively. Antihormonal treatment (AHT) was not applied in 9% (24/274) of the study population. The 5-year LRFS was 99% and 84.9% (exact $p = 0.0087$; 99% confidence interval, 0.0079–0.0094) in favor of the patients who received AHT. Lobular histology (45/274) was not associated with worse local control compared with all other histologies (229/274). The 5-year LRFS rates were 97.6% and 97.8%, respectively.

Conclusions.—Local control at 5 years is excellent and comparable to therapeutic successes reported from corresponding whole-breast irradiation trials. Our data indicate that patients <50 years of age ought to be excluded from APBI protocols, and that patients with hormone-sensitive breast cancer should definitely receive adjuvant AHT when interstitial multicatheter APBI is performed. Lobular histology need not be an exclusion criterion for future APBI trials.

▶ Worldwide enthusiasm for APBI is growing as more centers gain experience and data accumulate showing that local control rates are comparable to those after whole breast irradiation in selected groups of patients with early-stage disease. Both the American Society for Radiation Oncology (ASTRO) and the Groupe Européen de Curiethérapie-European Society for Therapeutic Radiology and Oncology have published patient selection criteria for APBI based on consensus[1] and clinical evidence.[2] According to these criteria, patients are categorized as suitable, cautionary, or unsuitable on the basis of perceived risk of recurrence and the recognition that only whole breast irradiation has a proven track record of long-term effectiveness with minimal toxicity. Although these are generally accepted as prudent clinical guidelines, the ability to categorize patients into groups with distinct outcomes has been questioned. Vicini and colleagues reviewed their experience applying the ASTRO consensus guidelines to their patients and reported equally low local recurrence rates in all 3 groups.[3] This is not to say that caution should not be applied to the cautionary group or that the unsuitable group is routinely suitable for APBI but instead reflects the fact that more data are required to further refine our understanding of the risk of recurrence within subgroups of patients.

In this article, Ott and colleagues reviewed the outcomes of 274 selected patients with early-stage disease treated with APBI. They confirmed the prognostic significance of young age, questioned the exclusion of patients with lobular histology, and stressed the importance of hormonal therapy in appropriate patients. Although we must await the results of randomized trial data for definitive answers, for clinicians who treat patients with early-stage disease, these authors provide additional insight into the applicability of the consensus guidelines to their everyday patients. Young age is particularly associated with local failure, and any form of breast-conserving therapy needs to be discussed at length with younger patients. Until more data are available, many of the other characteristics included in the consensus guidelines continue to serve as a framework for further clinical investigation.

M. T. Ballo, MD
V. K. Reed, MD

References

1. Smith BD, Arthur DW, Buchholz TA, et al. Accelerated partial breast irradiation consensus statement from the American Society for Radiation Oncology (ASTRO). *J Am Coll Surg*. 2009;209:269-277.
2. Polgár C, Van Limbergen E, Pötter R, et al; GEC-ESTRO breast cancer working group. Patient selection for accelerated partial-breast irradiation (APBI) after breast-conserving surgery: recommendations of the Groupe Européen de Curiethérapie-European Society for Therapeutic Radiology and Oncology (GEC-ESTRO) breast cancer working group based on clinical evidence (2009). *Radiother Oncol.* 2010;94:264-273.
3. Vicini F, Arthur D, Wazer D, et al. Limitations of the American Society of Therapeutic Radiology and Oncology Consensus Panel guidelines on the use of accelerated partial breast irradiation. *Int J Radiat Oncol Biol Phys.* 2011;79:977-984.

Accelerated partial breast irradiation: 5-year results of the German-Austrian multicenter phase II trial using interstitial multicatheter brachytherapy alone after breast-conserving surgery

Strnad V, Hildebrandt G, Pötter R, et al (Univ Hosp Erlangen, Germany; Univ Hosp Leipzig, Germany; Univ Hosp AKH Vienna, Austria; et al)
Int J Radiat Oncol Biol Phys 80:17-24, 2011

Purpose.—To evaluate the impact of accelerated partial breast irradiation on local control, side effects, and cosmesis using multicatheter interstitial brachytherapy as the sole method for the adjuvant local treatment of patients with low-risk breast cancer.

Methods and Materials.—274 patients with low-risk breast cancer were treated on protocol. Patients were eligible for the study if the tumor size was <3 cm, resection margins were clear by at least 2 mm, no lymph node metastases existed, age was >35 years, hormone receptors were positive, and histologic grades were 1 or 2. Of the 274 patients, 175 (64%) received pulse-dose-rate brachytherapy ($D_{ref} = 50$ Gy). and 99 (36%) received high-dose-rate brachytherapy ($D_{ref} = 32.0$ Gy).

Results.—Median follow-up was 63 months (range, 9—103). Only 8 of 274 (2.9%) patients developed an ipsilateral in-breast tumor recurrence at the time of analysis. The 5-year actuarial local recurrence-free survival probability was 98%. The 5- year overall and disease-free survival probabilities of all patients were 97% and 96%, respectively. Contralateral in-breast malignancies were detected in 2 of 274 (0.7%) patients, and distant metastases occurred in 6 of 274 (2.2%). Late side effects ≥Grade 3 (*i.e.*, breast tissue fibrosis and telangiectasia) occurred in 1 patient (0.4%,

95% CI: 0.0-2.0%) and 6 patients (2.2%, 95% CI: 0.8-4.7%), respectively. Cosmetic results were good to excellent in 245 of 274 patients (90%).

Conclusions.—The long-term results of this prospective Phase II trial confirm that the efficacy of accelerated partial breast irradiation using multicatheter brachytherapy is comparable with that of whole breast irradiation and that late side effects are negligible.

► The German-Austrian multi-institutional trial is the largest published multicatheter accelerated partial breast irradiation (APBI) experience. After 63 months, 8 (2.9%) of 274 patients had an ipsilateral breast tumor recurrence (IBTR). Only 3 of these patients were classified as having a true recurrence. These results are consistent with those observed in the American Society of Breast Surgeons (ASBS) MammoSite registry trial, in which 2.6% of patients had an IBTR after 54 months.[1] Unlike the ASBS trial, in which negative estrogen receptor (ER) status was associated with IBTR, this analysis revealed no association between any tumor parameter (tumor size, grade, lobular vs nonlobular histology, or ER status) and local control, disease-free survival, or overall survival.

Treatment was well tolerated, and excellent or good overall cosmesis was observed in over 90% of patients. It is important to note that the incidences of both telangiectasia and fibrosis, the most common late effects, increased with time. In fact, the incidences of these effects did not stabilize until after 6 years of follow-up. Overall cosmesis also changed over time for patients treated in the ASBS trial.

The results also showed that the dose nonuniformity ratio (DNR) may have been associated with local recurrence-free survival, but this association only approached statistical significance ($P = .1$). The DNR is an indicator of brachytherapy implant quality and is defined as the ratio of the high-dose volume to the reference-dose volume, with the optimal dose distribution achieved at the minimum DNR value. The authors noted that the quality of the implants could be important and, therefore, should be respected.

This large, prospective trial adds to the growing body of evidence demonstrating excellent local control and acceptable toxicity after APBI. I agree with the authors that it is not unfounded to conclude that we can expect results after APBI to be similar to those yielded by standard whole-breast irradiation. Clinicians should be aware, however, that the late effects of APBI do not stabilize until at least 5 years after treatment. The results of this trial also emphasize that, as has been observed with whole-breast irradiation, the quality of radiotherapy matters.

L. W. Cuttino, MD

Reference

1. Vicini F, Beitsch P, Quiet C, et al. Five-year analysis of treatment efficacy and cosmesis by the American Society of Breast Surgeons MammoSite Breast Brachytherapy Registry Trial in patients treated with accelerated partial breast irradiation. *Int J Radiat Oncol Biol Phys.* 2011;79:808-817.

Age, Comorbidity, and Breast Cancer Severity: Impact on Receipt of Definitive Local Therapy and Rate of Recurrence among Older Women with Early-Stage Breast Cancer

Field TS, Bosco JLF, Prout MN, et al (Meyers Primary Care Inst, Worcester, MA; Boston Univ Med Ctr, MA; Boston Univ School of Public Health, MA; et al)

J Am Coll Surg 213:757-765, 2011

Background.—The definitive local therapy options for early-stage breast cancer are mastectomy and breast-conserving surgery followed by radiation therapy. Older women and those with comorbidities frequently receive breast-conserving surgery alone. The interaction of age and comorbidity with breast cancer severity and their impact on receipt of definitive therapy have not been well-studied.

Study Design.—In a cohort of 1,837 women aged 65 years and older receiving treatment for early-stage breast cancer in 6 integrated health care delivery systems in 1990–1994 and followed for 10 years, we examined predictors of receiving nondefinitive local therapy and assessed the impact on breast cancer recurrence within levels of severity, defined as level of risk for recurrence.

Results.—Age and comorbidity were associated with receipt of nondefinitive therapy. Compared with those at low risk, women at the highest risk were less likely to receive nondefinitive therapy (odds ratio = 0.32; 95% CI, 0.22–0.47), and women at moderate risk were about half as likely (odds ratio = 0.54; 95% CI, 0.35–0.84). Nondefinitive local therapy was associated with higher rates of recurrence among women at moderate (hazard ratio = 5.1; 95% CI, 1.9–13.5) and low risk (hazard ratio = 3.2; 95% CI, 1.1–8.9). The association among women at high risk was weak (hazard ratio = 1.3; 95% CI, 0.75–2.1).

Conclusions.—Among these older women with early-stage breast cancer, decisions about therapy partially balanced breast cancer severity against age and comorbidity. However, even among women at low risk, omitting definitive local therapy was associated with increased recurrence.

▶ Although radiation therapy (RT) after breast-conserving surgery (BCS) has been shown to improve local control and survival outcomes in multiple randomized controlled trials, the role of RT after BCS in older patients with breast cancer is more controversial. The most influential study focusing on an older population, the Cancer and Leukemia Group B 9343 trial,[1] showed that within a highly selected group of older patients, RT reduced the 10-year locoregional recurrence rate from 9% to 2%.[2] However, no associated improvements in mastectomy-free survival or overall survival were observed, thereby leading the investigators to question whether RT confers a clinically meaningful benefit in this population. Conversely, evidence from previous studies in the population-based setting suggested that the benefits of RT include a statistically significant improvement in mastectomy-free survival.[3,4]

Consistent with the existing literature, this interesting study by Field and colleagues also demonstrates an association between the omission of RT and an increased risk of breast cancer recurrence. Furthermore, this study provides important data to help determine why certain patients may not receive RT. Interestingly, among the 23% of patients in their BCS cohort who did not receive RT, 83% were never referred to a radiation oncologist. In contrast, 97% of patients referred to a radiation oncologist, and for whom RT was recommended, went on to begin RT. These findings suggest that a crucial step toward compliance with recommended RT is actual consultation with a radiation oncologist.

Older patients with breast cancer are a very heterogeneous group, so it is not prudent to make generalized treatment recommendations based simply on 1 variable, such as age, comorbid conditions, or disease stage. Considering the well-documented challenges of predicting life expectancy in this patient population[5] and the variability in the expected benefit from RT based on patient and disease characteristics,[3,4] the decision concerning whether a particular patient should receive RT requires a nuanced conversation with the patient about the balance of recurrence risk, potential benefit from RT, and risk of death before recurrence. In light of the results of this study and previous research, we believe it is important for older women to receive individualized risk assessment from their oncology team and to discuss treatment options with a knowledgeable radiation oncologist.

J. M. Albert, MD
B. D. Smith, MD

References

1. Hughes KS, Schnaper LA, Berry D, et al. Lumpectomy plus tamoxifen with or without irradiation in women 70 years of age or older with early breast cancer. *N Engl J Med.* 2004;351:971-977.
2. Hughes KS, Schnaper LA, Cirrincione C, et al. Lumpectomy plus tamoxifen with or without irradiation in women age 70 or older with early breast cancer. *J Clin Oncol.* 2010;28:507A.
3. Smith BD, Gross CP, Smith GL, Galusha DH, Bekelman JE, Haffty BG. Effectiveness of radiation therapy for older women with early breast cancer. *J Natl Cancer Inst.* 2006;98:681-690.
4. Albert JM, Pan IW, Shih YC, et al. Effectiveness of radiation for prevention of mastectomy in older breast cancer patients treated with conservative surgery. *Cancer.* in press.
5. Yourman LC, Lee SJ, Schonberg MA, Widera EW, Smith AK. Prognostic indices for older adults: a systematic review. *JAMA.* 2012;307:182-192.

Early-stage young breast cancer patients: Impact of local treatment on survival

Bantema-Joppe EJ, De Munck L, Visser O, et al (Univ of Groningen, The Netherlands; Comprehensive Cancer Ctr North East, Groningen/Enschede, The Netherlands; Comprehensive Cancer Ctr Amsterdam, The Netherlands)
Int J Radiat Oncol Biol Phys 81:e553-e559, 2011

Purpose.—In young women, breast-conserving therapy (BCT), *i.e.*, lumpectomy followed by radiotherapy, has been associated with an increased risk of local recurrence. Still, there is insufficient evidence that BCT impairs survival. The aim of our study was to compare the effect of BCT with mastectomy on overall survival (OS) in young women with early-stage breast cancer.

Methods and Materials.—From two Dutch regional population-based cancer registries (covering 6.2 million inhabitants) 1,453 women < 40 years with pathologically T1N0–1M0 breast cancer were selected. Cox regression survival analysis was used to study the effect of local treatment (BCT vs. mastectomy) stratified for nodal stage on survival and corrected for tumor size, age, period of diagnosis, and use of adjuvant systemic therapy.

Results.—With a median follow-up of 9.6 years, 10-year OS was 83% after BCT and 78% after mastectomy, respectively (unadjusted hazard ratio [HR], 1.37; 95% confidence interval [CI], 1.09–1.72). In N0-patients, 10-year OS was 84% after BCT and 81% after mastectomy and local treatment was not associated with differences in OS (HR 1.19; 95% CI, 0.89–1.58; $p = 0.25$). Within the N1-patient group, OS was better after BCT compared with mastectomy, 79% vs. 71% at 10 years (HR 1.91; 95% CI, 1.28–2.84; $p = 0.001$) and in patients treated with adjuvant hormonal therapy (HR 0.34; 95% CI, 0.18–0.66; $p = 0.001$).

Conclusions.—In this large population-based cohort of early-stage young breast cancer patients, 10-year OS was not impaired after BCT compared with mastectomy. Patients with 1 to 3 positive lymph nodes had better prognosis after BCT than after mastectomy.

▶ Although breast conservation therapy is a well-established standard treatment for appropriately selected patients with early-stage breast cancer, there has been reluctance to apply this treatment to young women (variably defined as less than 30 to 50 years old). As evidence of this, a recent US patterns of care analysis revealed that not only do young women have a higher mastectomy rate, but also the mastectomy rate among young women—in contrast to older women—increased during the past decade.[1] Young women not only present with more aggressive tumors—with higher grade, lymphovascular space invasion, and estrogen and progesterone receptor negativity—but also have worse outcomes compared to older women, regardless of the local therapy. Although the initial randomized trials that established the efficacy of breast conservation therapy included women of all ages, young women represented a relatively small proportion of the patients on these trials. Several studies have since compared outcomes for young women undergoing either breast conservation therapy or mastectomy for breast cancer. Although some of these studies have suggested worse local control with breast conservation therapy, it is not clear whether the resultant higher local recurrence rate translates into a survival detriment for these patients.

In this context, Bantema-Joppe and colleagues investigated whether the type of local treatment affects survival in young women with early-stage breast cancer. Using 2 Dutch population-based cancer registries, they identified 1453 young women less than 40 years old with pT1 N0-1 M0 breast cancer treated by either breast conservation therapy or mastectomy between 1989 and 2005. They compared overall survival according to the type of local treatment using univariate and multivariate approaches. Because of an interaction between the type of local treatment and nodal stage, they analyzed patients with node-negative and node-positive disease separately. Among patients who had node-negative disease, they found no difference in survival according to the type of local treatment. With a median follow-up of 9.6 years, they found 10-year overall survival rates of 84% after breast conservation therapy and 81% after mastectomy ($P = .26$). This lack of survival difference was verified on multivariate analysis ($P = .25$). Interestingly, among patients with node-positive disease, breast conservation therapy resulted in improved survival. The 10-year survival rate after breast conservation therapy was 79%, compared with 71% after mastectomy ($P = .014$). Again, multivariate analysis confirmed the survival difference seen on univariate analysis ($P = .001$).

The strengths of this study include its relatively large sample size, despite restricting the analysis to patients less than 40 years old with pT1 N0-1 M0 disease, who are almost universally candidates for breast conservation therapy. As with any retrospective analysis, however, this study was limited by potential selection bias and a lack of information regarding known prognostic factors. Specifically, the study failed to incorporate important pathologic characteristics, such as tumor grade, lymphovascular space invasion, estrogen receptor, progesterone receptor, and HER2 status, and the numbers of positive and examined lymph nodes. Although the authors state that these tumor-related prognostic factors likely did not contribute to the choice of surgical procedure because they were assessed postoperatively, their conclusions would have been strengthened had they shown that these factors did not vary by the type of local treatment. Moreover, this study failed to account for important patient characteristics, such as race and genetic predisposition, as well as treatment variables such as the type of systemic therapy and whether regional radiotherapy was administered. Without further information regarding such patient, tumor, and treatment characteristics, one must view the improved survival among node-positive patients who underwent breast conservation therapy with caution.

What can more reliably be concluded, however, is that breast conservation therapy likely does not worsen survival for young women with early-stage breast cancer. This finding is in line with our soon-to-be published study in which we evaluated survival outcomes among 14 764 young women aged 20 to 39 years with T1-2 N0-1 M0 breast cancer who were identified via the Surveillance, Epidemiology, and End Results database.[2] In our study, both multivariable and matched pair analyses demonstrated no difference in overall or cause-specific survival by type of local treatment.

Taken together, these studies add to the growing body of literature suggesting that the increasing utilization of mastectomy in young women may not be justified, at least not on the basis of a perceived improvement in survival. Young women with early-stage breast cancer should be counseled appropriately regarding their treatment options—preferably in a multidisciplinary setting—and should not choose a mastectomy on the basis of the assumption that it will improve survival. Continued study of this unique patient population is, nonetheless, warranted.

U. Mahmood, MD

References

1. Habermann EB, Abbott A, Parsons HM, Virnig BA, Al-Refaie WB, Tuttle TM. Are mastectomy rates really increasing in the United States? *J Clin Oncol.* 2010;28: 3437-3441.
2. Mahmood U, Morris C, Neuner G, et al. Similar survival with breast conservation therapy or mastectomy in the management of young women with early stage breast cancer [published online ahead of print January 31, 2012]. *Int J Radiat Oncol Biol Phys.* 10.1016/j.ijrobp.2011.10.075.

Fractionation for whole breast irradiation: An American Society for Radiation Oncology (ASTRO) evidence-based guideline

Smith BD, Bentzen SM, Correa CR, et al (Univ of Texas, MD Anderson Cancer Ctr, Houston; Univ of Wisconsin School of Medicine and Public Health, Madison; Univ of Michigan, Ann Arbor; et al)

Int J Radiat Oncol Biol Phys 81:59-68, 2011

Purpose.—In patients with early-stage breast cancer treated with breast-conserving surgery, randomized trials have found little difference in local control and survival outcomes between patients treated with conventionally fractionated (CF-) whole breast irradiation (WBI) and those receiving hypofractionated (HF)-WBI. However, it remains controversial whether these results apply to all subgroups of patients. We therefore developed an evidence-based guideline to provide direction for clinical practice.

Methods and Materials.—A task force authorized by the American Society for Radiation Oncology weighed evidence from a systematic literature review and produced the recommendations contained herein.

Results.—The majority of patients in randomized trials were aged 50 years or older, had disease Stage pT1-2 pN0, did not receive chemotherapy, and were treated with a radiation dose homogeneity within ±7% in the central axis plane. Such patients experienced equivalent outcomes with either HF-WBI or CF-WBI. Patients not meeting these criteria were relatively underrepresented, and few of the trials reported subgroup analyses. For patients not receiving a radiation boost, the task force favored a dose schedule of 42.5 Gy in 16 fractions when HF-WBI is planned. The task force also recommended that the heart should be excluded from the primary treatment fields (when HF-WBI is used) due to lingering uncertainty regarding late effects of HF-WBI on cardiac function. The task force could not agree on the appropriateness of a tumor bed boost in patients treated with HF-WBI.

Conclusion.—Data were sufficient to support the use of HF-WBI for patients with early-stage breast cancer who met all the aforementioned criteria. For other patients, the task force could not reach agreement either for or against the use of HF-WBI, which nevertheless should not be interpreted as a contraindication to its use.

▶ Multiple randomized trials have demonstrated that WBI following breast-conserving surgery (BCS) reduces the risk of local recurrence in patients with early-stage breast cancer.[1] These trials used conventional fractionation (CF) for WBI consisting of a total dose of 45-50 Gy delivered in 25-28 daily fractions of 1.8-2.0 Gy per fraction. Over the past 2 decades, interest has increased among clinicians and patients in HF-WBI, defined as daily doses exceeding 2.0 Gy, to reduce overall treatment time, improve patient compliance, ease geographic constraints and transportation issues, and potentially reduce the cost of treatment.

In this article, ASTRO assembled a task force to undertake a systematic literature review in an effort to develop evidence-based recommendations for the use of HF-WBI. Four important clinical points were addressed: identifying the patients most appropriate for HF-WBI and determining the role of a tumor-bed boost, the appropriate dosing regimens, and the characteristics of an acceptable plan for delivering HF-WBI. The evidence for the guidelines was largely derived from 4 randomized trials (Canadian, START A, START B, and Royal Marsden Hospital/Gloucestershire Oncology Centre) that evaluated HF-WBI and CF-WBI regimens in more than 7000 patients with median follow-up times ranging from 5 to 12 years.[2-7] Using these data, the task force concluded that HF-WBI is a safe and effective treatment option that renders local control rates and survival outcomes that are equivalent to those of CF-WBI. Given the favorable results for HF-WBI, several intriguing questions have emerged regarding patient selection, particularly because these trials largely included older women who did not have nodal involvement and did not receive adjuvant chemotherapy. Indeed, 1 of the main clinical questions this article addressed is whether the equivalent results for HF-WBI and CF-WBI in the randomized trials extend to all subgroups of patients.

Ultimately, this question remains unanswered. The ASTRO task force validated the equivalence of HF-WBI to CF-WBI for patients 50 years or older with pathologic stage T1-2, node-negative disease treated with BCS without adjuvant chemotherapy. For patients who did not satisfy all of these criteria, the task force could not reach a consensus to make recommendations either for or against HF-WBI. The significance of this article is undeniable, as it helps guide treatment decisions regarding HF-WBI following BCS, but questions still remain as to the appropriateness of HF-WBI in certain patient subgroups. For instance, with respect to HF-WBI in younger women, the authors noted that only approximately 20% to 25% of patients included in the 4 randomized trials were younger than 50 years. Although the Canadian trial stratified patients by age and demonstrated equivalent results in patients younger and older than 50 years, the task force did not reach a consensus regarding the role of HF-WBI in younger women, as the available data were deemed insufficient to warrant routine recommendation of HF-WBI in these women.

Further questions remain unanswered regarding the addition of a radiation boost to the surgical cavity, the use of adjuvant chemotherapy, and the use of regional nodal irradiation along with HF-WBI. Although most patients included in these randomized trials had low-risk disease, HF-WBI was found to be equally effective in some subsets of patients with higher-risk disease.[8] One of the challenges facing the task force was to make recommendations for subgroups of patients who were not represented in the aforementioned clinical trials in sufficient numbers to allow for evidence-based conclusions.

Importantly, the article discusses possible late effects of HF-WBI given the potential deleterious effects that a higher dose per fraction could have on surrounding normal tissues. The overall rates of ischemic heart disease, pneumonitis, and symptomatic lung fibrosis were low in all of the trials, with no detectable difference between the HF-WBI and CF-WBI treatment groups. Rates of acute toxicity were largely equivalent between these groups as well, but whether acute toxicity can predict late toxicity will require longer follow-up. With the exception of the Canadian study, the trials had median follow-up times of less than 10 years, which may be too short to see the important long-term effects of radiation therapy.

Several unanswered questions remain, in light of the limited data regarding various subsets of patients for which the expert panel could not reach a consensus. Beyond the guidelines, 1 main contribution of this report is the identification of areas in which further research is needed, particularly with respect to the role of a tumor bed radiation boost in patients treated with HF-WBI and the appropriate dosing regimen. Longer follow-up of the existing randomized trials and additional prospective trials are necessary to answer the challenging questions that remain.

C. E. Fasola, MD, MPH
K. Horst, MD

References

1. Clarke M, Collins R, Darby S, et al. Effects of radiotherapy and of differences in the extent of surgery for early breast cancer on local recurrence and 15-year survival: an overview of the randomised trials. *Lancet.* 2005;366:2087-2106.
2. Whelan T, MacKenzie R, Julian J, et al. Randomized trial of breast irradiation schedules after lumpectomy for women with lymph node-negative breast cancer. *J Natl Cancer Inst.* 2002;94:1143-1150.
3. Whelan TJ, Pignol JP, Levine MN, et al. Long-term results of hypofractionated radiation therapy for breast cancer. *N Engl J Med.* 2010;362:513-520.
4. START Trialists' Group; Bentzen SM, Agrawal RK, Aird EG, et al. The UK Standardisation of Breast Radiotherapy (START) Trial A of radiotherapy hypofractionation for treatment of early breast cancer: a randomised trial. *Lancet Oncol.* 2008; 9:331-341.
5. START Trialists' Group; Bentzen SM, Agrawal RK, Aird EG, et al. The UK Standardisation of Breast Radiotherapy (START) Trial B of radiotherapy hypofractionation for treatment of early breast cancer: a randomised trial. *Lancet.* 2008;371: 1098-1107.
6. Yarnold J, Ashton A, Bliss JM, et al. Fractionation sensitivity and dose response of late adverse effects in the breast after radiotherapy for early breast cancer: long-term results of a randomised trial. *Radiother Oncol.* 2005;75:9-17.
7. Owen JR, Ashton A, Bliss JM, et al. Effect of radiotherapy fraction size on tumour control in patients with early-stage breast cancer after local tumour excision: long-term results of a randomised trial. *Lancet Oncol.* 2006;7:467-471.
8. Théberge V, Whelan T, Shaitelman S, Vicini FA. Altered fractionation: rationale and justification for whole and partial breast hypofractionated radiotherapy. *Semin Radiat Oncol.* 2011;21:55-65.

Irradiation effect after mastectomy on breast cancer recurrence in patients presenting with locally advanced disease

Taras AR, Thorpe JD, Morris AD, et al (Swedish Med Ctr, Seattle, WA; Fred Hutchinson Cancer Res Ctr, Seattle, WA)

Am J Surg 201:605-610, 2011

Background.—Current guidelines recommend postmastectomy irradiation (PMI) for patients with tumors >5 cm and/or ≥4 positive lymph nodes. This study evaluates the effect of PMI on recurrence and survival within tumor size and node status groups.

Methods.—Locoregional and distant recurrences and survival for different tumor and treatment characteristics were analyzed in 2,797 patients with invasive breast cancer treated with mastectomy.

Results.—Tumor size, positive nodes, extranodal extension, lymphatic/vascular invasion, estrogen receptor/progesterone negative, HER-2 positive, and high grade were associated with significantly increased recurrence. In patients with ≥4 positive nodes and patients with tumors >5 cm and positive nodes, PMI decreased local and distant recurrence (overall 53% vs 24%, $P < .001$) and increased disease-free survival ($P < .001$) but not overall survival. In patients with less disease, a benefit from PMI irradiation could not be identified.

Conclusions.—PMI is indicated for patients with ≥4 positive nodes or patients with tumors >5 cm and positive nodes.

► The importance of PMI for stage I or II disease continues to be debated. The authors of this article have presented the results of a large retrospective review of 2797 patients who underwent mastectomy with or without PMI. Similar to other studies published previously, their data support the use of PMI for tumors larger than 5 cm and in patients with 4 or more positive lymph nodes, but not in patients with N1 disease or early breast cancer.

The authors' conclusions, however, must be read with caution. These results do not stem from a prospective randomized trial, as PMI was administered on the basis of the providers' preferences and the perceptions of disease risk at their institution. In fact, when assessed as a whole, patients who received PMI had a significantly higher recurrence rate than those who did not (18% vs 10%, $P < .001$), which contradicts the findings reported in most prospective studies of PMI. Retrospective subgroup analyses were also performed on data from the patients treated at the Swedish Cancer Institute, although there are significant statistical limitations to performing multiple unplanned subgroup analyses.[1-3]

In this study, 427 patients with "low-risk" disease underwent PMI. Several of these patients had T1N0 or T2N0 disease and no clear or standard indication for PMI. Approximately 40% (168/427) had T2N1 disease, and despite the addition of PMI, no benefit was seen in this cohort either. Their study does support the notion that certain patients with T2N1 disease may not need PMI, a finding that is also supported by other retrospective series.[4-6] However, 3 prospective randomized trials of PMI all revealed a local control and survival benefit of PMI in patients with N1 disease.[7-9] Although these studies admittedly had limitations, a more recent study published in abstract only (the MA.20), included modern treatment practices and also strongly supported the use of radiation in women with N1 disease.[10] In the MA.20 study, patients underwent breast conservation therapy and were randomized to comprehensive regional nodal and breast irradiation or whole-breast irradiation alone. Patients who were treated comprehensively had significantly higher rates of isolated locoregional disease-free survival (DFS), and distant DFS, although these patients would have been considered "low risk" in the study presented by the Swedish Cancer Institute. In summary, this retrospective study supports the use of PMI in patients with high-risk disease but suggests that there may be a subgroup of patients with small node-positive tumors who do not benefit from PMI.

W. A. Hall, MD
M. A. Torres, MD

References

1. Lagakos SW. The challenge of subgroup analyses—reporting without distorting. *N Engl J Med.* 2006;354:1667-1669.
2. Pocock SJ, Assmann SE, Enos LE, Kasten LE. Subgroup analysis, covariate adjustment and baseline comparisons in clinical trial reporting: current practice and problems. *Stat Med.* 2002;21:2917-2930.
3. Wang R, Lagakos SW, Ware JH, Hunter DJ, Drazen JM. Statistics in medicine—reporting of subgroup analyses in clinical trials. *N Engl J Med.* 2007;357: 2189-2194.
4. Buchholz TA, Tucker SL, Masullo L, et al. Predictors of local-regional recurrence after neoadjuvant chemotherapy and mastectomy without radiation. *J Clin Oncol.* 2002;20:17-23.
5. Huang EH, Tucker SL, Strom EA, et al. Postmastectomy radiation improves local-regional control and survival for selected patients with locally advanced breast cancer treated with neoadjuvant chemotherapy and mastectomy. *J Clin Oncol.* 2004;22:4691-4699.
6. Huang EH, Tucker SL, Strom EA, et al. Predictors of locoregional recurrence in patients with locally advanced breast cancer treated with neoadjuvant chemotherapy, mastectomy, and radiotherapy. *Int J Radiat Oncol Biol Phys.* 2005;62: 351-357.
7. Overgaard M, Hansen PS, Overgaard J, et al. Postoperative radiotherapy in high-risk premenopausal women with breast cancer who receive adjuvant chemotherapy. Danish Breast Cancer Cooperative Group 82b Trial. *N Engl J Med.* 1997;337:949-955.
8. Overgaard M, Jensen MB, Overgaard J, et al. Postoperative radiotherapy in high-risk postmenopausal breast-cancer patients given adjuvant tamoxifen: Danish Breast Cancer Cooperative Group DBCG 82c randomised trial. *Lancet.* 1999; 353:1641-1648.
9. Ragaz J, Olivotto IA, Spinelli JJ, et al. Locoregional radiation therapy in patients with high-risk breast cancer receiving adjuvant chemotherapy: 20-year results of the British Columbia randomized trial. *J Natl Cancer Inst.* 2005;97:116-126.
10. Whelan TJ, Olivotto I, Ackerman I, et al. NCIC-CTG MA.20: an intergroup trial of regional nodal irradiation in early breast cancer [abstr LBA1003]. *J Clin Oncol.* 2011;29.

Surgical Treatment

Liver resection and local ablation of breast cancer liver metastases – A systematic review

Bergenfeldt M, Jensen BV, Skjoldbye B, et al (Univ of Copenhagen, Herlev, Denmark)

Eur J Surg Oncol 37:549-557, 2011

Aim.—To analyze surgical treatment of breast cancer liver metastases (BCLM) regarding selection criteria, outcome and prognostic parameters.

Methods.—We searched Embase and Medline for all studies published 1999–2010.

Results.—Resection was associated with a median survival (MOS) of 20–67 months and 5-year survival of 21–61%. Local ablation also had a favorable outcome; MOS was 30–60 months and 5-year survival 27–41%. Regarding selection, no specific limits regarding the number and size of BCLM can be given. Features of the primary breast cancer (BC) were not significant for the prognosis. Microscopically radical (R0) resection is a positive prognostic factor, while the effects of disease interval, hormone receptor status and response to preoperative chemotherapy were divergent. The presence of EHD had a negative effect on survival in some studies, but failed to have so in other studies.

Conclusions.—Surgical therapy may benefit a subset of patients with BCLM. Resection may be indicated, if an RO-resection can be done with a low risk of mortality. Liver resection in the presence of extrahepatic disease remains controversial, while patients with BCLM and bone metastases could possibly be managed differently than other EHD.

▶ Although breast cancer survival rates have improved each of the last several decades, with all-stage 5-year overall survival (OS) rates now approaching 90%, this is still a devastating and relentless disease in its advanced stages. Breast cancer patients with liver metastases are unlikely to live more than 2 years, and liver insufficiency resulting from tumor replacing the liver parenchyma and/or biliary obstruction often contributes to their deaths. In this patient population, local therapy, even if considered palliative, can have meaningful benefits if it can be performed with minimal morbidity and mortality.

The authors of this comprehensive review article should be congratulated on a thorough and well-written review of reported outcomes of patients treated for BCLM. Their work addresses 3 local treatment modalities: surgical resection, laser induced interstitial thermotherapy, and more traditional ablative technologies (eg, radiofrequency ablation). They nicely summarize a disparate number of mainly small-volume, single-institution, retrospective studies published over the past 3 decades on this topic. Given the constraints on the data, several specific questions remain unanswered at the conclusion of this article.

First, how can we integrate these data into our daily practice and into patient selection for local therapy? To start, we must remember that this is a systemic disease, and even at cancer centers with elite multidisciplinary teams treating the most optimal candidates, recurrence after local therapy is almost universal. The authors of this article astutely note that when the data from each of the studies reporting on this topic were pooled, recurrence rates increased proportionally with the duration of clinical follow-up. As such, surgery must be considered an adjuvant to systemic therapy, and the goal should be to prolong the progression-free interval.

The second issue is tumor biology. In clinical practice, particularly in cases with clinically apparent extrahepatic disease but also in cases with unifocal liver metastases, 2 dominant prognostic factors emerge. From an overall disease biology standpoint, hormone receptor status is a global prognostic marker. Patients with estrogen/progesterone receptor–negative primary tumors tend to be premenopausal and to have a more aggressive tumor biology. Several studies, including an analysis from The University of Texas MD Anderson Cancer Center of 86 patients, have confirmed that OS is closely associated with hormone receptor status (estrogen receptor– and progesterone receptor–negative primary breast cancers: median OS, 28.3 months vs estrogen receptor– or progesterone receptor–positive breast cancers: median OS, 76.8 months; OR 3.3).[1] Despite this general association, outcomes for selected patients with resected double-receptor–negative primary tumors are superior to those for medically treated patients, thus indicating that hormone receptor status should not be used as an absolute contraindication to surgical therapy.

A more specific prognostic marker is response to preoperative systemic cytotoxic and/or hormonal therapy. In contrast to hormone receptor status (a more population-based prognostic marker) response to systemic therapy is a more individualized, "patient-centric" prognostic factor. The MD Anderson experience corroborates this finding. Their data indicate that disease progression during preoperative therapy was the strongest predictor of poor outcome following hepatectomy (disease progression: median OS, 22.9 months vs treatment response/stable disease: median OS, 79.4 months; OR 3.8).[1] In practice, this becomes a clinically relevant decision-making tool. For example, I would much prefer to suggest surgery to a patient with triple-negative breast cancer who had significant radiologic response to preoperative systemic therapy than to a patient with a triple-positive pattern but progression during preoperative antihormonal therapy.

Third, which of the increasingly varied arrows do we pull from our quill to launch at this pattern of breast malignancy? This review reports on 3 categories of liver-directed therapy and suggests equivalence among them. However, this is an illusion based on bias in the literature. The authors borrow from reported experiences with ablative technologies applied to colorectal liver metastases and correctly caution against the use of this technology for treating tumors greater than 3 centimeters in diameter. It is also clear that ablation is anatomically restricted to selected "safe" areas in the liver. Several types of nonsurgical, transcatheter, intra-arterial therapy are on the horizon, but their efficacy in this setting is currently unproven.

Given that surgical resection performed in hepatobiliary centers by dedicated liver surgeons can be safely used to treat liver lesions in any segment or area of the liver (and can now frequently be performed using minimally invasive approaches), it should be regarded as the gold standard for liver-directed therapy.

We must remember that nonsurgical therapeutic approaches are not the only techniques with the potential to improve. Surgical approaches are constantly evolving toward increased safety and efficacy. Our most recent BCLM resection was of a synchronous liver metastasis. Despite a triple-negative receptor profile, the primary and metastatic disease responded well to induction chemotherapy. The patient underwent a simultaneous laparoscopic hepatectomy and modified radical mastectomy with reconstruction. The liver specimen revealed a complete pathologic response; the patient was discharged 3 days after surgery (hospitalization was extended at the request of Plastic Surgery) and was ready to resume systemic therapy after 3 weeks.

Breast cancer will always strike a fundamental emotional chord for physicians, and liver surgeons are no less susceptible. In turn, the difficult clinical problem of BCLM has been addressed by the giants in the field of liver surgery, including Pocard, Seifert, Bismuth (who proposed neoadjuvant chemotherapy followed by surgical resection as early as the 1980s), Makuuchi, Capussotti, Blumgart, Adam, Elias, Vauthey, and many others. Their combined experience clearly indicates that liver surgery can provide benefit for a selected group of patients with BCLM—mainly those with limited disease that is responsive to systemic therapy and treated with skilled and complete liver resection.

T. A. Aloia, MD

Reference

1. Abbott D, Brouquet A, Mittendorf E, et al. Resection of liver metastases from breast cancer: estrogen receptor status and response to chemotherapy before metastasectomy define outcome. *Surgery.* 2012;151:710-716.

Phase III randomized equivalence trial of early breast cancer treatments with or without axillary clearance in post-menopausal patients results after 5 years of follow-up

Avril A, On behalf of the AXIL95 Group (Institut Bergonié, Bordeaux Cedex, France; et al)

Eur J Surg Oncol 37:563-570, 2011

Background.—Axillary lymph node clearance (ALNC) improves locoregional control and provides prognostic information for early breast cancer treatment, but effects on survival are controversial. This multicentre, randomized pragmatic equivalence trial compares outcomes for post menopausal early invasive breast cancer patients after locoregional treatment with ALNC and adjuvant therapies to outcomes after locoregional treatment without ALNC and adjuvant therapies.

Methods.—From 1995–2005, women aged ≥50 years with early breast cancer (tumor ≤10 mm) and clinically-negative axillary nodes were randomized to receive treatment with ALNC (Ax) or without (no-Ax). Adjuvant therapies were prescribed according to hormonal receptor status and individual histological results. The primary endpoint was overall survival

(OS); secondary endpoints were event-free survival (EFS) and functional outcomes. The trial was terminated due to lack of equivalence and low accrual after first interim analyses. Trial registration NCT00210236.

Results.—Of 625 patients, 297 no-Ax and 310 Ax patients were maintained for final per-protocol analyses. OS and EFS at five years were not equivalent (Ax vs. no-Ax: 98% vs. 94% and 96% vs. 90% respectively). Recurrence was higher for no-Ax, particularly in the first five years after surgery. Axillary nodes were positive for 14% Ax patients but only 2% no-Ax patients experienced axillary node recurrence. Functional impairments were greater after ALNC.

Conclusion.—Our results fail to demonstrate equivalence of outcomes when ALNC is omitted from post-menopausal early breast cancer patient treatment. However the low locoregional recurrence rates warrant further examination over a longer duration, in particular to consider whether these would impact on survival.

▶ Before the introduction of sentinel lymph node biopsy (SLNB) into standard breast cancer treatment, several studies were initiated with the aim of identifying a subgroup of clinically node-negative breast cancer patients with favorable primary tumor characteristics for whom axillary lymph node dissection (ALND) might be safely omitted.[1-3] Most of these studies involved smaller tumors (T1a, T1b, or T1c) in older women, with the expectation of minimal impact on locoregional disease and OS. The National Surgical Adjuvant Breast and Bowel Project (NSABP) B-04 trial underpinned the belief that ALND conferred no significant survival advantage in the absence of overt or progressive axillary disease. Nonetheless, this seminal trial was confounded by salvage mastectomy and had a power of only 70% and 40% to detect survival differences of 7% and 5%, respectively.[4] Meta-analyses can partially overcome the problems of small patient populations and underpowering, but they cannot readily distinguish between the effects of removing nodal tissue per se and the influence of adjuvant treatments (radiotherapy and systemic therapies) on clinical outcomes. A large meta-analysis of 6 trials involving 3000 patients claimed a survival benefit of 5.4% with ALND,[5] whereas another meta-analysis drew the opposite conclusion.[6] Even though a clear survival advantage had not been demonstrated for ALND, it remained the standard treatment until the advent of SLNB. Omission of ALND was highly selective and based on clinician discretion; it was an attempt to reduce potential upper-limb morbidity when there were few perceived benefits of ALND in terms of survival, regional control, and choice of adjuvant therapy.

In this study, Avril and colleagues published results of a now-outmoded randomized equivalence trial conducted to assess whether omission of ALND in postmenopausal women with small (≤1 cm) clinically node-negative cancers impairs survival outcomes. The trial was started in 1995 and terminated 10 years later after failure to accrue its target of 1600 patients and consequent to provisional results rejecting equivalence. A total of 625 patients were recruited, most of whom were protocol compliant. The period of recruitment coincided not only with the introduction of SLNB but also with the widespread use of tamoxifen as adjuvant systemic hormonal therapy, which improves OS rates and reduces locoregional recurrence rates by one-third.

The authors concluded that the equivalence of outcomes between ALND and observation alone had not been demonstrated, with the implication that it cannot be claimed that the latter is not inferior to ALND. However, there were serious flaws in the execution and interpretation of this study, and a type I error seems likely. The statistical calculations for this study were based on 1612 patients and a predicted 90% power to detect noninferiority at 5 years with an equivalence margin of 3%. If the OS rate in the observation arm was not less than 92%, equivalence was upheld. This outcome measure was 94% for the observation arm when censored at 5 years and 92% after follow-up was completed. Moreover, the OS rate (98%) in the ALND group was higher than expected. Despite a hazard ratio of 3.07, there were wide confidence intervals, a *P* value of 1.0, and a trend toward equivalence when noncensored data were included.

This trial provides some reassuring data on axillary relapse; the predicted rate of nodal involvement in the observation arm was 14%, but the rate of axillary relapse was only 2%. The average tumor size in the observation group was only 7 mm, which accounts for the low rate of node positivity. This low rate of axillary recurrence is comparable to rates of locoregional relapse reported in the American College of Surgeons Oncology Group Z0011 trial for SLNB-positive patients at a median follow-up of 6.3 years.[7] Patients with a negative SLNB have been shown to have a low likelihood of any residual disease within the axilla for a technique that has a false-negative rate of 5% to 10%.[8,9] Furthermore, these low rates of axillary relapse are unlikely to translate into any meaningful decrease in OS, even with more prolonged follow-up. It should be noted that about 40% of patients were node positive in the NSABP B-04 study, and an axillary relapse rate of 18% did not affect survival after 25 years of follow-up.[4] Moreover, the NSABP B-32 study evaluating SLNB alone versus SLNB with completion ALND reported a small number of nodal recurrences within each group, which was consistent with an axillary relapse rate of less than 1% at 5 years. Despite almost twice as many regional recurrences in the SLNB-only arm (14 vs 8 events), no significant differences in the primary end points of OS, disease-free survival, and regional control were found at a median follow-up of 96 months.[10,11]

Improvements in the efficacy of adjuvant treatments have attenuated the therapeutic impact of axillary surgery in recent years. Tangential fields used to deliver radiation to the breast often include the lower axilla, which may contribute to regional control and indirectly influence OS by eliminating a potential source of distant metastasis. Axillary radiotherapy was administered to 14% of patients in the observation group and 19% in the ALND group. This would promote the equivalence of event-free survival outcomes but enhance any disparity in functional outcomes. Though adjuvant hormonal therapies can be associated with thromboembolism and adverse cardiovascular/cerebrovascular events, all-cause mortality is reduced by both tamoxifen and aromatase inhibitors. Most patients in this study presumably received tamoxifen only and had a relatively low risk of disease recurrence. It is inconceivable that poorer OS in the observation group could be attributable to a higher proportion (91%) of patients receiving hormonal therapy compared with the ALND arm, in which only two-thirds had tamoxifen and many for less than 5 years. The authors are correct, however, in concluding that the administration of chemotherapy in 8% of patients undergoing ALND was unlikely to account for any survival advantage for this group in which absolute benefits were modest.

The statistical limitations of this study notwithstanding, it does provide an important reminder that omission of an axillary staging procedure is still appropriate in the era of SLNB. Most of the deaths in the observation group were not breast cancer specific, and older patients have competing causes of mortality. Rates of axillary relapse at 5 years of follow-up have been reported to be only 2% after omission of axillary surgery in a group of patients with mainly T1a and T1b clinically node-negative tumors but exceed 10% for T1c and T2 lesions.[12] These low rates are likely to appertain to older patients with smaller (≤1 cm), non—high-grade tumors for whom any net benefit of SLNB may be more difficult to justify when balanced against the risks, including seroma formation and lymphedema. There are potential concerns about pathologic upstaging, but regardless of the tumor load within the SLN, this is likely to be relevant and clinically meaningful in only a small proportion of cases. A flexible policy for axillary management based on the probability of nodal involvement, the quality of life, and competing causes of death seems appropriate.

J. R. Benson, MA, DM (Oxon), MD (Cantab), FRCS

References

1. Silverstein MJ, Gierson ED, Waisman JR, Senofsky GM, Colburn WJ, Gamagami P. Axillary lymph node dissection for T1a breast carcinoma. Is it indicated? *Cancer.* 1994;73:664-667.
2. White RE, Vezeridis MP, Konstadoulakis M, Cole BF, Wanebo HJ, Bland KI. Therapeutic options and results for the management of minimally invasive carcinoma of the breast: influence of axillary dissection for treatment of T1a and T1b lesions. *J Am Coll Surg.* 1996;183:575-582.
3. della Rovere GQ, Bonomi R, Ashley S, Benson JR. Axillary staging in women with small invasive breast tumours. *Eur J Surg Oncol.* 2006;32:733-737.
4. Fisher B, Jeong JH, Anderson S, Bryant S, Fisher ER, Wolmark N. Twenty-five-year follow-up of a randomized trial comparing radical mastectomy, total mastectomy, and total mastectomy followed by irradiation. *N Eng J Med.* 2002;347:567-575.
5. Orr RK. The impact of prophylactic axillary node dissection on breast cancer survival—a Bayesian meta-analysis. *Ann Surg Oncol.* 1999;6:109-116.
6. Sanghani M, Balk EM, Cady B. Impact of axillary lymph node dissection on breast cancer outcome in clinically node negative patients: a systematic review and meta-analysis. *Cancer.* 2009;115:1613-1620.
7. Giuliano AE, Hunt KK, Ballman KV, et al. Axillary dissection vs no axillary dissection in women with invasive breast cancer and sentinel node metastases: a randomized clinical trial. *JAMA.* 2011;305:569-575.
8. Naik AM, Fey J, Gemignani M, et al. The risk of axillary relapse after sentinel lymph node biopsy for breast cancer is comparable with that of axillary lymph node dissection: a follow-up study of 4008 procedures. *Ann Surg.* 2004;240: 462-468. discussion 468—471.
9. Veronesi U, Galimberti V, Paganelli G, et al. Axillary metastases in breast cancer patients with negative sentinel nodes: a follow-up of 3548 cases. *Eur J Cancer.* 2009;45:1381-1388.
10. Krag DN, Anderson SJ, Julian TB, et al. Sentinel lymph node resection compared with conventional axillary-lymph node dissection in clinically node-negative patients with breast cancer: overall survival findings from the NSABP B-32 randomised phase 3 trial. *Lancet Oncol.* 2010;11:927-933.

11. Benson JR. An alternative to initial axillary-lymph node dissection. *Lancet Oncol.* 2010;11:908-909.
12. Greco M, Agresti R, Cascinelli N, et al. Breast cancer patients treated without axillary surgery: clinical implications and biologic analysis. *Ann Surg.* 2000; 232:1-7.

Subsets of women with close or positive margins after breast-conserving surgery with high local recurrence risk despite breast plus boost radiotherapy

Lupe K, Truong PT, Alexander C, et al (British Columbia Cancer Agency, Vancouver, Canada; et al)
Int J Radiat Oncol Biol Phys 81:e561-e568, 2011

Purpose.—(1) To examine the effect of surgical margin status on local recurrence (LR) and survival following breast-conserving therapy; (2) To identify subsets with close or positive margins with high LR risk despite whole breast radiotherapy (RT) plus boost.

Methods and Materials.—Subjects were 2,264 women with pT1−3, any N, M0 invasive breast cancer, treated with breast-conserving surgery and whole breast ± boost RT. Five-year Kaplan-Meier (KM) LR, breast cancer–specific and overall survival (BCSS and OS) were compared between cohorts with negative ($n = 1{,}980$), close ($n = 222$), and positive ($n = 62$) margins. LR rates were analyzed according to clinicopathologic characteristics. Multivariable Cox regression modeling and matched analysis of close/positive margin cases and negative margin controls were performed.

Results.—Median follow-up was 5.2 years. Boost RT was used in 92% of patients with close or positive margins. Five-year KM LR rates in the negative, close and positive margin cohorts were 1.3%, 4.0%, and 5.2%, respectively ($p = 0.001$). BCSS and OS were similar in the three margin subgroups. In the close/positive margin cohort, LR rates were 10.2% with age <45 years, 11.8% with Grade III, 11.3% with lymphovascular invasion (LVI), and 26.3% with ≥4 positive nodes. Corresponding rates in the negative margin cohort were 2.3%, 2.4%, 1.0%, and 2.4%, respectively. On Cox regression analysis of the entire cohort, close or positive margin, Grade III histology, ≥4 positive nodes, and lack of systemic therapy were significantly associated with higher LR risk. When close/positive margin cases were matched to negative margin controls, the difference in 5-year LR remained significant (4.25% vs. 0.7%, $p < 0.001$)

Conclusions.—On univariable analysis, subsets with close or positive margins, in combination with age <45 years, Grade III, LVI, and ≥4 positive nodes, have 5-year LR >10% despite whole breast plus boost RT. These patients should be considered for more definitive surgery.

▶ Margin status appears to be the single most important prognostic factor for the risk of local recurrence following breast-conserving surgery and RT.[1] Nonetheless, there is no consensus regarding what constitutes an "adequate" margin among radiation oncologists[2] or surgeons,[3] despite more than 2 decades of study. The most important reason for this is that a multitude of patient-, tumor-, and treatment-related factors may modulate the impact of margin status. Combinations of prognostic factors are, therefore, likely to be more useful than a single variable in defining subgroups of patients at increased risk of local failure. However, few studies have examined local failure rates in relation to margin width in combination with even a single additional variable. The current study by Lupe and colleagues is an important exception.

Of particular interest was the authors' finding of how small the absolute risk of local recurrence was, and how little difference there was between subgroups, among the 1980 patients with "negative" margins (defined as 2 mm or more) treated in the "modern" era. The 5-year local failure rates were 1% to 3%, regardless of tumor size (except for the 12 patients with T3 lesions), the number of involved nodes, tumor histology (except for the 12 patients with "other" histologies), extent of disease (unifocal or multifocal), estrogen receptor status, grade, the presence of lymphovascular invasion, the use of a boost, or the use of systemic therapy (Table 3). However, they did not perform a multivariate analysis restricted solely to patients with negative margins or look at absolute failure rates in subgroups of patients with negative margins defined by more than 1 variable simultaneously (eg, both high grade and lymphovascular invasion present).

Their second important result was that there was no difference in local failure rates between patients with "close" margins of 0.1-1 mm (4%, or 6/170 patients) and of 1.1-2 mm (4%, or 2/52 patients), which confirms findings from 2 previous studies that examined such narrow divisions of margin width.[4,5] Lupe and colleagues also found no differences in outcome for patients with close margins in relation to other variables. For example, the crude risk of local recurrence for patients with close margins who were younger than 45 years was 3% (1/33), compared to 4% (7/189) for older patients. However, a study from Tufts Medical Center in Boston contradicts these findings. Among patients with close margins (2 mm or less), with a median follow-up of 121 months, 28 patients age 45 years or younger had a 19% failure rate, compared to a 5% failure rate for 71 older patients.[6]

Lastly, Lupe and colleagues found that the 5-year local failure rate for the 62 patients with positive margins was only 5%. Most studies of this subgroup have reported local failure rates of 20% to 30% or more.[1] Perhaps this is because only 5 patients in the current study had more than 1 involved margin (and none of these 5 patients had local failure). In a study from Marseille, France, with a median follow-up of 72 months, the risk of local failure was 14% (10/70) for patients with a single positive margin, compared to 36% (17/47) for patients with multiple involved margins.[7] Lupe and colleagues also found hints that some patient subgroups may be more affected by having positive margins than others. For example, the crude risk of local recurrence for patients younger than 45 years with positive margins was 27% (3/11), compared to 0% (0/51) for patients age 45 years or older. Similarly, the series from Tufts Medical Center found a 12-year actuarial failure rate for patients with positive margins of 24% for 25 patients younger than age 45, compared to 14% for 81 older patients.[6]

There are several issues that must be kept in mind when interpreting the results of this important study. Findings regarding subgroups must always be

TABLE 3.—Five-Year Kaplan-Meier Local Recurrence According to Margin Status and Clinicopathologic Characteristics

Variable	Negative Margin ($n = 1{,}980$) LR% (SE)	p Value	Close/Positive Margin ($n = 284$) LR% (SE)	p Value	Crude LR Rates (%) Close n (%)	Crude LR Rates (%) Positive n (%)
Age (years)						
<45	2.3 (1.0)	0.158	10.2 (4.8)	0.041	1 (3.0)	3 (27.3)
≥45	1.1 (0.3)		3.2 (1.2)		7 (3.7)	0
Tumor stage						
T1	1.1 (0.3)	0.010	3.8 (1.6)	0.843	6 (4.2)	0 (0)
T2	1.7 (0.6)		5.0 (2.2)		2 (2.6)	3 (9.7)
T3	11.1 (10.5)		0		0	0
No. positive nodes						
0	1.4 (0.3)	0.262	1.4 (1.0)	<0.001	2 (1.4)	0 (0.0)
1–3	0.5 (0.4)		5.8 (2.8)		2 (3.5)	2 (14.3)
≥4	2.4 (1.7)		26.3 (10.2)		4 (22.2)	1 (20.0)
Histology						
Ductal	1.2 (0.3)	0.074	4.7 (1.4)	0.545	8 (4.0)	3 (5.2)
Lobular	1.6 (1.1)		0		0 (0)	0 (0)
Other	8.3 (8.0)		0		0 (0)	0 (0)
Extent						
Unifocal	1.3 (0.3)	0.345	4.8 (1.4)	0.229	8 (4.1)	3 (5.4)
Multifocal	0		0		0 (0)	0
ER status						
Positive	0.9 (0.2)	0.009	3.5 (1.3)	0.176	5 (2.9)	2 (3.9)
Negative	2.8 (1.0)		7.3 (3.5)		3 (6.0)	1 (9.1)
Grade						
I–II	0.8 (0.3)	0.009	0.6 (0.6)	<0.001	0 (0)	1 (2.7)
III	2.4 (0.7)		11.8 (3.5)		8 (11.2)	2 (8.0)
LVI						
Negative	1.4 (0.3)	0.713	1.7 (1.0)	<0.001	2 (1.3)	1 (2.3)
Positive	1.0 (0.6)		11.3 (3.8)		6 (9.7)	2 (11.1)
RT volume						
Breast	1.2 (0.3)	0.424	2.1 (1.1)	0.001	3 (1.8)	1 (2.0)
Breast/nodes	1.7 (0.7)		11.7 (4.2)		5 (9.4)	2 (16.7)
RT boost use						
Boost	1.4 (0.5)	0.683	4.6 (1.4)	0.336	8 (3.9)	3 (5.2)
No boost	1.2 (0.3)		0		0	0
Systemic therapy						
Yes	1.0 (0.3)	0.048	4.9 (1.4)	0.205	8 (4.1)	3 (5.5)
No	2.5 (0.9)		0		0	0

Abbreviations: ER = estrogen receptor; LR = local recurrence; LVI = lymphovascular invasion; RT = radiation therapy.
*Log rank statistics performed on known values only.

viewed cautiously until they are reproduced by several other studies, particularly when the subgroups are very small. The median follow-up time of 5.2 years for this study means that the findings regarding the effects of tumor grade and other variables related to proliferation may change substantially with time, as patients with more slowly proliferating tumors will have later local failures.

Unfortunately, the authors did not provide information about the extent of margin involvement or the amount of disease near the margin for patients with close margins. In a study from the Joint Center for Radiation Therapy in Boston, with a median follow-up time of 127 months, the crude 8-year local failure rate was 14% for 122 patients with "focal" margin involvement (defined as ductal carcinoma in situ and invasive cancer across all examined slides that could be encompassed by 3 or fewer low-power microscopic fields); however, for 66 patients with "extensive" margin involvement, the rate was 27%.[4] Furthermore, the 45 patients with focally positive margins who received systemic therapy had a 7% local recurrence rate, compared with 18% for the 77 patients who did not receive systemic therapy. A study from William Beaumont Hospital found that having a substantial amount of tumor in the zone within 2 mm of the inked margin was associated with a high risk of local recurrence.[5]

Lupe and colleagues also did not examine their results in relation to the surgery-to-radiotherapy interval. In the "upfront-outback" trial performed at the Joint Center for Radiation Therapy in Boston and affiliated institutions from 1984 to 1992, patients with clinical stage I or II breast carcinoma were randomized to receive 4 cycles of chemotherapy at 3-week intervals, either before or after RT.[8] With a median follow-up time of 135 months, local failure rates did not differ significantly in the RT-first (13%) and chemotherapy-first (6%) arms for the 123 patients with margins greater than 1 mm in width, but the respective failure rates in the 2 arms were 4% and 32% for the 47 patients with close margins. This may in part account for why local failure rates in the current study were higher for patients with close margins and 4 or more positive nodes (22%, 4/18 patients) than for those with 1-3 positive nodes (4%, 2/57) or negative nodes (1%, 2/147), although the proportions of patients in these 3 subgroups receiving chemotherapy and its sequencing with RT were not reported.

Despite these caveats, Lupe and colleagues give us important additional information for the continuing debate about the meaning of margin status and when reexcision should be recommended. Above all, they show that the risk of local recurrence following breast-conserving therapy can be made very low for nearly all patients treated in a largely community-based healthcare system. This is a testimony to the hard work of the dedicated individuals involved in guideline development, standardization of practice, and quality control at the British Columbia Cancer Agency.

A. Recht, MD

References

1. Recht A. Breast cancer: stages I and II. In: Gunderson LL, Tepper JE, eds. *Clinical Radiation Oncology.* 3rd ed. New York: Elsevier; 2011:1321-1338.
2. Taghian A, Jagsi R, Makris A, et al. Results of a survey regarding irradiation of internal mammary chain in patients with breast cancer: practice is culture driven rather than evidence based. *Int J Radiat Oncol Biol Phys.* 2004;60:706-714.
3. Azu M, Abrahamse P, Katz SJ, Jagsi R, Morrow M. What is an adequate margin for breast-conserving surgery? Surgeon attitudes and correlates. *Ann Surg Oncol.* 2010;17:558-563.
4. Park CC, Mitsumori M, Nixon A, et al. Outcome at 8 years after breast-conserving surgery and radiation therapy for invasive breast cancer: influence of margin status and systemic therapy on local recurrence. *J Clin Oncol.* 2000;18:1668-1675.
5. Goldstein NS, Kestin L, Vicini F. Factors associated with ipsilateral breast failure and distant metastases in patients with invasive breast carcinoma treated with breast-conserving therapy. A clinicopathologic study of 607 neoplasms from 583 patients. *Am J Clin Pathol.* 2003;120:500-527.
6. Neuschatz AC, DiPetrillo T, Safaii H, et al. Long-term follow-up of a prospective policy of margin-directed radiation dose escalation in breast-conserving therapy. *Cancer.* 2003;97:30-39.

7. Cowen D, Houvenaeghel G, Bardou V, et al. Local and distant failures after limited surgery with positive margins and radiotherapy for node-negative breast cancer. *Int J Radiat Oncol Biol Phys.* 2000;47:305-312.
8. Bellon JR, Come SE, Gelman RS, et al. Sequencing of chemotherapy and radiation therapy in early-stage breast cancer: updated results of a prospective randomized trial. *J Clin Oncol.* 2005;23:1934-1940.

Tumor Biology

Effect of Very Small Tumor Size on Cancer-Specific Mortality in Node-Positive Breast Cancer

Wo JY, Chen K, Neville BA, et al (Harvard Radiation Oncology Program, Boston, MA; Massachusetts General Hosp, Boston; Harvard Med School, Boston, MA)

J Clin Oncol 29:2619-2627, 2011

Purpose.—Traditionally, larger tumor size and increasing lymph node (LN) involvement have been considered independent predictors of increased breast cancer–specific mortality (BCSM). We sought to characterize the interaction between tumor size and LN involvement in determination of BCSM. In particular, we evaluated whether very small tumor size may predict for increased BCSM relative to larger tumors in patients with extensive LN involvement.

Patients and Methods.—Using Surveillance, Epidemiology and End Results registry data, we identified 50,949 female patients diagnosed between 1990 and 2002 with nonmetastatic T1/T2 invasive breast cancer treated with surgery and axillary LN dissection. Primary study variables were tumor size, degree of LN involvement, and their corresponding interaction term. Kaplan-Meier methods, adjusted Cox proportional hazards models with interaction terms, and a linear trend test across nodal categories were performed.

Results.—Median follow-up was 99 months. In multivariable analysis, there was significant interaction between tumor size and LN involvement ($P < .001$). Using T1aN0 as reference, T1aN2+ conferred significantly higher BCSM compared with T1bN2+ (hazard ratio [HR], 20.66 *v* 12.53; $P = .02$). A similar pattern was seen among estrogen receptor (ER)–negative patients with T1aN2+ compared with T1bN2+ (HR, 24.16 *v* 12.67; $P = .03$), but not ER-positive patients ($P = .52$). The effect of very small tumor size on BCSM was intermediate among N1 cancers, between that of N0 and N2+ cancers.

Conclusion.—Very small tumors with four positive LNs may predict for higher BCSM compared with larger tumors. In extensive node-positive disease, very small tumor size may be a surrogate for biologically aggressive disease. These results should be validated in future database studies.

▶ Using the National Cancer Institute's Surveillance, Epidemiology, and End Results (SEER) database, Wo and colleagues performed a retrospective analysis of 50 949 patients with a history of stage I-III unilateral invasive ductal carcinoma of the breast, evaluating the interaction between tumor size and LN status, as well as the effects of year of diagnosis, age, race, histologic grade, ER status, progesterone receptor status, number of LNs dissected, degree of LN involvement, and tumor size on BCSM. They described a phenomenon in which patients with extremely small tumors (T1a, 1-5 mm) and extensive nodal involvement (N2, ≥4 positive LNs) demonstrated poorer BCSM than those with larger tumors (T1b). This study demonstrated the disconnection between tumor size and prognosis, highlighting the link between mortality and tumor biology, rather than tumor size. Because of the nature of the SEER database, this study was limited by lack of significant tumor characteristics and treatment information, including human epidermal growth factor receptor 2/neu status, presence or absence of lymphovascular invasion, and type of cancer therapy. However, given the importance of nodal status in determining treatment, it would be unlikely that cancer treatment would differ widely for such extensively node-positive disease. Furthermore, use of the SEER database provided a large patient population and long-term follow-up, which were essential in obtaining the statistical power to make these determinations. Importantly, Wo and colleagues' study pinpoints the importance of tumor biology, which usurps anatomic staging in this setting, in determining BCSM, suggesting the importance of adequate cancer therapy for even the smallest tumors in the presence of nodal involvement.

P. K. Morrow, MD

Axillary Management

Axillary Dissection vs No Axillary Dissection in Women With Invasive Breast Cancer and Sentinel Node Metastasis: A Randomized Clinical Trial

Giuliano AE, Hunt KK, Ballman KV, et al (John Wayne Cancer Inst at Saint John's Health Ctr, Santa Monica, CA; M. D. Anderson Cancer Ctr, Houston, TX; Mayo Clinic Rochester, MN; et al)

JAMA 305:569-575, 2011

Context.—Sentinel lymph node dissection (SLND) accurately identifies nodal metastasis of early breast cancer, but it is not clear whether further nodal dissection affects survival.

Objective.—To determine the effects of complete axillary lymph node dissection (ALND) on survival of patients with sentinel lymph node (SLN) metastasis of breast cancer.

Design, Setting, and Patients.—The American College of Surgeons Oncology Group Z0011 trial, a phase 3 noninferiority trial conducted at 115 sites and enrolling patients from May 1999 to December 2004. Patients were women with clinical T1-T2 invasive breast cancer, no palpable adenopathy, and 1 to 2 SLNs containing metastases identified by frozen section, touch preparation, or hematoxylin-eosin staining on permanent section. Targeted enrollment was 1900 women with final analysis after 500 deaths, but the trial closed early because mortality rate was lower than expected.

Interventions.—All patients underwent lumpectomy and tangential whole-breast irradiation. Those with SLN metastases identified by SLND were randomized to undergo ALND or no further axillary treatment. Those randomized to ALND underwent dissection of 10 or more nodes. Systemic therapy was at the discretion of the treating physician.

Main Outcome Measures.—Overall survival was the primary end point, with a noninferiority margin of a 1-sided hazard ratio of less than 1.3 indicating that SLND alone is noninferior to ALND. Disease-free survival was a secondary end point.

Results.—Clinical and tumor characteristics were similar between 445 patients randomized to ALND and 446 randomized to SLND alone. However, the median number of nodes removed was 17 with ALND and 2 with SLND alone. At a median follow-up of 6.3 years (last follow-up, March 4, 2010), 5-year overall survival was 91.8% (95% confidence interval [CI], 89.1%-94.5%)with ALND and 92.5% (95% CI, 90.0%-95.1%) with SLND alone; 5-year disease-free survival was 82.2% (95% CI, 78.3%-86.3%) with ALND and 83.9% (95% CI, 80.2%-87.9%) with SLND alone. The hazard ratio for treatment-related overall survival was 0.79 (90% CI, 0.56-1.11) without adjustment and 0.87 (90% CI, 0.62-1.23) after adjusting for age and adjuvant therapy.

Conclusion.—Among patients with limited SLN metastatic breast cancer treated with breast conservation and systemic therapy, the use of SLND alone compared with ALND did not result in inferior survival.

Trial Registration.—clinicaltrials.gov Identifier: NCT00003855.

▶ The development of sentinel lymph node dissection and its use in identifying women with breast cancer who do not need an axillary lymph node dissection has saved thousands of women the significant toxicities of axillary lymph node dissection. It is well documented that axillary lymph node dissection results in a significant risk of complications from seroma and infection to lymphedema. Thus, the use of axillary lymph node dissection needs to be justified given the potential debilitating toxicities.

Although patients with negative sentinel lymph node dissection clearly do not need axillary lymph node dissection, it has been the standard of care to perform axillary lymph node dissection on patients with positive sentinel lymph nodes. These authors have performed a phase III randomized trial to question whether these positive sentinel lymph node patients in fact need the axillary lymph node dissection. Their results have shown no benefit to the axillary lymph node dissection over sentinel lymph node dissection alone at 5 years. Yet it is important to realize that these results only apply to patients who receive lumpectomy and postoperative irradiation to the whole breast (supine position), which usually will result in radiation to the low axilla. Patients who had mastectomy, prone radiation after lumpectomy, or partial breast irradiation were not part of this trial. Applying these results to the appropriate breast cancer population is critical in its correct usage.

C. Lawton, MD

Hormonal Therapy

Timing of radiotherapy and outcome in patients receiving adjuvant endocrine therapy

Karlsson P, for the International Breast Cancer Study Group (Sahlgrenska Univ Hosp, Gothenburg, Sweden; et al)

Int J Radiat Oncol Biol Phys 80:398-402, 2011

Purpose.—To evaluate the association between the interval from breast-conserving surgery (BCS) to radiotherapy (RT) and the clinical outcome among patients treated with adjuvant endocrine therapy.

Patients and Methods.—Patient information was obtained from three International Breast Cancer Study Group trials. The analysis was restricted to 964 patients treated with BCS and adjuvant endocrine therapy. The patients were divided into two groups according to the median number of days between BCS and RT and into four groups according to the quartile of time between BCS and RT. The endpoints were the interval to local recurrence, disease-free survival, and overall survival. Proportional hazards regression analysis was used to perform comparisons after adjustment for baseline factors.

Results.—The median interval between BCS and RT was 77 days. RT timing was significantly associated with age, menopausal status, and estrogen receptor status. After adjustment for these factors, no significant effect of a RT delay ≤20 weeks was found. The adjusted hazard ratio for RT within 77 days vs. after 77 days was 0.94 (95% confidence interval [CI], 0.47–1.87) for the interval to local recurrence, 1.05 (95% CI, 0.82–1.34) for disease-free survival, and 1.07 (95% CI, 0.77–1.49) for overall survival. For the interval to local recurrence the adjusted hazard ratio for ≤48, 49–77, and 78–112 days was 0.90 (95% CI, 0.34–2.37), 0.86 (95% CI, 0.33–2.25), and 0.89 (95% CI, 0.33–2.41), respectively, relative to ≥113 days.

Conclusion.—A RT delay of ≤20 weeks was significantly associated with baseline factors such as age, menopausal status, and estrogen-receptor status. After adjustment for these factors, the timing of RT was not significantly associated with the interval to local recurrence, disease-free survival, or overall survival.

▶ The past 2 decades have witnessed an increase both in the use of RT and in the wait times prior to the initiation of RT.[1-4] Waiting lists for RT are now common in many parts of the world.[4-8] What constitutes a safe interval between surgery and the initiation of RT for breast cancer has been the subject of much debate. A trial randomizing patients to different wait times after surgery would provide the most definitive evidence regarding the effect of the surgery-to-RT interval on local recurrence in breast cancer, but this would be unethical. Some previous retrospective studies did not find an association between time to RT and local recurrence after BCS,[9-11] whereas others reported increased recurrence among patients with longer intervals.[12-15]

In this article, Karlsson and colleagues examined the effect of the interval between BCS and RT initiation among 964 women treated with adjuvant endocrine therapy in International Breast Cancer Study Group (IBCSG) trials VII, VIII, and IX. They found that the median time to RT was 77 days in their cohort and that the timing of RT was not significantly associated with the interval to local recurrence, disease-free survival, or overall survival after adjusting for baseline factors.

The lack of a disease-free or overall survival difference in this study is not surprising, given the relatively few patients analyzed. A meta-analysis of over 7000 patients treated with BCS was required to detect a survival difference for the comparison of RT and no RT.[16] In this study, where differences in local recurrence are expected to be much smaller, as the comparison is between RT intervals and not the use or nonuse of RT, many more patients would be needed to detect any survival benefit from early RT, should it exist.

The relatively small number of patients in this study may also account for the lack of difference in local recurrence rates. Because local recurrence after BCS and RT is relatively uncommon, the inconsistency in local recurrence rates across this and other studies may reflect variable power to detect a difference. A strength of this study could have been the analysis of results by surgical margin width and radiation dose, which many population-based studies of RT interval are unable to perform.[17] However, the authors did not report the status of the margins or describe the doses of radiation delivered.

In addition, despite demonstrating in a previously published report of the IBCSG trials[18] that the duration of chemotherapy does not affect local recurrence risk, the authors included some women in this study who had received chemotherapy. These women had longer intervals to RT, as analyzed in the current report, but the authors' previous study and others[19] have confirmed that radiation delay due to chemotherapy use does not significantly affect the risk of local recurrence, perhaps because the use of chemotherapy may itself reduce local recurrence. The inclusion of patients who received chemotherapy, with the interval calculated as time from surgery instead of time from completion of chemotherapy, may have obscured the results.

It is especially critical to have a clear answer regarding whether interval to RT affects local recurrence, given that meta-analyses of randomized studies have now demonstrated unequivocally a link between local recurrence and decreased survival in patients with breast cancer.[16] Given the large numbers of women with breast cancer treated with RT, it is important that studies of RT interval are carefully conducted and analyzed.

R. S. Punglia, MD, MPH

References

1. Jack RH, Davies EA, Robinson D, Sainsbury R, Møller H. Radiotherapy waiting times for women with breast cancer: a population-based cohort study. *BMC Cancer.* 2007;7:71.
2. Mikeljevic JS, Haward R, Johnston C, et al. Trends in postoperative radiotherapy delay and the effect on survival in breast cancer patients treated with conservation surgery. *Br J Cancer.* 2004;90:1343-1348.
3. Johnston GM, MacGarvie VL, Elliott D, Dewar RA, MacIntyre MM, Nolan MC. Radiotherapy wait times for patients with a diagnosis of invasive cancer, 1992–2000. *Clin Invest Med.* 2004;27:142-156.

4. Mackillop WJ, Fu H, Quirt CF, Dixon P, Brundage M, Zhou Y. Waiting for radiotherapy in Ontario. *Int J Radiat Oncol Biol Phys.* 1994;30:221-228.
5. Dodwell D, Crellin A. Waiting for radiotherapy. *BMJ.* 2006;332:107-109.
6. Schäfer C, Nelson K, Herbst M. Waiting for radiotherapy a national call for ethical discourse on waiting lists in radiotherapy: findings from a preliminary survey. *Strahlenther Onkol.* 2005;181:9-19.
7. Lim KS, Vinod SK, Bull C, O'Brien P, Kenny L. Prioritization of radiotherapy in Australia and New Zealand. *Australas Radiol.* 2005;49:485-488.
8. Mackillop WJ. Killing time: the consequences of delays in radiotherapy. *Radiother Oncol.* 2007;84:1-4.
9. Cèfaro GA, Genovesi D, Marchese R, et al. The effect of delaying adjuvant radiation treatment after conservative surgery for early breast cancer. *Breast J.* 2007; 13:575-580.
10. Froud PJ, Mates D, Jackson JS, et al. Effect of time interval between breast-conserving surgery and radiation therapy on ipsilateral breast recurrence. *Int J Radiat Oncol Biol Phys.* 2000;46:363-372.
11. Livi L, Borghesi S, Saieva C, et al. Radiotherapy timing in 4,820 patients with breast cancer: University of Florence experience. *Int J Radiat Oncol Biol Phys.* 2009;73:365-369.
12. Olivotto IA, Lesperance ML, Truong PT, et al. Intervals longer than 20 weeks from breast-conserving surgery to radiation therapy are associated with inferior outcome for women with early-stage breast cancer who are not receiving chemotherapy. *J Clin Oncol.* 2009;27:16-23.
13. Huang J, Barbera L, Brouwers M, Browman G, Mackillop WJ. Does delay in starting treatment affect the outcomes of radiotherapy? A systematic review. *J Clin Oncol.* 2003;21:555-563.
14. Chen Z, King W, Pearcey R, Kerba M, Mackillop WJ. The relationship between waiting time for radiotherapy and clinical outcomes: a systematic review of the literature. *Radiother Oncol.* 2008;87:3-16.
15. Hébert-Croteau N, Freeman CR, Latreille J, Rivard M, Brisson J. A population-based study of the impact of delaying radiotherapy after conservative surgery for breast cancer. *Breast Cancer Res Treat.* 2004;88:187-196.
16. Clarke M, Collins R, Darby S, et al; Early Breast Cancer Trialists' Collaborative Group (EBCTCG). Effects of radiotherapy and of differences in the extent of surgery for early breast cancer on local recurrence and 15-year survival: an overview of the randomised trials. *Lancet.* 2005;366:2087-2106.
17. Punglia RS, Saito AM, Neville BA, Earle CC, Weeks JC. Impact of interval from breast conserving surgery to radiotherapy on local recurrence in older women with breast cancer: retrospective cohort analysis. *BMJ.* 2010;340:c845.
18. Wallgren A, Bernier J, Gelber RD, et al. Timing of radiotherapy and chemotherapy following breast-conserving surgery for patients with node-positive breast cancer. International Breast Cancer Study Group. *Int J Radiat Oncol Biol Phys.* 1996;35:649-659.
19. Bellon JR, Come SE, Gelman RS, et al. Sequencing of chemotherapy and radiation therapy in early-stage breast cancer: updated results of a prospective randomized trial. *J Clin Oncol.* 2005;23:1934-1940.

Intraductal Cancer

Adjuvant Tamoxifen Reduces Subsequent Breast Cancer in Women With Estrogen Receptor–Positive Ductal Carcinoma in Situ: A Study Based on NSABP Protocol B-24

Allred DC, Anderson SJ, Paik S, et al (Natl Surgical Adjuvant Breast and Bowel Project (NSABP), St Louis, MO; et al)

J Clin Oncol 30:1268-1273, 2012

Purpose.—The NSABP (National Surgical Adjuvant Breast and Bowel Project) B-24 study demonstrated significant benefit with adjuvant tamoxifen in patients with ductal carcinoma in situ (DCIS) after lumpectomy and radiation. Patients were enrolled without knowledge of hormone receptor status. The current study retrospectively evaluated the relationship between receptors and response to tamoxifen.

Patients and Methods.—Estrogen (ER) and progesterone receptors (PgR) were evaluated in 732 patients with DCIS (41% of original study population). An experienced central laboratory determined receptor status in all patient cases with available paraffin blocks (n = 449) by immunohistochemistry (IHC) using comprehensively validated assays. Results for additional patients (n = 283) determined by various methods (primarily IHC) were available from enrolling institutions. Combined results were evaluated for benefit of tamoxifen by receptor status at 10 years and overall follow-up (median, 14.5 years).

Results.—ER was positive in 76% of patients. Patients with ER-positive DCIS treated with tamoxifen (*v* placebo) showed significant decreases in subsequent breast cancer at 10 years (hazard ratio [HR], 0.49; $P < .001$) and overall follow-up (HR, 0.60; $P = .003$), which remained significant in multivariable analysis (overall HR, 0.64; $P = .003$). Results were similar, but less significant, when subsequent ipsilateral and contralateral, invasive and noninvasive, breast cancers were considered separately. No significant benefit was observed in ER-negative DCIS. PgR and either receptor were positive in 66% and 79% of patients, respectively, and in general, neither was more predictive than ER alone.

Conclusion.—Patients in NSABP B-24 with ER-positive DCIS receiving adjuvant tamoxifen after standard therapy showed significant reductions in subsequent breast cancer. The use of adjuvant tamoxifen should be considered for patients with DCIS.

▶ The National Surgical Adjuvant Breast and Bowel Project (NSABP) B24 study randomized patients with ductal carcinoma in situ (DCIS) treated with lumpectomy plus radiation to either tamoxifen or placebo. Prior reports of NSABP B24 showed an advantage for the use of tamoxifen in these patients. This article reports subset analyses of those patients according to estrogen receptor status. These analyses show a clear reduction in the incidence of both ipsilateral and contralateral subsequent breast cancers in those patients with estrogen receptor (ER)–positive DCIS. The results are not so clear for patients with ER-negative

DCIS. Trends show no difference between tamoxifen and placebo in regard to ipsilateral subsequent breast cancers, but trends also suggest there may be a reduction in the incidence of subsequent contralateral breast cancers. In evaluating these observations, the reader must remember two facts: First, these are unplanned subset analyses and thus cannot be regarded as definitive observations. Second, the number of contralateral breast cancers is extremely small and thus does not permit definitive conclusions. It would seem, however, that it would be reasonable to continue to use tamoxifen in all these patients until it is clear that patients with ER-negative DCIS do not benefit from a reduction in subsequent contralateral breast cancers.

J. T. Thigpen, MD

Non-Invasive Cancer

Ductal Carcinoma In Situ Treated With Breast-Conserving Surgery and Radiotherapy: A Comparison With ECOG Study 5194

Motwani SB, Goyal S, Moran MS, et al (UMDNJ/Robert Wood Johnson Med School, New Brunswick, NJ; Yale Univ School of Medicine, New Haven, CT; et al)

Cancer 117:1156-1162, 2011

Background.—Recent data from Eastern Cooperative Oncology Group (ECOG) Study 5194 (E5194) prospectively defined a low-risk subset of ductal carcinoma in situ (DCIS) patients where radiation therapy was omitted after lumpectomy alone. The purpose of the study was to determine the ipsilateral breast tumor recurrence (IBTR) in DCIS patients who met the criteria of E5194 treated with lumpectomy and adjuvant whole breast radiation therapy (RT).

Methods.—A total of 263 patients with DCIS were treated between 1980 and 2009 who met the enrollment criteria for E5194: 1) low to intermediate grade (LIG) with size >0.3 cm but <2.5 cm and margins >3 mm (n = 196), or 2) high grade (HG), size <1 cm and margins >3 mm (n = 67). All patients were treated with lumpectomy and whole breast RT with a boost to a median total tumor bed dose of 6400 cGy. Standard statistical analyses were performed with SAS (v. 9.2).

Results.—The average follow-up time was 6.9 years. The 5-year and 7-year IBTR for the LIG cohort in this study was 1.5% and 4.4% compared with 6.1% and 10.5% in E5194, respectively. The 5-year and 7-year IBTR for the HG cohort was 2.0% and 2.0% in this study compared with 15.3% and 18% in E5194, respectively.

Conclusions.—Adjuvant whole breast radiation therapy reduced the rate of local recurrence by more than 70% in patients with DCIS who met the criteria of E5194 (6.1% to 1.5% in the LIG cohort and 15.3% to 2% in the HG cohort). Additional follow-up is necessary given that 70% of IBTRs occurred after 5 years.

▶ This article by Motwani and colleagues evaluating adjuvant whole breast irradiation (WBI) after breast-conserving surgery (BCS) and the companion study published in the same issue of *Cancer* addressing the benefit of adjuvant accelerated partial breast irradiation (APBI) in patients with DCIS[1] are quite thought provoking in the era of health care reform. Both studies were retrospective in nature. However, they both demonstrated a significant decrease in IBTR with the use of adjuvant RT, whether WBI or APBI, in well-selected patients with small lesions of DCIS who met the same selection criteria as the ECOG 5194 study where patients were treated with BCS without RT.[2] It is obvious from all 3 studies that adjuvant RT is necessary for HG DCIS, as demonstrated by a recurrence rate of 15.3% at 5 years in the ECOG trial.[2] However, the question still arises concerning the necessity of WBI or APBI after BCS for small, low-grade DCIS lesions removed with generously clear margins. On the surface, although RT reduced the rate of local recurrence by more than 70%, the absolute recurrence rate without RT in the ECOG trial was only 6.1% at 5 years. More concerning was the continued rise in the IBTR rate to 10.5% at 7 years.[2] Therefore, a very thorough discussion with the patient is warranted about the role of adjuvant RT, using either WBI or APBI techniques, for LIG, mammographically detected, small DCIS lesions in terms of efficacy, toxicity, surveillance, and treatment in the setting of recurrence. Some patients would still elect for observation and would have a 90% chance of being recurrence free at 7 years. Others would choose to maximize their chances of not dealing with breast cancer for a second time. Since a survival advantage of adjuvant RT has not been demonstrated for DCIS,[3-5] an individualized discussion of risks versus benefits of adjuvant RT is still required.

E. S. Bloom, MD

References

1. Goyal S, Vicini F, Beitsch PD, et al. Ductal carcinoma in situ treated with breast-conserving surgery and accelerated partial breast irradiation: comparison of the Mammosite registry trial with intergroup study E5194. *Cancer.* 2011;117: 1149-1155.
2. Hughes LL, Wang M, Page DL, et al. Local excision alone without irradiation for ductal carcinoma in situ of the breast: a trial of the Eastern Cooperative Oncology Group. *J Clin Oncol.* 2009;27:5319-5324.
3. Bijker N, Meijnen P, Peterse JL, et al; EORTC Breast Cancer Cooperative Group, EORTC Radiotherapy Group. Breast-conserving treatment with or without radiotherapy in ductal carcinoma-in-situ: ten-year results of European Organisation for Research and Treatment of Cancer randomized phase III trial 10853—a study by the EORTC Breast Cancer Cooperative Group and EORTC Radiotherapy Group. *J Clin Oncol.* 2006;24:3381-3387.
4. Fisher B, Land S, Mamounas E, Dignam J, Fisher ER, Wolmark N. Prevention of invasive breast cancer in women with ductal carcinoma in situ: an update of the National Surgical Adjuvant Breast and Bowel Project experience. *Semin Oncol.* 2001;28:400-418.
5. Houghton J, George WD, Cuzick J, Duggan C, Fentiman IS, Spittle M; UK Coordinating Committee on Cancer Research, Ductal Carcinoma in situ Working Party, DCIS trialists in the UK, Australia, and New Zealand. Radiotherapy and tamoxifen in women with completely excised ductal carcinoma in situ of the breast in the UK, Australia, and New Zealand: randomised controlled trial. *Lancet.* 2003;362: 95-102.

Advanced

Everolimus in Postmenopausal Hormone-Receptor–Positive Advanced Breast Cancer

Baselga J, Campone M, Piccart M, et al (Harvard Med School, Boston, MA; Institut de Cancérologie de l'Ouest/René Gauducheau, France; Inst Jules Bordet, Brussels, Belgium; et al)

N Engl J Med 366:520-529, 2012

Background.—Resistance to endocrine therapy in breast cancer is associated with activation of the mammalian target of rapamycin (mTOR) intracellular signaling pathway. In early studies, the mTOR inhibitor everolimus added to endocrine therapy showed antitumor activity.

Methods.—In this phase 3, randomized trial, we compared everolimus and exemestane versus exemestane and placebo (randomly assigned in a 2:1 ratio) in 724 patients with hormone-receptor–positive advanced breast cancer who had recurrence or progression while receiving previous therapy with a nonsteroidal aromatase inhibitor in the adjuvant setting or to treat advanced disease (or both). The primary end point was progression-free survival. Secondary end points included survival, response rate, and safety. A preplanned interim analysis was performed by an independent data and safety monitoring committee after 359 progression-free survival events were observed.

Results.—Baseline characteristics were well balanced between the two study groups. The median age was 62 years, 56% had visceral involvement, and 84% had hormone-sensitive disease. Previous therapy included letrozole or anastrozole (100%), tamoxifen (48%), fulvestrant (16%), and chemotherapy (68%). The most common grade 3 or 4 adverse events were stomatitis (8% in the everolimus-plus-exemestane group vs. 1% in the placebo-plus-exemestane group), anemia (6% vs. <1%), dyspnea (4% vs. 1%), hyperglycemia (4% vs. <1%), fatigue (4% vs. 1%), and pneumonitis (3% vs. 0%). At the interim analysis, median progression-free survival was 6.9 months with everolimus plus exemestane and 2.8 months with placebo plus exemestane, according to assessments by local investigators (hazard ratio for progression or death, 0.43; 95% confidence interval [CI], 0.35 to 0.54; $P < 0.001$). Median progression-free survival was 10.6 months and 4.1 months, respectively, according to central assessment (hazard ratio, 0.36; 95% CI, 0.27 to 0.47; $P < 0.001$).

Conclusions.—Everolimus combined with an aromatase inhibitor improved progression-free survival in patients with hormone-receptor–positive advanced breast cancer previously treated with nonsteroidal aromatase inhibitors. (Funded by Novartis; BOLERO-2 ClinicalTrials.gov number, NCT00863655.)

▶ Everolimus is 1 of a number of agents known as mammalian target of rapamycin (mTOR) inhibitors that target the mTOR intracellular signaling pathway. The class of agents has demonstrated activity in a number of human cancers, most notably renal cell carcinoma. Because breast cancers that develop resistance to hormonal therapy demonstrate an activation of this pathway, the use of mTOR inhibitors is an attractive therapeutic option. In this particular study, 724 patients with positive hormone receptors who had developed progression or recurrence while receiving a nonsteroidal aromatase inhibitor were randomized to exemestane (a steroidal aromatase inhibitor) and the mTOR inhibitor everolimus. The primary endpoint of the trial was progression-free survival (PFS). The exemestane/everolimus combination demonstrated a substantial increase in PFS with a more than doubling of PFS at the median and a hazard ratio of 0.36. Toxicity was not substantially different, although previous reports in at least 1 other cancer (endometrial carcinoma) had shown an increase in deep venous thrombosis, a problem not observed in this series. These data suggest that everolimus has a role to play in the management of breast cancer.

J. T. Thigpen, MD

Loss of Human Epidermal Growth Factor Receptor 2 (HER2) Expression in Metastatic Sites of HER2-Overexpressing Primary Breast Tumors

Niikura N, Liu J, Hayashi N, et al (The Univ of Texas MD Anderson Cancer Ctr, Houston; et al)

J Clin Oncol 30:593-599, 2012

Purpose.—We evaluated whether patients with human epidermal growth factor receptor 2 (HER2) –positive primary breast tumors had metastatic tumors that were HER2 positive (concordant) or HER2 negative (discordant). We then evaluated whether treatment with trastuzumab or chemotherapy before biopsy of the metastasis had any effect on the rate of HER2 discordance. We also compared the overall survival durations of patients with HER2-concordant and -discordant tumors.

Patients and Methods.—We retrospectively identified all patients who initially had been diagnosed with HER2-positive (immunohistochemistry 3+ and/or fluorescent in situ hybridization positive) primary breast cancer between 1997 and 2008 at MD Anderson Cancer Center who also had metastatic tumor biopsy results available for review.

Results.—We included 182 patients who met our criteria. Forty-three (24%) of the 182 patients with HER2-positive primary tumors had HER2-negative metastatic tumors. The HER2 discordance rates differed significantly on the basis of whether patients received chemotherapy ($P = .022$) but not on the basis of whether patients received trastuzumab ($P = .296$). Patients with discordant HER2 status had shorter overall survival than did patients with concordant HER2 status (hazard ratio [HR], 0.43; $P = .003$). A survival difference remained among the 67 patients who received trastuzumab (HR, 0.56; $P = .083$) and 101 patients who did not (HR, 0.53; $P = .033$) before their metastasis biopsies.

Conclusion.—We confirmed that loss of HER2-positive status in metastatic tumors can occur in patients with primary HER2-positive breast cancer. Our data strongly support the need for biopsies of metastatic lesions to accurately determine patient prognosis and appropriate use of targeted therapy.

▶ Overexpression of human epidermal growth factor 2 (HER2)-neu occurs in about 25% of breast cancer patients and is associated with biologically more aggressive cancers. With the introduction of trastuzumab, a monoclonal antibody directed against the receptor, the outcome of patients with HER2 positive tumors has improved substantially. It is now considered essential to include agents such as trastuzumab and lapatinib in the management scheme for patients with HER2-overexpressing cancers in order to improve outcome. This study seeks to determine whether one can reliably predict that recurrences in patients with HER2 overexpressing cancers will still be HER2-overexpressing and thus still require the use of these agents directed against the receptor. The study makes 2 very interesting observations with treatment implications. First, there is a discordance rate of about 25%, which suggests that these 25% of patients will, without a biopsy of the new disease, be overtreated with either trastuzumab or lapatinib. This strongly suggests that new disease should be biopsied. Second, discordance appears to relate to prior treatment with chemotherapy, not with trastuzumab. The bottom line of this study is that, when patients with HER2 positive tumors recur, biopsies of the recurrent disease should be a part of the evaluation to determine whether the patient still requires anti-HER2 therapy.

J. T. Thigpen, MD

Pertuzumab plus Trastuzumab plus Docetaxel for Metastatic Breast Cancer

Baselga J, for the CLEOPATRA Study Group (Massachusetts General Hosp Cancer Ctr and Harvard Med School, Boston; et al)

N Engl J Med 366:109-119, 2012

Background.—The anti–human epidermal growth factor receptor 2 (HER2) humanized monoclonal antibody trastuzumab improves the outcome in patients with HER2-positive metastatic breast cancer. However, most cases of advanced disease eventually progress. Pertuzumab, an anti-HER2 humanized monoclonal antibody that inhibits receptor dimerization, has a mechanism of action that is complementary to that of trastuzumab, and combination therapy with the two antibodies has shown promising activity and an acceptable safety profile in phase 2 studies involving patients with HER2-positive breast cancer.

Methods.—We randomly assigned 808 patients with HER2-positive metastatic breast cancer to receive placebo plus trastuzumab plus docetaxel (control group) or pertuzumab plus trastuzumab plus docetaxel (pertuzumab group) as first-line treatment until the time of disease progression or the development of toxic effects that could not be effectively managed. The primary end point was independently assessed progression-free survival. Secondary end points included overall survival, progression-free survival as assessed by the investigator, the objective response rate, and safety.

Results.—The median progression-free survival was 12.4 months in the control group, as compared with 18.5 months in the pertuzumab group (hazard ratio for progression or death, 0.62; 95% confidence interval, 0.51 to 0.75; $P < 0.001$). The interim analysis of overall survival showed a strong trend in favor of pertuzumab plus trastuzumab plus docetaxel. The safety profile was generally similar in the two groups, with no increase in left ventricular systolic dysfunction; the rates of febrile neutropenia and diarrhea of grade 3 or above were higher in the pertuzumab group than in the control group.

Conclusions.—The combination of pertuzumab plus trastuzumab plus docetaxel, as compared with placebo plus trastuzumab plus docetaxel, when used as first-line treatment for HER2-positive metastatic breast cancer, significantly prolonged progression-free survival, with no increase in cardiac toxic effects. (Funded by F. Hoffmann–La Roche/Genentech; ClinicalTrials.gov number, NCT00567190.)

▶ This randomized phase III study evaluated the effects of pertuzumab, an anti-HER2 humanized monoclonal antibody with a mechanism of action (inhibition of receptor dimerization) that should be complementary to trastuzumab. A total of 808 patients with metastatic breast cancer were randomly assigned to docetaxel/trastuzumab plus either placebo or pertuzumab. The primary endpoint of the trial was progression-free survival. The addition of pertuzumab substantially increased progression-free survival at the median from 12.4 months to 18.5 months (HR = 0.62). This gain was bought for a modest increase in diarrhea and febrile neutropenia. No increase in cardiac toxicity was observed. This led to the recent approval of pertuzumab for use with trastuzumab plus docetaxel in patients with breast cancers that are HER2+.

J. T. Thigpen, MD

Miscellaneous

Management of hot flashes in patients who have breast cancer with venlafaxine and clonidine: a randomized, double-blind, placebo-controlled trial

Boekhout AH, Vincent AD, Dalesio OB, et al (The Netherlands Cancer Inst-Antoni van Leeuwenhoek Hosp, Amsterdam)

J Clin Oncol 29:3862-3868, 2011

Purpose.—Therapies for breast cancer may induce hot flashes that can affect quality of life. We undertook a double-blind, placebo-controlled trial with the primary objective of comparing the average daily hot flash scores in the twelfth week among patients treated with venlafaxine, clonidine, and placebo. Additional analyses of the hot flash score over the full 12 weeks of treatment were performed.

Patients and Methods.—In all, 102 patients with a history of breast cancer were randomly assigned (2:2:1) to venlafaxine 75 mg, clonidine 0.1 mg, or placebo daily for 12 weeks. Questionnaires at baseline and during treatment assessed daily hot flash scores, sexual function, sleep quality, anxiety, and depression.

Results.—After 12 weeks, a total of 80 patients were evaluable for the primary end point. During week 12, hot flash scores were significantly lower in the clonidine group versus placebo ($P = .03$); for venlafaxine versus placebo, the difference was borderline not significant ($P = .07$). However, hot flash scores were equal in the clonidine and venlafaxine groups. Over the course of 12 weeks, the differences between both treatments and placebo were significant ($P < .001$ for venlafaxine v placebo; $P = .045$ for clonidine v placebo). Frequencies of treatment-related adverse effects of nausea ($P = .02$), constipation ($P = .04$), and severe appetite loss were higher in the venlafaxine group.

Conclusion.—Venlafaxine and clonidine are effective treatments in the management of hot flashes in patients with breast cancer. Venlafaxine resulted in a more immediate reduction of hot flash scores when compared with clonidine; however, hot flash scores at week 12 were lower in the clonidine group than in the venlafaxine group.

▶ Hot flashes as a result of treatment for women with breast cancer and men with prostate cancer are a debilitating complication. Methods to mitigate this toxicity are important.

These authors report a significant randomized, placebo-controlled trial of 2 agents frequently used to treat hot flashes, venlafaxine and clonidine. Their results are somewhat mixed in that venlafaxine caused a more immediate reduction in hot flash scores, yet the clonidine had better hot flash scores at 12 weeks (the endpoint of the study).

So there are 2 important messages regarding this research: The first is that while the effects of hot flash scores were mixed for these drugs, both cause significant reduction in hot flash scores overall. The second message is that we need more data in larger trials (there were only 102 patients on this study) to validate these data and to consider other medications to help treat this challenging toxicity for some breast and prostate cancer patients.

C. Lawton, MD

Nodal status and clinical outcomes in a large cohort of patients with triple-negative breast cancer

Hernandez-Aya LF, Chavez-Macgregor M, Lei X, et al (The Univ of Texas MD Anderson Cancer Ctr, Houston)

J Clin Oncol 29:2628-2634, 2011

Purpose.—To evaluate the clinical outcomes and relationship between tumor size, lymph node status, and prognosis in a large cohort of patients with confirmed triple receptor-negative breast cancer (TNBC).

Patients and Methods.—We reviewed 1,711 patients with TNBC diagnosed between 1980 and 2009. Patients were categorized by tumor size and nodal status. Kaplan-Meier product limit method was used to calculate overall survival (OS) and relapse-free survival (RFS). A Sidak adjustment was used for multiple group comparisons. Cox proportional hazards models were fit to determine the association of tumor size and nodal status with survival outcomes after adjustment for other patient and disease characteristics.

Results.—Median age was 48 years (range, 21 to 87 years). At a median follow-up of 53 months (range, 0.7 to 317 months), there were 614 deaths and 747 recurrences. The 5-year OS was 80% for node-negative patients (N0), 65% for one to three positive lymph nodes (N1), 48% for four to nine positive lymph nodes (N2), and 44% for ≥10 positive lymph nodes (N3; $P < .0001$). The 5-year RFS rates were 67% for N0, 52% for N1, 36% for N2, and 33% for N3 ($P < .0001$). Pairwise comparison by nodal status showed that when comparing N0 with node-positive disease, there was a significant difference in OS and RFS ($P < .001$ all comparisons). However, when comparing N1 with N2 and N3 disease regardless of tumor size, there were no significant differences in OS or RFS.

Conclusion.—In patients with TNBC, once there is evidence of lymph node metastasis, the prognosis may not be affected by the number of positive lymph nodes.

▶ Breast cancer remains a serious problem in our country, despite years of research and encouraging results. It has long been understood that increasing tumor size and number of positive lymph nodes in patients with this diagnosis portends for poorer outcomes. Yet many other factors have been shown to play prognostic roles in this disease, with receptor status being just one of them.

The development of targeted therapy such as trastuzumab for human epidermal growth factor receptor 2 (HER2)—positive patients has lead to markedly improved outcomes for these patients. This is in addition to the previously well-documented benefit of tamoxifen for estrogen receptor—positive breast cancer patients. Yet for patients who are estrogen receptor, progesterone receptor, and HER2 negative (ie, triple negative), the results are unquestionably poorer. The clear relationship between tumor size and number of lymph nodes involved and outcomes may not be well correlated in patients with triple-negative tumors.

These authors have evaluated the question of lymph node status and outcome for over 1000 patients in the MD Anderson Cancer Center database. Their results support the well-known effect of lymph node positivity on outcomes, but the increasing number of lymph nodes involved did not appear to worsen the outcome.

These data support the need for significant research for triple-negative breast cancer patients, as they appear to have a uniquely separate biology from nontriple-negative breast cancer tumors.

C. Lawton, MD

6 Genitourinary

Prostate

10-year experience with I-125 prostate brachytherapy at the Princess Margaret Hospital: results for 1,100 patients

Crook J, Borg J, Evans A, et al (Princess Margaret Hosp, Toronto, Ontario, Canada)

Int J Radiat Oncol Biol Phys 80:1323-1329, 2011

Purpose.—To report outcomes for 1,111 men treated with iodine-125 brachytherapy (BT) at a single institution.

Methods and Materials.—A total of 1,111 men (median age, 63) were treated with iodine-125 prostate BT for low- or intermediate-risk prostate cancer between March 1999 and November 2008. Median prostate-specific antigen (PSA) level was 5.4 ng/ml (range, 0.9—26.1). T stage was T1c in 66% and T2 in 34% of patients. Gleason score was 6 in 90.1% and 7 or 8 in 9.9% of patients. Neoadjuvant hormonal therapy (2—6 months course) was used in 10.1% of patients and combined external radiotherapy (45 Gy) with BT (110 Gy) in 4.1% ($n = 46$) of patients. Univariate and multivariate Cox proportional hazards were used to determine predictors of failure.

Results.—Median follow-up was 42 months (range, 6—114), but for biochemical freedom from relapse, a minimum PSA test follow-up of 30 months was required (median 54; $n = 776$). There were 27 failures, yielding an actuarial 7-year disease-free survival rate of 95.2% (96 at risk beyond 84 months). All failures underwent repeat 12-core transrectal ultrasound -guided biopsies, confirming 8 local failures. On multivariate analysis, Gleason score was the only independent predictor of failure ($p = 0.001$; hazard ratio, 4.8 (1.9—12.4). Median International Prostate Symptom score from 12 to 108 months ranged between 3 and 9. Of the men reporting baseline potency, 82.8% retained satisfactory erectile function beyond 5 years.

Conclusion.—Iodine-125 prostate BT is a highly effective treatment option for favorable- and intermediate-risk prostate cancer and is associated with maintenance of good urinary and erectile functions.

▶ Prostate cancer remains the most common nonskin malignancy in US men. The vast majority of patients diagnosed with the disease have organ-confined disease for which there are multiple treatment options. Certainly active surveillance (AS) remains an excellent alternative for patients with low-risk disease (ie, prostate-specific antigen [PSA] less than 10, Gleason score less than 6, and clinical T1b to T2a disease), especially if they are elderly or have significant comorbidities that are likely to affect longevity. But for the thousands of patients with organ-confined disease who do not fall into the AS category, definitive treatment is likely appropriate.

Curative treatment for these patients comes in many forms from surgery (open vs robotic) to radiation (external beam irradiation vs low-dose rate brachytherapy vs high-dose rate brachytherapy). Head-to-head randomized comparisons of these different treatment options are lacking. Yet one can safely say that all work well in terms of PSA control and, therefore, cancer control.

The important aspect of low-dose rate brachytherapy, as seen for this dataset, is that it is a onetime procedure that is safe, effective, and from a cost perspective compares very favorably with the other treatments. These data are an excellent addition to the other large datasets that support the use of I-125 low-dose rate brachytherapy for localized prostate cancer. With these data and the others like it, there is no question that this treatment is an excellent option for most of these patients.

C. Lawton, MD

American Society for Radiation Oncology (ASTRO) and American College of Radiology (ACR) practice guideline for the transperineal permanent brachytherapy of prostate cancer

Rosenthal SA, Bittner NH, Beyer DC, et al (Radiological Associates of Sacramento, CA; Tacoma/Valley Radiation Oncology Ctrs, WA; Arizona Oncology Services, Scottsdale; et al)

Int J Radiat Oncol Biol Phys 79:335-341, 2011

Transperineal permanent prostate brachytherapy is a safe and efficacious treatment option for patients with organ-confined prostate cancer. Careful adherence to established brachytherapy standards has been shown to improve the likelihood of procedural success and reduce the incidence of treatment-related morbidity. A collaborative effort of the American College of Radiology (ACR) and American Society for Therapeutic Radiation Oncology (ASTRO) has produced a practice guideline for permanent prostate brachytherapy.

The guideline defines the qualifications and responsibilities of all the involved personnel, including the radiation oncologist, physicist and dosimetrist. Factors with respect to patient selection and appropriate use of supplemental treatment modalities such as external beam radiation and androgen suppression therapy are discussed. Logistics with respect to the brachtherapy implant procedure, the importance of dosimetric parameters, and attention to radiation safety procedures and documentation are presented. Adherence to these practice guidelines can be part of ensuring quality and safety in a successful prostate brachytherapy program.

▶ Over the past year, there has been extensive media coverage on the poor quality prostate seed implants (transperineal permanent brachytherapy of the prostate) performed at the veterans hospital in Pennsylvania. It has resulted in a questioning of the quality of prostate seed implants performed across the United States. In addition, multiple Veterans Administration prostate seed implant programs have been closed. The positive result of this media attention is that many programs have improved the rigor of the evaluation of the seed implants performed, which can improve outcomes. The downside of this attention has been a limitation on available sites for patients (especially veterans) to have seed implants performed.

Given the excellent results in terms of quality of life and prostate cancer control for patients treated with prostate seed implants, we must develop methods to improve the quality of them. This article is an excellent example of exactly how to do this. The emphasis on a dedicated team of physicians and physicists and careful patient selection as well as postimplant dosimetry can and will result in better outcomes for patients treated with prostate seed implants for localized prostate cancer.

C. Lawton, MD

Behavioral Therapy With or Without Biofeedback and Pelvic Floor Electrical Stimulation for Persistent Postprostatectomy Incontinence: A Randomized Controlled Trial

Goode PS, Burgio KL, Johnson TM II, et al (Birmingham–Atlanta Geriatric Res, GA; et al)

JAMA 305:151-159, 2011

Context.—Although behavioral therapy has been shown to improve postoperative recovery of continence, there have been no controlled trials of behavioral therapy for postprostatectomy incontinence persisting more than 1 year.

Objective.—To evaluate the effectiveness of behavioral therapy for reducing persistent postprostatectomy incontinence and to determine whether the technologies of biofeedback and pelvic floor electrical stimulation enhance the effectiveness of behavioral therapy.

Design, Setting, and Participants.—A prospective randomized controlled trial involving 208 community-dwelling men aged 51 through 84 years with incontinence persisting 1 to 17 years after radical prostatectomy was conducted at a university and 2 Veterans Affairs continence clinics (2003-2008) and included a 1-year follow-up after active treatment. Twenty-four percent of the men were African American; 75%, white.

Interventions.—After stratification by type and frequency of incontinence, participants were randomized to 1 of 3 groups: 8 weeks of behavioral therapy (pelvic floor muscle training and bladder control strategies);

behavioral therapy plus in-office, dual-channel electromyograph biofeedback and daily home pelvic floor electrical stimulation at 20 Hz, current up to 100 mA (behavior plus); or delayed treatment, which served as the control group.

Main Outcome Measure.—Percentage reduction in mean number of incontinence episodes after 8 weeks of treatment as documented in 7-day bladder diaries.

Results.—Mean incontinence episodes decreased from 28 to 13 per week (55% reduction; 95% confidence interval [CI], 44%-66%) after behavioral therapy and from 26 to 12 (51% reduction; 95% CI, 37%-65%) after behavior plus therapy. Both reductions were significantly greater than the reduction from 25 to 21 (24% reduction; 95% CI, 10%-39%) observed among controls (*P*=.001 for both treatment groups). However, there was no significant difference in incontinence reduction between the treatment groups (*P*=.69). Improvements were durable to 12 months in the active treatment groups: 50% reduction (95% CI, 39.8%-61.1%; 13.5 episodes per week) in the behavioral group and 59% reduction (95% CI, 45.0%-73.1%; 9.1 episodes per week) in the behavior plus group (*P*=.32).

Conclusions.—Among patients with postprostatectomy incontinence for at least 1 year, 8 weeks of behavioral therapy, compared with a delayed-treatment control, resulted in fewer incontinence episodes. The addition of biofeedback and pelvic floor electrical stimulation did not result in greater effectiveness.

Trial Registration.—clinicaltrials.gov Identifier: NCT00212264.

▶ For patients with prostate cancer who choose surgery as their definitive treatment, the 2 major toxicities and concerns for these patients are sexual dysfunction and incontinence. Although patients clearly do not want to have to deal with either of these potential side effects, most men would rate incontinence as more of a quality of life issue than sexual dysfunction.

For patients who suffer from postprostatectomy incontinence, there are options for treatment. One very effective option is the surgical placement of an artificial sphincter. But many men do not want to have another surgery. Thus, nonsurgical approaches need to be evaluated thoroughly. These authors have done an excellent job in evaluating both behavioral therapy and biofeedback with pelvic floor stimulation in this randomized controlled trial. Their results show a clear benefit to 8 weeks of behavioral therapy (including pelvic floor muscle exercises, bladder control techniques, and fluid management) that is helpful information for this population of patients. Equally useful in these data was that the addition of the biofeedback and pelvic floor electrical stimulation to the behavioral therapy did not result in better continence. Behavioral therapy needs to be offered to patients who have suffered from postprostatectomy incontinence for at least 1 year.

C. Lawton, MD

Comparison of Health-Related Quality of Life 5 Years After SPIRIT: Surgical Prostatectomy Versus Interstitial Radiation Intervention Trial

Crook JM, Gomez-Iturriaga A, Wallace K, et al (Univ of Toronto, Ontario, Canada)

J Clin Oncol 29:362-368, 2011

Purpose.—The American College of Surgeons Oncology Group phase III Surgical Prostatectomy Versus Interstitial Radiation Intervention Trial comparing radical prostatectomy (RP) and brachytherapy (BT) closed after 2 years due to poor accrual. We report health-related quality of life (HRQOL) at a mean of 5.3 years for 168 trial-eligible men who either chose or were randomly assigned to RP or BT following a multidisciplinary educational session.

Patients and Methods.—After initial lack of accrual, a multidisciplinary educational session was introduced for eligible patients. In all, 263 men attended 47 sessions. Of those, 34 consented to random assignment, 62 chose RP, and 94 chose BT. Five years later, these 190 men underwent HRQOL evaluation by using the cancer-specific 50-item Expanded Prostate Cancer Index Composite, the Short Form 12 Physical Component Score, and Short Form 12 Mental Component Score. Response rate was 88.4%. The Wilcoxon rank sum test was used to compare summary scores between the two interventions.

Results.—Of 168 survey responders, 60.7% had BT (9.5% randomly assigned) and 39.3% had RP (9.5% randomly assigned). Median age was 61.4 years for BT and 59.4 for RP ($P = .05$). Median follow-up was 5.2 years (range, 3.2 to 6.5 years). For BT versus RP, there was no difference in bowel or hormonal domains, but men treated with BT scored better in urinary (91.8 *v* 88.1; $P = .02$) and sexual (52.5 *v* 39.2; $P = .001$) domains, and in patient satisfaction (93.6 *v* 76.9; $P < .001$).

Conclusion.—Although treatment allocation was random in only 19%, all patients received identical information in a multidisciplinary setting before selecting RP, BT, or random assignment. HRQOL evaluated 3.2 to 6.5 years after treatment showed an advantage for BT in urinary and sexual domains and in patient satisfaction.

▶ Prostate cancer remains the most common nonskin cancer diagnosed in US men. The majority of patients are diagnosed by an increased prostate-specific antigen (PSA) level, prompting a biopsy. This increase in early detection has resulted in an increase in the diagnosis of localized prostate cancer since PSA was introduced in the late 1980s and early 1990s.

It is now well understood that many of these patients who are diagnosed with low-risk disease (eg, PSA <10, GS <6, and clinical T1c–T2a) require no treatment at all and often are best served with watchful waiting. Yet there is a cohort of patients with localized disease who do need treatment, and for those patients, the treatment options can be overwhelming: surgery (open vs robotic/laparoscopic), radiation (seed implants vs external beam), and on and on.

To try to understand the relative merits of some of these treatments for localized prostate cancer, the American College of Surgeons developed the SPIRIT Trial (surgical prostatectomy vs interstitial radiation intervention trial). Patients in this trial had low-risk prostate cancer and were randomly assigned to surgery versus brachytherapy (seed implant). Unfortunately, the trial closed after 2 years due to poor accrual—a sad reality for sure.

For the patients who were accrued, a subset agreed to quality-of-life (QOL) evaluations. This report of the results of that QOL evaluation showed an advantage for brachytherapy in terms of urinary and sexual domains and patient satisfaction. Given the early closure of this trial for lack of accrual and randomized assignment of treatment in only 19% of patients reported, we have to take these data cautiously. Yet these patient-reported outcomes are precisely what we need to help patients navigate the extensive options before them when diagnosed with localized prostate cancer.

C. Lawton, MD

Cost-Effectiveness of Prostate Specific Antigen Screening in the United States: Extrapolating From the European Study of Screening for Prostate Cancer

Shteynshlyuger A, Andriole GL (Washington Univ School of Medicine, St Louis, MO)

J Urol 185:828-832, 2011

Purpose.—Preliminary results of the European Randomized Study of Screening for Prostate Cancer showed a decrease in prostate cancer specific mortality associated with prostate specific antigen screening. We evaluated the cost-effectiveness of prostate specific antigen screening using data from the European Randomized Study of Screening for Prostate Cancer protocol when extrapolated to the United States.

Materials and Methods.—We used previously reported Surveillance, Epidemiology and End Results-Medicare data and a nationwide sample of employer provided estimates of costs of care for patients with prostate cancer. The European data were used in accordance with the study protocol to determine the costs and cost-effectiveness of prostate specific antigen screening.

Results.—The lifetime cost of screening with prostate specific antigen, evaluating abnormal prostate specific antigen and treating identified prostate cancer to prevent 1 death from prostate cancer was $5,227,306 based on the European findings and extrapolated to the United States. If screening achieved a similar decrease in overall mortality as the decrease in prostate cancer specific mortality in the European study, such intervention would cost $262,758 per life-year saved. Prostate specific antigen screening reported in the European study would become cost effective when the lifelong treatment costs were below $1,868 per life-year, or when the number needed to treat was lowered to 21 or fewer men.

Conclusions.—The lifelong costs of screening protocols are determined by the cost of treatment with an insignificant contribution from screening costs. We established a model that predicts the minimal requirements that would make screening a cost-effective measure for population based implementation.

► Prostate cancer claims the lives of over 32 000 US males annually, and unfortunately, it is too often thought of as an indolent disease that requires little concern much less treatment or screening. Breast cancer in women, on the other hand, claims the lives of approximately 40 000 US women annually and is considered an epidemic that must be stopped at all cost, with mammography screening and breast examinations remaining imperative. Given this disproportional concern, the role of prostate-specific antigen (PSA) screening for prostate cancer is constantly evaluated and often debunked as too expensive, given that virtually no one dies of this disease!

Since thousands of men do die of this disease, it is important that we continue to evaluate the role of digital rectal examination and PSA screening for prostate cancer. The goal is to define a population of men for which digital rectal examinations and PSA help diagnose those prostate cancers that do impact survival. These authors suggest such a model, which takes into account the age of the patient, life expectancy, and costs of evaluating men in the age range of 50 to 80 years. We simply must work with models like this to establish the role of digital rectal examinations and PSA screening so as to decrease the risk of prostate cancer deaths in the United States, which are second only to lung cancer deaths.

C. Lawton, MD

Definition of medical event is to be based on the total source strength for evaluation of permanent prostate brachytherapy: A report from the American Society for Radiation Oncology

Nag S, Demanes DJ, Hagan M, et al (Northern California Kaiser Permanente, Santa Clara, CA; Univ of California Los Angeles; Virginia Commonwealth Univ, Richmond; et al)

Pract Radiat Oncol 1:218-223, 2011

Purpose.—The Nuclear Regulatory Commission deems it to be a medical event (ME) if the total dose delivered differs from the prescribed dose by 20% or more. A dose-based definition of ME is not appropriate for permanent prostate brachytherapy as it generates too many spurious MEs and thereby creates unnecessary apprehension in patients, and ties up regulatory bodies and the licensees in unnecessary and burdensome investigations. A more suitable definition of ME is required for permanent prostate brachytherapy.

Methods and Materials.—The American Society for Radiation Oncology (ASTRO) formed a working group of experienced clinicians to review the literature, assess the validity of current regulations, and make specific recommendations about the definition of an ME in permanent prostate brachytherapy.

Results.—The working group found that the current definition of ME in §35.3045 as "the total dose delivered differs from the prescribed dose by 20 percent or more" was not suitable for permanent prostate brachytherapy since the prostate volume (and hence the resultant calculated prostate dose) is dependent on the timing of the imaging, the imaging modality used, the observer variability in prostate contouring, the planning margins used, inadequacies of brachytherapy treatment planning systems to calculate tissue doses, and seed migration within and outside the prostate. If a dose-based definition for permanent implants is applied strictly, many properly executed implants would be improperly classified as an ME leading to a detrimental effect on brachytherapy. The working group found that a source strength-based criterion, of >20% of source strength prescribed in the post-procedure written directive being implanted outside the planning target volume is more appropriate for defining ME in permanent prostate brachytherapy.

Conclusions.—ASTRO recommends that the definition of ME for permanent prostate brachytherapy should not be dose based but should be based upon the source strength (air-kerma strength) administered.

▶ Safe treatment of patients using radiation has been a serious concern of physicians, patients, insurers, and the state and federal government. At the national level, it is the Nuclear Regulatory Commission (NRC) that monitors "safe" use of radioactive materials and defines a medical event for the user (eg, the physician in the case of the medical use of radioactive materials). Yet the NRC is very careful to say that medical consequences of what they term a medical event (previously called a misadministration) is not their concern, but resides with the treating physician. This "jargon dancing" does not negate the fact that if a medical event occurs as defined by the NRC, a cascade of procedures has to be performed, including telling the patient and the referring physician.

Thus, careful definition of a real medical event is critically important, for safety reasons most importantly, and to avoid inappropriately scaring patients and referring physicians. The American Society for Radiation Oncology group, who defined a medical event for permanent prostate brachytherapy, is to be commended for its work. This group has carefully and systematically addressed this issue and developed a definition that is clear and, most importantly, will identify medical events in this area, which really are medical events for which the patient and both treating and referring physicians need to be aware of so that corrective action, if needed, can be performed.

C. Lawton, MD

Does hormone therapy reduce disease recurrence in prostate cancer patients receiving dose-escalated radiation therapy? An analysis of Radiation Therapy Oncology Group 94-06

Valicenti RK, Bae K, Michalski J, et al (Univ of California–Davis School of Medicine; Radiation Therapy Oncology Group, Philadelphia, PA; Washington Univ, St Louis, MO; et al)

Int J Radiat Oncol Biol Phys 79:1323-1329, 2011

Purpose.—The purpose of this study was to evaluate the effect on freedom from biochemical failure (bNED) or disease-free survival (DFS) by adding hormone therapy (HT) to dose-escalated radiation therapy (HDRT).

Methods and Materials.—We used 883 analyzable prostate cancer patients who enrolled on Radiation Therapy Oncology Group (RTOG) 94-06, a Phase I/II dose escalation trial, and whose mean planning target volume dose exceeded 73.8 Gy (mean, 78.5 Gy; maximum, 84.3 Gy). We defined biochemical failure according to the Phoenix definition.

Results.—A total of 259 men started HT 2 to 3 months before HDRT, but not longer than 6 months, and 66 men with high-risk prostate cancer received HT for a longer duration. At 5 years, the biochemical failure rates after HDRT alone were 12%, 18%, and 29% for low-, intermediate-, and high-risk patients, respectively ($p < 0.0001$). Cox proportional hazards regression analysis adjusted for covariates revealed that pretreatment PSA level was a significant factor, whereas risk group, Gleason score, T-stage, and age were not. When the patients were stratified by risk groups, the Cox proportion hazards regression model (after adjusting for pretreatment PSA, biopsy Gleason score, and T stage) did not reveal a significant effect on bNED or DFS by adding HT to HDRT.

Conclusion.—The addition of HT did not significantly improve bNED survival or DFS in all prostate cancer patients receiving HDRT, but did approach significance in high-risk patient subgroup. The result of this study is hypothesis generating and requires testing in a prospective randomized trial.

▶ Dose escalation in the treatment of localized prostate cancer has become a standard. Multiple clinical trials have found a benefit in terms of biochemical disease-free survival (bNED), especially in patients with intermediate-risk disease. In addition, both the National Cancer Institute through the Radiation Therapy Oncology Group (RTOG) and the European Cooperative Group have found a benefit to the addition of hormone therapy in prostate cancer patients especially those with locally advanced disease (eg, T3 and T4) or high-risk disease (eg, Gleason Score 8–10 or prostate-specific antigen < 20).

Just how both dose escalation and hormone therapy may work to further improve outcomes has not been tested prospectively. This trial was a first shot at looking at the addition of hormone therapy to dose-escalated radiation therapy. While the goal of this phase I/II study was to determine the MTD (maximally tolerated radiation dose), 259 men of the 883 accrued also received hormone therapy.

Interestingly, the addition of the hormone therapy was not associated with an increase bNED survival for patients on this trial but did approach significance for patients in the high-risk group. These data are, of course, hypothesis generating. It clearly supports the need for randomized clinical trials for patients with localized prostate cancer receiving dose-escalated external beam radiation therapy to see whether the addition of a short course of hormone therapy can further improve dose-escalated outcomes. Currently, RTOG trial 08-15 is asking this very question and we anxiously await the results.

C. Lawton, MD

Dose escalation and quality of life in patients with localized prostate cancer treated with radiotherapy: long-term results of the Dutch randomized dose-escalation trial (CKTO 96-10 Trial)

Al-Mamgani A, van Putten WLJ, van der Wielen GJ, et al (Erasmus MC—Daniel den Hoed Cancer Ctr, Rotterdam, The Netherlands)

Int J Radiat Oncol Biol Phys 79:1004-1012, 2011

Purpose.—To assess the impact of dose escalation of radiotherapy on quality of life (QoL) in prostate cancer patients.

Patients and Methods.—Three hundred prostate cancer patients participating in the Dutch randomized trial (CKTO 69-10) comparing 68 Gy with 78 Gy were the subject of this analysis. These patients filled out the SF-36 QoL questionnaire before radiotherapy (baseline) and 6, 12, 24, and 36 months thereafter. Changes in QoL over time of ≥10 points were considered clinically relevant. Repeated-measures regression analyses were applied to estimate and test the QoL changes over time, the differences between the two arms, and for association with a number of covariates.

Results.—At 3-year follow-up, the summary score physical health was 73.2 for the 68-Gy arm vs. 71.6 for the 78-Gy arm ($p = 0.81$), and the summary score mental health was 76.7 for the 68-Gy arm vs. 76.1 for the 78-Gy arm ($p = 0.97$). Statistically significant ($p < 0.01$) deterioration in QoL scores over time was registered in both arms in six scales. The deterioration over time was more pronounced in the high-dose arm for most scales. However, clinically relevant deterioration (>10 points) was seen for only two scales. None of the tested covariates were significantly correlated with QoL scores.

Conclusion.—Dose escalation did not result in significant deterioration of QoL in prostate cancer patients. In both randomization arms, statistically significant decreases in QoL scores over time were seen in six scales. The deterioration of QoL was more pronounced in the physical than in the mental health domain and in some scales more in the high- than in the low-dose arm, but the differences between arms were not statistically significant.

▶ Dose escalation for patients with localized prostate cancer has become routine, given multiple randomized trials showing a benefit to dose escalation especially in patients with intermediate risk disease (eg, patients with prostate-specific antigen

[PSA] greater than 10, or Gleason score of 7, or clinical T2b or clinical T2c disease). Improvement in PSA endpoints is the basis for these recommendations, not overall survival or disease-specific survival.

In light of these "nonsurvival" improvements, issues of impact on quality of life become very important. The standard clinician-reported quality of life outcomes are fraught with inaccuracies, and patient-reported quality of life outcomes are the important endpoints that we as oncologists need to focus on.

The results of this Dutch randomized trial of 68 versus 78 Gy radiotherapy dose reported in this article are especially important for 2 reasons: First, these are patient-reported outcomes and 75% of patients filled out at least 1 questionnaire. Second, there did not appear to be a decrement in quality of life with the use of the increased dose, as might be expected. There was, however, a decrease in quality of life overall (ie, in all patients) regardless of dose, and with longer follow-up (given that these are only 3-year data), one might see further changes in quality of life. In addition, one might also see a difference in these potential changes in quality of life that correlate with increasing dose. We await more of these excellent patient-reported quality-of-life data with longer follow-up.

C. Lawton, MD

Fifteen-year biochemical relapse-free survival, cause-specific survival, and overall survival following I^{125} prostate brachytherapy in clinically localized prostate cancers: Seattle experience

Sylvester JE, Grimm PD, Wong J, et al (Lakewood Ranch Oncology, FL; Prostate Cancer Treatment Ctr, Seattle, WA; Univ California, Irvine, et al)
Int J Radiat Oncol Biol Phys 81:376-381, 2011

Purpose.—To report 15-year biochemical relapse–free survival (BRFS), cause-specific survival (CSS), and overall survival (OS) outcomes of patients treated with I^{125} brachytherapy monotherapy for clinically localized prostate cancer early in the Seattle experience.

Methods and Materials.—Two hundred fifteen patients with clinically localized prostate cancer were consecutively treated from 1988 to 1992 with I^{125} monotherapy. They were prospectively followed as a tight cohort. They were evaluated for BRFS, CSS, and OS. Multivariate analysis was used to evaluate outcomes by pretreatment clinical prognostic factors. BRFS was analyzed by the Phoenix (nadir + 2 ng/mL) definition. CSS and OS were evaluated by chart review, death certificates, and referring physician follow-up notes. Gleason scoring was performed by general pathologists at a community hospital in Seattle. Time to biochemical failure (BF) was calculated and compared by Kaplan-Meier plots.

Results.—Fifteen-year BRFS for the entire cohort was 80.4%. BRFS by D'Amico risk group classification cohort analysis was 85.9%, 79.9%, and 62.2% for low, intermediate, and high-risk patients, respectively. Follow-up ranged from 3.6 to 18.4 years; median follow-up was 15.4 years for biochemically free of disease patients. Overall median follow-up was 11.7 years. The median time to BF in those who failed was 5.1 years.

CSS was 84%. OS was 37.1%. Average age at time of treatment was 70 years. There was no significant difference in BRFS between low and intermediate risk groups.

Conclusion.—I^{125} monotherapy results in excellent 15-year BRFS and CSS, especially when taking into account the era of treatment effect.

▶ Treatment options for organ-confined prostate cancer, especially those patients with low or intermediate risk disease, are numerous. Surgery is available robotically or as an open procedure. Watchful waiting or active surveillance is appropriate for many low-risk patients (eg, <clinical T2a, <Gleason Score 6, and <prostate-specific antigen 10). Radiation is available as external beam or brachytherapy, both low-dose rate (LDR) and high-dose rate.

The team of physicians from Seattle who pioneered the resurgence of I-125 LDR brachytherapy for these patients has reported their results with 15-year follow-up. This report is important for a number of reasons: First, it confirms that the long-term outcome in terms of disease control for these patients is very good. Second, it confirms that many patients with intermediate-risk disease are also very appropriate candidates for LDR brachytherapy. Third, it shows that patients who fail generally do so within 8 to 10 years. Finally, although a thorough review of toxicity is not available in this article, there were no treatment-related deaths or other serious complications, such deep venous thrombosis or strokes. The take-home message here is that this option for patients with low- or intermediate-risk prostate cancer should be offered, as it appears to be effective and certainly is cost effective.

C. Lawton, MD

Phase I dose-escalation study of stereotactic body radiation therapy for low and intermediate-risk prostate cancer

Boike TP, Lotan Y, Cho LC, et al (Univ of Texas Southwestern, Dallas)

J Clin Oncol 29:2020-2026, 2011

Purpose.—To evaluate the tolerability of escalating doses of stereotactic body radiation therapy in the treatment of localized prostate cancer.

Patients and Methods.—Eligible patients included those with Gleason score 2 to 6 with prostate-specific antigen (PSA) $\leq$ 20, Gleason score 7 with PSA $\leq$ 15, $\leq$ T2b, prostate size $\leq$ 60 cm^3, and American Urological Association (AUA) score $\leq$ 15. Pretreatment preparation required an enema and placement of a rectal balloon. Dose-limiting toxicity (DLT) was defined as grade 3 or worse GI/genitourinary (GU) toxicity by Common Terminology Criteria of Adverse Events (version 3). Patients completed quality-of-life questionnaires at defined intervals.

Results.—Groups of 15 patients received 45 Gy, 47.5 Gy, and 50 Gy in five fractions (45 total patients). The median follow-up is 30 months (range, 3 to 36 months), 18 months (range, 0 to 30 months), and 12 months (range, 3 to 18 months) for the 45 Gy, 47.5 Gy, and 50 Gy groups, respectively. For all patients, GI grade $\geq$ 2 and grade $\geq$ 3 toxicity occurred in

18% and 2%, respectively, and GU grade ≥ 2 and grade ≥ 3 toxicity occurred in 31% and 4%, respectively. Mean AUA scores increased significantly from baseline in the 47.5-Gy dose level ($P = .002$) as compared with the other dose levels, where mean values returned to baseline. Rectal quality-of-life scores (Expanded Prostate Cancer Index Composite) fell from baseline up to 12 months but trended back at 18 months. In all patients, PSA control is 100% by the nadir + 2 ng/mL failure definition.

Conclusion.—Dose escalation to 50 Gy has been completed without DLT. A multicenter phase II trial is underway treating patients to 50 Gy in five fractions to further evaluate this experimental therapy.

▶ Traditionally prostate cancer is treated, from an external beam perspective, with small fractions (1.8 to 2.0 Gy) over 7 to 8 weeks or more. It was thought to be well understood that the alpha to beta ratio of the disease was relatively high, and thus small fraction sizes were appropriate for disease and toxicity control. Over the past decade, oncologists have come to understand that the real alpha to beta ratio is likely low, perhaps in the range of 1.0 to 3.0, and thus larger fraction sizes are most appropriate. Given our ability to conform radiation to the patient's anatomy, the toxicities should be reasonable as well.

Multiple studies have shown that moderate hypofractionation (fraction sizes of approximately 2.5 to 3.0 Gy) is safe and effective in the treatment of localized prostate cancer. Given the pervasiveness of the disease and cost associated with the number of fractions, a decrease in the fraction number is helpful from the economic and patient convenience perspectives. Thus the question of ultrafractionation in the form of stereotactic body radiation therapy is worth serious study.

The results of phase 1 trials such as the data presented here are exactly what we as treating radiation oncologists need to understand the best form of hypofractionation for localized prostate cancer patients. With a median follow-up of 30 months, 18 months, and 12 months for the 45 Gy, 47.5 Gy, and 50 Gy groups, respectively, we can say that acute toxicity was reasonable. We need much longer follow-up to comment on late toxicity. Clearly these data represent a start, and we need more of these types of trials to know the real benefit versus risk of this ultrahypofractionation option of our localized prostate cancer patients.

C. Lawton, MD

Progression From High-Grade Prostatic Intraepithelial Neoplasia to Cancer: A Randomized Trial of Combination Vitamin-E, Soy, and Selenium

Fleshner NE, Kapusta L, Donnelly R, et al (Univ Health Network, Toronto, Ontario, Canada; Credit Valley Hosp, Mississauga, Ontario, Canada; London Health Sciences Centre, UK; et al)

J Clin Oncol 29:2386-2390, 2011

Purpose.—High-grade prostatic intraepithelial neoplasia (HGPIN) is a putative precursor of invasive prostate cancer (PCa). Preclinical evidence suggests vitamin E, selenium, and soy protein may prevent progression of

HGPIN to PCa. This hypothesis was tested in a randomized phase III double-blind study of daily soy (40 g), vitamin E (800 U), and selenium (200 μg) versus placebo.

Patients and Methods.—Three hundred three men in 12 Canadian centers were analyzed. The main eligibility criterion was confirmed HGPIN in at least one of two biopsies within 18 months of random assignment. Treatment was administered daily for 3 years. Follow-up prostate biopsies occurred at 6, 12, 24, and 36 months postrandomization. The primary end point was time to development of invasive PCa. Kaplan-Meier plots and log-rank tests were used to compare two treatment groups for this end point.

Results.—For all patients, the median age was 62.8 years. The median baseline prostate-specific antigen (PSA; n = 302) was 5.41 ug/L; total testosterone (n = 291) was 13.4 nmol/L. Invasive PCa developed among 26.4% of patients. The hazard ratio for the nutritional supplement to prevent PCa was 1.03 (95% CI, 0.67 to 1.60; *P* =.88). Gleason score distribution was similar in both groups with 83.5% of cancers graded Gleason sum of 6. Baseline age, weight, PSA, and testosterone did not predict for development of PCa. The supplement was well tolerated with flatulence reported more frequently (27% *v* 17%) among men receiving micronutrients.

Conclusion.—This trial does not support the hypothesis that combination vitamin E, selenium, and soy prevents progression from HGPIN to PCa.

▶ Given that prostate cancer kills approximately 30 000 US men annually and that its increased incidence has been associated with countries with a high animal fat diet (such as the United States), it is of importance to try to understand factors that may help decrease the risk of the disease. It has been well established that high-grade prostatic intraepithelial neoplasia (PIN) can progress to prostate cancer. So 1 way to help decrease the risk of the disease potentially is to understand agents that may stop or lower the progression of high-grade PIN to prostate cancer.

These authors have evaluated the potential role of vitamin E, soy, and selenium in the prevention of the cascade of high-grade PIN to prostate cancer in a double-blind, placebo-controlled, phase III trial. The results do not support the hypothesis that combination vitamin E, soy, and selenium prevents progression of high-grade PIN to invasive prostate cancer. This is consistent with the findings of the SELECT trial (Selenium and Vitamin E cancer prevention trial), which evaluated vitamin E and selenium prospectively in the prevention of prostate cancer. Clearly more work is needed in the area of dietary research, as the data are clear that countries with lower animal fat diets (eg, Japan and African countries) have lower incidence of prostate cancer.

C. Lawton, MD

Radiotherapy and Short-Term Androgen Deprivation for Localized Prostate Cancer

Jones CU, Hunt D, McGowan DG, et al (Radiological Associates of Sacramento, CA; Radiation Therapy Oncology Group Statistical Ctr, Philadelphia, PA; Cross Cancer Inst, Edmonton, Alberta, Canada; et al)

N Engl J Med 365:107-118, 2011

Background.—It is not known whether short-term androgen-deprivation therapy (ADT) before and during radiotherapy improves cancer control and overall survival among patients with early, localized prostate adenocarcinoma.

Methods.—From 1994 through 2001, we randomly assigned 1979 eligible patients with stage T1b, T1c, T2a, or T2b prostate adenocarcinoma and a prostate-specific antigen (PSA) level of 20 ng per milliliter or less to radiotherapy alone (992 patients) or radiotherapy with 4 months of total androgen suppression starting 2 months before radiotherapy (radiotherapy plus short-term ADT, 987 patients). The primary end point was overall survival. Secondary end points included disease-specific mortality, distant metastases, biochemical failure (an increasing level of PSA), and the rate of positive findings on repeat prostate biopsy at 2 years.

Results.—The median follow-up period was 9.1 years. The 10-year rate of overall survival was 62% among patients receiving radiotherapy plus short-term ADT (the combined-therapy group), as compared with 57% among patients receiving radiotherapy alone (hazard ratio for death with radiotherapy alone, 1.17; $P = 0.03$). The addition of short-term ADT was associated with a decrease in the 10-year disease-specific mortality from 8% to 4% (hazard ratio for radiotherapy alone, 1.87; $P = 0.001$). Biochemical failure, distant metastases, and the rate of positive findings on repeat prostate biopsy at 2 years were significantly improved with radiotherapy plus short-term ADT. Acute and late radiation induced toxic effects were similar in the two groups. The incidence of grade 3 or higher hormone-related toxic effects was less than 5%. Reanalysis according to risk showed reductions in overall and disease-specific mortality primarily among intermediate-risk patients, with no significant reductions among low-risk patients.

Conclusions.—Among patients with stage T1b, T1c, T2a, or T2b prostate adenocarcinoma and a PSA level of 20 ng per milliliter or less, the use of short-term ADT for 4 months before and during radiotherapy was associated with significantly decreased disease-specific mortality and increased overall survival. According to post hoc risk analysis, the benefit was mainly seen in intermediate-risk, but not low-risk, men. (Funded by the National Cancer Institute; RTOG 94-08 ClinicalTrials.gov number, NCT00002597.)

▶ Improvements in the treatment of localized prostate cancer can help save the lives of thousands of men across the United States and therefore are important. Oncologists know that combining androgen deprivation with external beam radiation therapy is critical in obtaining the best results for high-risk patients. Previously, the Radiation Therapy Oncology Group (RTOG) protocol 86-10 showed a significant improvement in outcomes for high-risk patients with radiation therapy and 4 months of total androgen suppression (starting 2 months neoadjuvant to the radiation therapy and concurrent with the radiation therapy). Therefore, exploring this in patients with localized disease makes obvious sense.

To examine this, the RTOG conducted a prospective randomized trial on patients with localized prostate cancer (clinical T2b or less and prostate-specific antigen <20 ng/mL). Patients were randomized to radiation therapy alone versus 4 months of total androgen suppression starting 2 months neoadjuvant to the radiation therapy and concurrent with radiation therapy.

The results reported here show a clear benefit in terms of overall survival and disease-specific survival with the addition of 4 months of total androgen suppression to radiation therapy.

But there are at least 2 very important points to remember regarding these data: The first point is that the benefit was not seen in low-risk patients, despite the low dose of radiation therapy used (66.6 Gy to isocenter). The second point is that this benefit has to be tempered since the dose of radiation used was clearly low by today's standards. It has been well documented in randomized trials of organ-confined prostate cancer that 66.6 Gy is not an adequate radiation dose to obtain the best results, especially for intermediate-risk patients. What impact 4 months of total androgen suppression has on localized prostate cancer treated to appropriate doses of approximately 75 to 80 Gy remains to be seen. RTOG 08-15 will address this important question.

C. Lawton, MD

Radical Prostatectomy versus Watchful Waiting in Early Prostate Cancer

Bill-Axelson A, for the Scandinavian Prostate Cancer Group Study No. 4 (Univ Hosp, Uppsala, Sweden; et al)

N Engl J Med 352:1977-1984, 2005

Background.—In 2002, we reported the initial results of a trial comparing radical prostatectomy with watchful waiting in the management of early prostate cancer. After three more years of follow-up, we report estimated 10-year results.

Methods.—From October 1989 through February 1999, 695 men with early prostate cancer (mean age, 64.7 years) were randomly assigned to radical prostatectomy (347 men) or watchful waiting (348 men). The follow-up was complete through 2003, with blinded evaluation of the causes of death. The primary end point was death due to prostate cancer; the secondary end points were death from any cause, metastasis, and local progression.

Results.—During a median of 8.2 years of follow-up, 83 men in the surgery group and 106 men in the watchful-waiting group died ($P=0.04$). In 30 of the 347 men assigned to surgery (8.6 percent) and 50 of the 348 men assigned to watchful waiting (14.4 percent), death was due to prostate cancer. The difference in the cumulative incidence of death due to prostate cancer increased from 2.0 percentage points after 5 years to 5.3 percentage points after 10 years, for a relative risk of 0.56 (95 percent confidence interval, 0.36 to 0.88; $P = 0.01$ by Gray's test). For distant metastasis, the corresponding increase was from 1.7 to 10.2 percentage points, for a relative risk in the surgery group of 0.60 (95 percent confidence interval, 0.42 to 0.86; $P = 0.004$ by Gray's test), and for local progression, the increase was from 19.1 to 25.1 percentage points, for a relative risk of 0.33 (95 percent confidence interval, 0.25 to 0.44; $P < 0.001$ by Gray's test).

Conclusions.—Radical prostatectomy reduces disease-specific mortality, overall mortality, and the risks of metastasis and local progression. The absolute reduction in the risk of death after 10 years is small, but the reductions in the risks of metastasis and local tumor progression are substantial.

► With the advent of prostate-specific antigen (PSA) as a screening tool, many patients have been diagnosed with prostate cancer at a very early stage (ie, often low-risk disease). Whether treatment is really necessary for many of these patients is not known. Furthermore, there are multiple datasets that support active surveillance or watchful waiting as a monitor of these cases, with a plan of definitive treatment if significant change in the PSA or clinical examination occurs.

Yet oncologists are often worried about patients who receive either too much treatment or too little. This concern is well addressed in this Scandinavian randomized trial where patients with early prostate cancer were randomized to watchful waiting versus radical retropubic prostatectomy. The median follow-up is long (12.8 years) and therefore the results have significant meaning. Given the statistical improvement in death from prostate cancer with upfront surgery over watchful waiting, it behooves us as oncologists to offer curative treatment to our patients. This is not to say that watchful waiting is inappropriate. We must continue to evaluate each patient and offer the options that we feel are best suited to the particular situation.

C. Lawton, MD

Vitamin E and the Risk of Prostate Cancer: The Selenium and Vitamin E Cancer Prevention Trial (SELECT)

Klein EA, Thompson IM Jr, Tangen CM, et al (Cleveland Clinic, OH; Univ of Texas Health Science Ctr, San Antonio; Fred Hutchinson Cancer Res Ctr, Seattle, WA; et al)

JAMA 306:1549-1556, 2011

Context.—The initial report of the Selenium and Vitamin E Cancer Prevention Trial (SELECT) found no reduction in risk of prostate cancer with either selenium or vitamin E supplements but a statistically nonsignificant increase in prostate cancer risk with vitamin E. Longer follow-up and more prostate cancer events provide further insight into the relationship of vitamin E and prostate cancer.

Objective.—To determine the long-term effect of vitamin E and selenium on risk of prostate cancer in relatively healthy men.

Design, Setting, and Participants.—A total of 35 533 men from 427 study sites in the United States, Canada, and Puerto Rico were randomized between August 22, 2001, and June 24, 2004. Eligibility criteria included a prostate-specific antigen (PSA) of 4.0 ng/mL or less, a digital rectal examination not suspicious for prostate cancer, and age 50 years or older for black men and 55 years or older for all others. The primary analysis included 34 887 men who were randomly assigned to 1 of 4 treatment groups: 8752 to receive selenium; 8737, vitamin E; 8702, both agents, and 8696, placebo. Analysis reflect the final data collected by the study sites on their participants through July 5, 2011.

Interventions.—Oral selenium (200 μg/d from *L*-selenomethionine) with matched vitamin E placebo, vitamin E (400 IU/d of all *rac*-α-tocopheryl acetate) with matched selenium placebo, both agents, or both matched placebos for a planned follow-up of a minimum of 7 and maximum of 12 years.

Main Outcome Measures.—Prostate cancer incidence.

Results.—This report includes 54 464 additional person-years of follow-up and 521 additional cases of prostate cancer since the primary report. Compared with the placebo (referent group) in which 529 men developed prostate cancer, 620 men in the vitamin E group developed prostate cancer (hazard ratio [HR], 1.17; 99% CI, 1.004-1.36, $P = .008$); as did 575 in the selenium group (HR, 1.09; 99% CI, 0.93-1.27; $P = .18$), and 555 in the selenium plus vitamin E group (HR, 1.05; 99% CI, 0.89-1.22, $P = .46$). Compared with placebo, the absolute increase in risk of prostate cancer per 1000 person-years was 1.6 for vitamin E, 0.8 for selenium, and 0.4 for the combination.

Conclusion.—Dietary supplementation with vitamin E significantly increased the risk of prostate cancer among healthy men.

Trial Registration.—Clinicaltrials.gov Identifier: NCT00006392.

▶ Prostate cancer prevention, given the 16% lifetime risk for the average US male, is important. SELECT, which randomized over 35 000 North American men to supplemental vitamin E, selenium, or both, showed no decrease in the risk of prostate cancer with those supplements. It also asked whether the vitamin E alone group may actually have had an increase in prostate cancer diagnoses.

This follow-up article is exceedingly important in that it has shown a statistically significant increase in the risk of prostate cancer in patients randomized to 400 IU of vitamin E alone (selenium placebo). Patients receiving both vitamin E and selenium did not have an increased risk of prostate cancer.

This study reinforces the absolute need to study supplements in general. Patients are always looking for ways to improve their health, and vitamins are often thought to be a simple, innocuous way to do so. These data show us that we can do serious harm to our patients if we do not study the potential effects (good and bad) of vitamins and other over-the-counter supplements.

C. Lawton, MD

Testis

Association of diagnostic radiation exposure and second abdominal-pelvic malignancies after testicular cancer

van Walraven C, Fergusson D, Earle C, et al (Univ of Ottawa, Ontario, Canada)

J Clin Oncol 29:2883-2888, 2011

Purpose.—The evidence associating cancer risk with diagnostic radiation exposure is unclear. Men recovering from low-grade testicular cancer frequently undergo serial abdominal-pelvic computerized tomography (CT) scanning to monitor for recurrent disease.

Methods.—We used population-based administrative data sets to identify every incident case of testicular cancer between 1991 and 2004 in Ontario, Canada. We excluded those with previous cancer, concurrent radiation therapy, retroperitoneal lymph node dissection, or fewer than 5 years observation. Patients were observed until the occurrences of death or development of a second abdominal-pelvic malignancy or until December 31, 2009.

Results.—A total of 2,569 men (mean age, 34.7 years; standard deviation, 10.2) were observed for a median of 11.2 years (interquartile range [IQR], 8.3 to 14.3). During the first 5 years after diagnosis, men underwent a median of 10 computed tomography (CT) scans (IQR, 4 to 18) of the abdominal-pelvic area, and they were exposed to a median of 110 mSv of radiation from radiologic investigations (IQR, 44 to 190). After this, 14 men were diagnosed with a second abdominal-pelvic malignancy (rate, five per 10,000 patient-years observation, 95% CI, three to eight); the most common diagnoses were colorectal and kidney malignancies. Radiation exposure was not associated with an excess risk of second cancers (hazard ratio per 10 mSv increase, 0.99; 95% CI, 0.95 to 1.04). This association did not change if men observed for fewer than 5 years were included in the analysis (hazard ratio, 1.00; 95% CI, 0.96 to 1.04).

Conclusion.—Second malignancies of the abdomen-pelvis are uncommon in men with low-grade testicular cancer. In this study, the risk of second cancer was not associated with the amount of diagnostic radiation exposure.

▶ Patients with low-stage testicular cancer are routinely monitored with CT scans as often as every 2 to 4 months in the first few years following their diagnosis and then somewhat less often thereafter, but continuing for upward of 7 to 10 years. The benefit of close monitoring is clear in that it allows for early diagnosis of potential recurrences and therefore increases the likelihood of eradicating recurrent disease.

Yet there is always the concern that this exposure to radiation could cause secondary cancers. These authors have tried to evaluate this risk by looking at the Ontario Cancer Registry. They identified over 2500 men who were observed for over 10 years (11.2 years median) with a median of 10 CTs of the abdomen and pelvis and found no increase in secondary malignancies.

These results, of course, do not rule out the possibility that serial CT scanning could cause a secondary cancer, but they certainly are comforting. The risk of developing a secondary malignancy based on these data is very low and supports continued use of CT monitoring of these patients.

C. Lawton, MD

Management of Seminomatous Testicular Cancer: A Binational Prospective Population-Based Study From the Swedish Norwegian Testicular Cancer Study Group

Tandstad T, Smaaland R, Solberg A, et al (St Olavs Univ Hosp, Trondheim, Norway; Stavanger Univ Hosp, Norway; Haukeland Hosp, Bergen, Norway; et al)

J Clin Oncol 29:719-725, 2011

Purpose.—A binational, population-based treatment protocol was established to prospectively treat and follow patients with seminomatous testicular cancer. The aim was to standardize care for all patients with seminoma to further improve the good results expected for this disease.

Patients and Methods.—From 2000 to 2006, a total of 1,384 Norwegian and Swedish patients were included in the study. Treatment in clinical stage 1 (CS1) was surveillance, adjuvant radiotherapy, or adjuvant carboplatin. In metastatic disease, recommended treatment was radiotherapy in CS2A and cisplatin-based chemotherapy in CS2B or higher.

Results.—At a median follow-up of 5.2 years, 5-year cause-specific survival was 99.6%. In CS1, 14.3% (65 of 512) of patients relapsed following surveillance, 3.9% (seven of 188) after carboplatin, and 0.8% (four of 481) after radiotherapy. We could not identify any factors predicting relapse in CS1 patients who were subjected to surveillance only. In CS2A, 10.9% (three of 29) patients relapsed after radiotherapy compared with no relapses in CS2A/B patients (zero of 73) treated with chemotherapy ($P = .011$).

Conclusion.—An international, population-based treatment protocol for testicular seminoma is feasible with excellent results. Surveillance remains a good option for CS1 patients. No factors predicted relapse in CS1 patients on surveillance. Despite resulting in a lower rate of relapse than with adjuvant carboplatin, adjuvant radiotherapy has been abandoned in the Swedish and Norwegian Testicular Cancer Project (SWENOTECA) as a recommended treatment option because of concerns of induction of secondary cancers. The higher number of relapses in radiotherapy-treated CS2A patients when compared with chemotherapy-treated CS2A/B patients is of concern. Late toxicity of cisplatin-based chemotherapy versus radiotherapy must be considered in CS2A patients.

▶ Patients with testicular seminoma have multiple treatment options, especially for those presenting with clinically stage I (CSI) disease. Surveillance or radiation therapy has been the standard option for decades. With the recent updated results of the European carboplatin versus radiation therapy trial, carboplatin as adjuvant postorchiectomy treatment has gained widespread acceptance.

This study of the results of treatment for all stages of seminoma in Swedish and Norwegian men diagnosed in 2000 through 2006 is interesting in that it shows multiple outcomes. First, with a median follow-up of more than 5 years, 14.3% of the 512 CSI patients on surveillance experienced relapse with 1 relapsing at 7 years. This number is confirmatory to the standard perception that approximately 15% to 20% of patients will relapse on surveillance and that follow-up is required to at least 10 years. Second, only 0.8% of the 481 patients treated with adjuvant radiation therapy experienced relapse, and 3.9% of the 189 patients treated with adjuvant carboplatin had relapse. Despite this statistical difference in relapse rates favoring radiation, there is a trend toward increasing the use of carboplatin and decreased use of radiation in these countries to the point that, although discussed as an option, adjuvant radiation therapy has essentially been abandoned. Secondary malignancies are the main reason for this recommendation. Only time will tell if this turns out to be the best decision. Secondary malignancies must be carefully evaluated over time in the carboplatin-treated patients as well.

C. Lawton, MD

Randomized Trial of Carboplatin Versus Radiotherapy for Stage I Seminoma: Mature Results on Relapse and Contralateral Testis Cancer Rates in MRC TE19/EORTC 30982 Study (ISRCTN27163214)

Oliver RTD, Mead GM, Rustin GJS, et al (St Bartholomews and the London Hosp, UK; Med Res Council Clinical Trials Unit, London; UK; Southampton General Hosp, UK; et al)

J Clin Oncol 29:957-962, 2011

Purpose.—Initial results of a randomized trial comparing carboplatin with radiotherapy (RT) as adjuvant treatment for stage I seminoma found carboplatin had a noninferior relapse-free rate (RFR) and had reduced contralateral germ cell tumors (GCTs) in the short-term. Updated results with a median follow-up of 6.5 years are now reported.

Patients and Methods.—Random assignment was between RT and one infusion of carboplatin dosed at 7 × (glomerular filtration rate +25) on the basis of EDTA (n = 357) and 90% of this dose if determined on the basis of creatinine clearance (n = 202). The trial was powered to exclude a doubling in RFRs assuming a 96-97% 2-year RFR after radiotherapy (hazard ratio [HR], approximately 2.0).

Results.—Overall, 1,447 patients were randomly assigned in a 3-to-5 ratio (carboplatin, n = 573; RT, n = 904). RFRs at 5 years were 94.7% for carboplatin and 96.0% for RT (RT-C 90% CI, 0.7% to 3.5%; HR, 1.25; 90% CI, 0.83 to 1.89). One death as a result of seminoma (in RT arm) occurred. Patients receiving at least 99% of the 7 × AUC dose had a 5-year RFR of 96.1% (95% CI, 93.4% to 97.7%) compared with 92.6% (95% CI, 88.0% to 95.5%) in those who received lower doses

(HR, 0.51; 95% CI, 0.24 to 1.07; P =.08). There was a clear reduction in the rate of contralateral GCTs (carboplatin, n = 2; RT, n = 15; HR, 0.22; 95% CI, 0.05 to 0.95; P =.03), and elevated pretreatment follicle-stimulating hormone (FSH) levels (>12 IU/L) was a strong predictor (HR, 8.57; 95% CI, 1.82 to 40.38).

Conclusion.—These updated results confirm the noninferiority of single dose carboplatin (at 7 × AUC dose) versus RT in terms of RFR and establish a statistically significant reduction in the medium term of risk of second GCT produced by this treatment.

▶ For decades, radiation has played a pivotal role in the treatment of patients with testicular tumors and in particular seminomas. With the advent of chemotherapy, the role of radiation nonseminomatous germ cell tumors was essentially replaced. Yet for seminomas testis cancers, given that most are stage I, postoperative irradiation has been the standard of care.

The volumes of the radiation field have also evolved from the "dog-leg" portals directing radiation to the periaortic lymph nodes and ipsilateral pelvic lymph nodes to the current periaortic lymph node radiation fields only for most patients.

This article updates the Medical Research Council trial comparing radiation therapy with single-dose carboplatin and potentially changes the treatment standard for stage I seminoma patients again. These data show that single-agent carboplatin appears to be equally effective as radiation, but with less risk of secondary malignancies. Yet it is imperative to remember that most patients with stage I seminoma should be treated expectantly with no upfront treatment and careful monitoring. This allows for treatment of only those patients who absolutely need it and avoids any negative secondary effects of both chemotherapy and radiation therapy from the majority of patients who will never need any treatment.

C. Lawton, MD

7 Gynecology

Ovarian

A Multicenter, Randomized, Phase 2 Clinical Trial to Evaluate the Efficacy and Safety of Combination Docetaxel and Carboplatin and Sequential Therapy With Docetaxel Then Carboplatin in Patients With Recurrent Platinum-Sensitive Ovarian Cancer

Secord AA, Berchuck A, Higgins RV, et al (Duke Univ Med Ctr, Durham, NC; Carolinas Med Ctr, Charlotte, NC; et al)

Cancer 118:3283-3293, 2012

Background.- The aim of this randomized clinical trial was to evaluate the efficacy and safety of combination (cDC) and sequential (sDC) weekly docetaxel and carboplatin in women with recurrent platinum-sensitive epithelial ovarian cancer (EOC).

Methods.—Participants were randomized to either weekly docetaxel 30 mg/m^2 on days 1 and 8 and carboplatin area under the curve (AUC) = 6 on day 1, every 3 weeks or docetaxel 30 mg/m^2 on days 1 and 8, every 3 weeks for 6 cycles followed by carboplatin AUC = 6 on day 1, every 3 weeks for 6 cycles or until disease progression. The primary endpoint was measurable progression-free survival (PFS).

Results.—Between January 2004 and March 2007, 150 participants were enrolled. The response rate was 55.4% and 43.2% for those treated with cDC and sDC, respectively. The median PFS was 13.7 months (95% confidence interval [CI], 9.9-16.8) for cDC and 8.4 months (95% CI, 7.1-11.0) for sDC. On the basis of an exploratory analysis, patients treated with sDC were at a 62% increased risk of disease progression compared to those treated with cDC (hazard ratio = 1.62; 95% CI, 1.08-2.45; P = .02). The median overall survival time was similar in both groups (33.2 and 30.1 months, P = .2). The incidence of grade 2 or 3 neurotoxicity and grade 3 or 4 neutropenia was higher with cDC than with sDC (11.7% vs 8.5%; 36.8% vs 11.3%). The sDC group demonstrated significant improvements in the Functional Assessment for Cancer Therapy-Ovarian, Quality of Life Trial Outcome Index scores compared with the combination cohort (P = .013).

Conclusions.—Both cDC and sDC regimens have activity in recurrent platinum-sensitive EOC with acceptable toxicity profiles. The cDC regimen may provide a PFS advantage over sDC.

▶ There are many who believe that sequential use of single agents as initial chemotherapy in ovarian carcinoma would yield results similar to those with combination chemotherapy with less toxicity. This belief is based on 2 facts. First, the Gynecologic Oncology Group (GOG) randomly assigned patients with advanced ovarian carcinoma to cisplatin, paclitaxel, or concurrent paclitaxel/cisplatin in GOG 132 and found no difference among the 3 arms after the group had shown a clear advantage for paclitaxel/cisplatin over cyclophosphamide/cisplatin in GOG 111. It turned out that patients on GOG 132 assigned to the single-agent regimens immediately got the opposite agent upon completion of their assigned regimen before progression had taken place in many instances. The study was thus effectively sequential versus concurrent therapy. Secondly, data from breast cancer suggest that sequential single-agent therapy is as good as combination chemotherapy. This article is the first attempt actually to randomly assign patients to either concurrent or sequential therapy with docetaxel and carboplatin. Although the study is a randomized phase II and thus underpowered for definitive answers, the data strongly suggest an advantage for the concurrent administration of the agents (combination chemotherapy, if you will). Based on these data, the current standard of care should remain surgery followed by combination chemotherapy consisting of paclitaxel plus carboplatin.

J. T. Thigpen, MD

A Phase 3 Trial of Bevacizumab in Ovarian Cancer

Perren TJ, for the ICON7 Investigators (St James's Univ Hosp, Leeds, UK; et al)

N Engl J Med 365:2484-2496, 2011

Background.—Angiogenesis plays a role in the biology of ovarian cancer. We examined the effect of bevacizumab, the vascular endothelial growth factor inhibitor, on survival in women with this disease.

Methods.—We randomly assigned women with ovarian cancer to carboplatin (area under the curve, 5 or 6) and paclitaxel (175 mg per square meter of body-surface area), given every 3 weeks for 6 cycles, or to this regimen plus bevacizumab (7.5 mg per kilogram of body weight), given concurrently every 3 weeks for 5 or 6 cycles and continued for 12 additional cycles or until progression of disease. Outcome measures included progression-free survival, first analyzed per protocol and then updated, and interim overall survival.

Results.—A total of 1528 women from 11 countries were randomly assigned to one of the two treatment regimens. Their median age was 57 years; 90% had epithelial ovarian cancer, 69% had a serous histologic type, 9% had high-risk early-stage disease, 30% were at high risk for progression, and 70% had stage IIIC or IV ovarian cancer. Progression-free survival (restricted mean) at 36 months was 20.3 months with standard therapy, as compared with 21.8 months with standard therapy plus bevacizumab (hazard ratio for progression or death with bevacizumab added, 0.81; 95% confidence interval, 0.70 to 0.94; $P = 0.004$ by the log-rank test). Nonproportional hazards were detected (i.e., the treatment effect was not consistent over time on the hazard function scale) ($P < 0.001$), with a maximum effect at 12 months, coinciding with the end of planned bevacizumab treatment and diminishing by 24 months. Bevacizumab was associated with more toxic effects (most often hypertension of grade 2 or higher) (18%, vs. 2% with chemotherapy alone). In the updated analyses, progression-free survival (restricted mean) at 42 months was 22.4 months without bevacizumab versus 24.1 months with bevacizumab ($P = 0.04$ by log-rank test); in patients at high risk for progression, the benefit was greater with bevacizumab than without it, with progression-free survival (restricted mean) at 42 months of 14.5 months with standard therapy alone and 18.1 months with bevacizumab added, with respective median overall survival of 28.8 and 36.6 months.

Conclusions.—Bevacizumab improved progression-free survival in women with ovarian cancer. The benefits with respect to both progression-free and overall survival were greater among those at high risk for disease progression. (Funded by Roche and others; ICON7 Controlled-Trials.com number, ISRCTN91273375.)

▶ This article presents the results of the second phase III trial of the addition of bevacizumab to paclitaxel/carboplatin in the treatment of patients with newly diagnosed advanced ovarian carcinoma (ICON 7). The study was designed as a 2-arm randomized phase III study: paclitaxel/carboplatin followed by no maintenance versus paclitaxel/carboplatin/bevacizumab followed by bevacizumab maintenance out to12 months. The trial involved more than 1500 patients and found a statistically significant superior progression-free survival (PFS) with the paclitaxel/carboplatin/bevacizumab followed by bevacizumab maintenance with a hazard ratio of 0.87. No difference in overall survival was observed, but this is not surprising when one considers that patients, upon progression, are treated with up to 8 additional lines of therapy chosen from among the more than 20 additional active agents in ovarian carcinoma. The only significantly increased adverse effects were hypertension and proteinuria. This trial is 1 of 2 large phase III studies evaluating bevacizumab added to chemotherapy in newly diagnosed advanced ovarian carcinoma. The major differences between the 2 studies were: inclusion of patients with stages I–II disease in this trial (ICON 7) and no blinding or placebo control in this study, and a lower dose of bevacizumab in this trial (7.5 mg/kg every 3 weeks in ICON 7 vs 15 mg/kg every 3 weeks in GOG 218). The results across these 2 trials are in addition to a third trial in platinum-sensitive recurrent disease (OCEANS) and a fourth trial in platinum-resistant recurrent disease (Aurelia). More than 4000 patients thus demonstrate the consistent improvement in PFS with the addition of bevacizumab to standard chemotherapy for ovarian carcinoma.

J. T. Thigpen, MD

A systematic review evaluating the relationship between progression free survival and post progression survival in advanced ovarian cancer

Sundar S, Wu J, Hillaby K, et al (City Hosp, UK; Univ of Birmingham, UK)

Gynecol Oncol 125:493-499, 2012

Objective.—Although overall survival is the ultimate goal of cancer therapy, many clinical and health economic decisions are taken when only progression free survival (PFS) data are available. This study evaluates the relationship between PFS and post progression survival (i.e. the time between disease progression and death) to estimate how many months a new drug for ovarian cancer might add to overall survival if the number of months the drug added to PFS (relative to a standard drug) was already known.

Methods.—A literature search was conducted over Medline for randomised controlled trials published between January 1990 and July 2010 that evaluated the effect of a drug treatment in comparison to alternative drug treatment in patients with either advanced stage primary or recurrent ovarian cancer. A systematic review of progression free and post progression survival (PPS) was performed. The relationship between PFS and PPS was evaluated by a graphical method and standard statistical tests.

Results.—Thirty-seven trials involving 15,850 patients met the inclusion criteria. The review found that increases in median PFS generally lead to little change in post-progression survival. Percentage gains in PFS are generally associated with no percentage gains or with very slight percentage gains or losses in post-progression survival.

Conclusion.—If the effect of a new drug treatment for ovarian cancer is to extend median PFS by x months, then it is reasonable to estimate that the treatment will also extend median overall survival by x months. This information will be useful for individual and collective decision making.

▶ The issue of endpoints in ovarian cancer has become an important and controversial issue over the past several years. The Food and Drug Administration (FDA) has generally taken the position that only overall survival (OS) will suffice as a regulatory endpoint in ovarian cancer for at least 2 stated reasons. First, they feel that progression-free survival (PFS) cannot be measured accurately because of the perceived difficulty in determining the point of progression. Second, they contend that PFS does not reflect patient benefit. This puts the FDA at odds with a number of other regulatory agencies worldwide that accept PFS as a valid regulatory endpoint. For ovarian cancers, this is a major problem. The patient with ovarian cancer has many options for further treatment upon progression, with the literature showing at least 22 agents with documented activity at least in phase II trials. In the United States, most patients receive multiple lines of additional therapy, including in many instances crossover to the experimental agent. This postprogression therapy blurs the survival endpoint and for practical purposes renders it uninterpretable. This study illustrates this with the observation that the changes in median PFS led to little change in postprogression survival. Prior to 1990, 13 of 15 phase III trials showed a clear correlation between PFS and OS with similar hazard ratios for both PFS and OS (see FDA website, 2006 endpoints in ovarian cancer conference). Given that very few options were available for the patient with progression of disease in that era, it seems clear that, in the absence of effective postprogression therapy, PFS and OS correlate. Furthermore, in 4 recent trials of bevacizumab added to chemotherapy (total patients over 4000), a very consistent PFS benefit is observed and suggests that PFS can be consistently and accurately measured. These facts argue for PFS as a valid regulatory endpoint and as an indicator of patient benefit.

J. T. Thigpen, MD

CA-125 can be part of the tumour evaluation criteria in ovarian cancer trials: experience of the GCIG CALYPSO trial

Alexandre J, Brown C, Coeffic D, et al (Université Paris Descartes, France; NHMRC Clinical Trials Centre, Sydney, Australia; Hôpital des Diaconesses, Paris, France; et al)

Br J Cancer 106:633-637, 2012

Background.—CA-125 as a tumour progression criterion in relapsing ovarian cancer (ROC) trials remains controversial. CALYPSO is a large randomised trial incorporating CA-125 (GCIG criteria) and symptomatic deterioration in addition to Response Evaluation Criteria in Solid Tumours (RECIST) criteria (radiological) to determine progression.

Methods.—In all, 976 patients with platinum-sensitive ROC were randomised to carboplatin–paclitaxel (C-P) or carboplatin-pegylated liposomal doxorubicin (C-PLD). CT-scan and CA-125 were performed every 3 months until progression.

Results.—In all, 832 patients (85%) progressed, with 60% experiencing a first radiological progression, 10% symptomatic progression, and 28% CA-125 progression without evidence of radiological or symptomatic progression. The benefit of C-PLD *vs* C-P in progression-free survival was not influenced by type of first progression (hazard ratio 0.85 (95% confidence interval (CI): 0.66–1.10) and 0.84 (95% CI: 0.72–0.98) for CA-125 and RECIST, respectively). In patients with CA-125 first progression who subsequently progressed radiologically, a delay of 2.3 months was observed between the two progression types. After CA-125 first progression, median time to new treatment was 2.0 months. In all, 81% of the patients with CA-125 or radiological first progression and 60% with symptomatic first progression received subsequent treatment.

Conclusion.—CA-125 and radiological tests performed similarly in determining progression with C-PLD or C-P. Additional follow-up with CA-125 measurements was not associated with overtreatment.

▶ The CALYPSO trial was a Gynecologic Cancer Intergroup study that randomized patients with platinum-sensitive recurrent ovarian carcinoma to treatment with carboplatin plus either paclitaxel or pegylated liposomal doxorubicin

(PLD). The final results of the study showed a small advantage for the PLD-containing regimen in terms of progression-free survival and no difference in overall survival. Because of the controversy over whether progression-free survival can be measured accurately in ovarian carcinoma, the investigators in this article look at determination of progression by scan as opposed to cancer antigen-125 (CA-125). The data suggest that both methods can accurately determine the onset of progression and that use of CA-125 as a criterion does not lead to overtreatment of the patients. As has been reported before, they also observed that CA-125 can determine the onset of progression a median of 2.3 months earlier in about 30% of the patients. This study is part of a growing body of evidence suggesting that progression-free survival can be an accurate endpoint for ovarian carcinoma trials and that CA-125 is a reliable marker of progression and thus can be a part of the approach to determining onset of progression.

J. T. Thigpen, MD

Evolution of surgical treatment paradigms for advanced-stage ovarian cancer: Redefining 'optimal' residual disease

Chang S-J, Bristow RE (Ajou Univ School of Medicine, Suwon, Republic of Korea; Univ of California, Orange)

Gynecol Oncol 125:483-492, 2012

Over the past 40 years, the survival of patients with advanced ovarian cancer has greatly improved due to the introduction of combination chemotherapy with platinum and paclitaxel as standard front-line treatment and the progressive incorporation of increasing degrees of maximal cytoreductive surgery. The designation of "optimal" surgical cytoreduction has evolved from residual disease ≤1 cm to no gross residual disease. There is a growing body of evidence that patients with no gross residual disease have better survival than those with optimal but visible residual disease. In order to achieve this, more radical cytoreductive procedures such as radical pelvic resection and extensive upper abdominal procedures are increasingly performed. However, some investigators still suggest that tumor biology is a major determinant in survival and that optimal surgery cannot fully compensate for tumor biology. The aim of this review is to outline the theoretical rationale and historical evolution of primary cytoreductive surgery, to re-evaluate the preferred surgical objective and procedures commonly required to achieve optimal cytoreduction in the platinum/taxane era based on contemporary evidence, and to redefine the concept of "optimal" residual disease within the context of future surgical developments and analysis of treatment outcomes.

▶ This is an excellent review of surgical studies that have led to the conclusion that surgical bulk reduction improves outcome in ovarian cancer. The review provides a solid rationale for evolving our understanding of what constitutes appropriate goals for bulk reduction. The authors present evidence that those patients who do best with surgical bulk reduction are those in whom all gross disease can be resected. Based on this, they suggest replacing the old terminology of optimal cytoreduction (defined in the literature initially as no residual disease greater than 2 cm diameter, then later as 1 cm) and suboptimal cytoreduction (> 2 cm disease remaining) with a newer classification with 3 categories (no gross residual, gross residual [GR] less than 1 cm or GR-1, and bulky gross residual or GR-B). These considerations were also discussed at the Fourth Ovarian Cancer Consensus Conference in Vancouver, Canada, by the Gynecologic Cancer InterGroup member groups with strong support for such a new classification. If accepted generally by the practicing community, this new understanding would mean the performance of more aggressive surgery to achieve no gross residual disease status. Such aggressive surgery is already done routinely in the United States by well-trained gynecologic oncologists, but such an understanding would represent for much of the rest of the world a relatively substantial departure from current practice. The article is well worth reading for a complete understanding of the problem.

J. T. Thigpen, MD

Final overall survival results of phase III GCIG CALYPSO trial of pegylated liposomal doxorubicin and carboplatin *vs* paclitaxel and carboplatin in platinum-sensitive ovarian cancer patients

Wagner U, Marth C, Largillier R, et al (Univ Hosp of Gießen and Marburg, Germany; Med Univ Innsbruck, Austria; Centre Azuréen de Cancérologie, Mougins, France; et al)

Br J Cancer 1-4, 2012

Background.—The CALYPSO phase III trial compared CD (carboplatin-pegylated liposomal doxorubicin (PLD)) with CP (carboplatin-paclitaxel) in patients with platinum-sensitive recurrent ovarian cancer (ROC). Overall survival (OS) data are now mature.

Methods.—Women with ROC relapsing > 6 months after first- or second-line therapy were randomised to CD or CP for six cycles in this international, open-label, non-inferiority trial. The primary endpoint was progression-free survival. The OS analysis is presented here.

Results.—A total of 976 patients were randomised (467 to CD and 509 to CP). With a median follow-up of 49 months, no statistically significant difference was observed between arms in OS (hazard ratio = 0.99 (95% confidence interval 0.85, 1.16); log-rank $P = 0.94$). Median survival times were 30.7 months (CD) and 33.0 months (CP). No statistically significant difference in OS was observed between arms in predetermined subgroups according to age, body mass index, treatment-free interval, measurable disease, number of lines of prior chemotherapy, or performance status. Post-study cross-over was imbalanced between arms, with a greater proportion of patients randomised to CP receiving post-study PLD (68%) than patients randomised to CD receiving post-study paclitaxel (43%; $P < 0.001$).

Conclusion.—Carboplatin-PLD led to delayed progression and similar OS compared with carboplatin-paclitaxel in platinum-sensitive ROC.

▶ Two previously reported phase III trials have established the value of carboplatin-based doublets over single-agent carboplatin for platinum-sensitive recurrent ovarian carcinoma: ICON4 (carboplatin paclitaxel) and AGO-OVAR2.5 (carboplatin gemcitabine). This study randomized patients with platinum-sensitive recurrent ovarian carcinoma to either paclitaxel/carboplatin or pegylated liposomal doxorubicin (PLD)/carboplatin. The study was conducted by the Gynecologic Cancer Intergroup and involved over 900 patients. The PLD-containing regimen demonstrated a superior progression-free survival in an earlier report. This article presents the overall survival data, which show no difference between the 2 regimens. The bottom line of this study is that oncologists can now choose any of the 3 carboplatin-based doublets as systemic therapy for the patient with platinum-sensitive recurrent ovarian carcinoma and be well within the standard of care. Given the small advantage of PLD/carboplatin in terms of progression-free survival, one could even argue that PLD/carboplatin would be preferred over paclitaxel/carboplatin; thus the choice becomes either PLD/carboplatin or gemcitabine/carboplatin based on available evidence.

J. T. Thigpen, MD

Incorporation of Bevacizumab in the Primary Treatment of Ovarian Cancer

Burger RA, for the Gynecologic Oncology Group (Fox Chase Cancer Ctr, Philadelphia, PA; et al)

N Engl J Med 365:2473-2483, 2011

Background.—Vascular endothelial growth factor is a key promoter of angiogenesis and disease progression in epithelial ovarian cancer. Bevacizumab, a humanized anti–vascular endothelial growth factor monoclonal antibody, has shown single-agent activity in women with recurrent tumors. Thus, we aimed to evaluate the addition of bevacizumab to standard front-line therapy.

Methods.—In our double-blind, placebo-controlled, phase 3 trial, we randomly assigned eligible patients with newly diagnosed stage III (incompletely resectable) or stage IV epithelial ovarian cancer who had undergone debulking surgery to receive one of three treatments. All three included chemotherapy consisting of intravenous paclitaxel at a dose of 175 mg per square meter of body-surface area, plus carboplatin at an area under the curve of 6, for cycles 1 through 6, plus a study treatment for cycles 2 through 22, each cycle of 3 weeks' duration. The control treatment was chemotherapy with placebo added in cycles 2 through 22; bevacizumab-initiation treatment was chemotherapy with bevacizumab (15 mg per kilogram of body weight) added in cycles 2 through 6 and placebo added in cycles 7 through 22. Bevacizumab-throughout treatment was chemotherapy with bevacizumab added in cycles 2 through 22. The primary end point was progression-free survival.

Results.—Overall, 1873 women were enrolled. The median progression-free survival was 10.3 months in the control group, 11.2 in the bevacizumab-initiation group, and 14.1 in the bevacizumab-throughout group. Relative to control treatment, the hazard ratio for progression or death was 0.908 (95% confidence interval [CI], 0.795 to 1.040; $P = 0.16$) with bevacizumab initiation and 0.717 (95% CI, 0.625 to 0.824; $P < 0.001$) with bevacizumab throughout. At the time of analysis, 76.3% of patients were alive, with no significant differences in overall survival among the three groups. The rate of hypertension requiring medical therapy was higher in the bevacizumab-initiation group (16.5%) and the bevacizumab-throughout group (22.9%) than in the control group (7.2%). Gastrointestinal-wall disruption requiring medical intervention occurred in 1.2%, 2.8%, and 2.6% of patients in the control group, the bevacizumab-initiation group, and the bevacizumab-throughout group, respectively.

Conclusions.—The use of bevacizumab during and up to 10 months after carboplatin and paclitaxel chemotherapy prolongs the median progression-free survival by about 4 months in patients with advanced epithelial ovarian cancer. (Funded by the National Cancer Institute and Genentech; ClinicalTrials.gov number, NCT00262847.)

▶ This article presents the results of the first phase III trial of the addition of bevacizumab to paclitaxel/carboplatin in the treatment of patients with newly diagnosed advanced ovarian carcinoma (GOG 218). The study was designed as a blinded placebo-controlled trial with 3 arms: paclitaxel/carboplatin/placebo followed by placebo maintenance out to 15 months, paclitaxel/carboplatin/bevacizumab followed by placebo maintenance out to15 months, or paclitaxel/carboplatin/bevacizumab followed by bevacizumab maintenance out to15 months. The trial involved more than 1800 patients and showed a statistically significant superior progression-free survival (PFS) with the paclitaxel/carboplatin/bevacizumab followed by bevacizumab maintenance with a hazard ratio of 0.71. No difference in overall survival was observed, but this is not surprising when one considers that patients, upon progression, are treated with up to 8 additional lines of therapy chosen from among the more than 20 additional active agents in ovarian carcinoma. The only significantly increased adverse effects were hypertension and proteinuria. This trial is 1 of 2 large phase III studies evaluating bevacizumab added to chemotherapy in newly diagnosed advanced ovarian carcinoma. The major differences between the 2 studies were inclusion of patients with stages I–II disease in the other trial (ICON 7) and no blinding or placebo control in ICON 7, and a lower dose of bevacizumab in ICON 7 (7.5 mg/kg every 3 weeks in ICON 7 vs 15 mg/kg every 3 weeks in GOG 218). The results across these 2 trials are in addition to a third trial in platinum-sensitive recurrent disease (OCEANS) and a fourth trial in platinum-resistant recurrent disease (Aurelia). More than 4000 patients thus show the consistent improvement in PFS with the addition of bevacizumab to standard chemotherapy for ovarian carcinoma.

J. T. Thigpen, MD

Is comprehensive surgical staging needed for thorough evaluation of early-stage ovarian carcinoma?

Garcia-Soto AE, Boren T, Wingo SN, et al (Univ of Texas Southwestern Med Ctr, Dallas)

Am J Obstet Gynecol 206:242.e1-242.e5, 2012

Objective.—Patients with ovarian cancer may have occult metastasis at the time of surgery. Our purpose was to determine the prevalence and sites of occult metastasis in epithelial ovarian cancer grossly confined to the ovary and examine the significance of routine omentectomy and peritoneal biopsies as part of a comprehensive staging procedure.

Study Design.—Data were retrospectively abstracted from patients presenting to University of Texas Southwestern Medical Center Hospitals from 1993 through 2009 with ovarian cancer without gross spread beyond the ovary who underwent comprehensive surgical staging.

Results.—A total of 86 patients with ovarian cancer grossly confined to the ovary who underwent complete surgical staging were identified. Of patients, 29% were upstaged following comprehensive surgical staging; 6% had metastatic disease in uterus and/or fallopian tubes, 6% in lymph nodes, and 17% in peritoneal, omental, or adhesion biopsies.

Conclusion.—Patients with epithelial ovarian cancer should continue to undergo comprehensive surgical staging, since it identifies occult metastasis in a significant number of patients.

▶ Limited stage (stages I to IIA) ovarian carcinoma accounts for only about 20% of epithelial carcinomas in the United States. From earlier trials, we have learned that these patients can be divided into 2 major groups: the first group at low risk for recurrence after surgery only (~10% recurrence and death rate) and the other at high risk for recurrence and death after surgery only (~40% recurrence rate if no further therapy is given). The recurrence rate in the high-risk group can be substantially reduced with adjuvant platinum-based chemotherapy. Therefore, identifying those at high risk and those with more advanced disease than suspected clinically through careful surgical staging becomes important to appropriate clinical decision making if the rate at which additional factors are discovered is sufficiently high.

This article looks at the frequency with which patients are upstaged with comprehensive surgical staging. Among 86 patients with apparently early disease, comprehensive surgical staging revealed more advanced disease than suspected in 29, a frequency high enough to justify comprehensive surgical staging as the standard approach for such patients.

J. T. Thigpen, MD

OCEANS: A Randomized, Double-Blind, Placebo-Controlled Phase III Trial of Chemotherapy With or Without Bevacizumab in Patients With Platinum-Sensitive Recurrent Epithelial Ovarian, Primary Peritoneal, or Fallopian Tube Cancer

Aghajanian C, Blank SV, Goff BA, et al (Memorial Sloan-Kettering Cancer Ctr and Weill Cornell Med College, NY; New York Univ School of Medicine; Univ of Washington School of Medicine, Seattle; et al)

J Clin Oncol 30:2039-2045, 2012

Purpose.—This randomized, multicenter, blinded, placebo-controlled phase III trial tested the efficacy and safety of bevacizumab (BV) with gemcitabine and carboplatin (GC) compared with GC in platinum-sensitive recurrent ovarian, primary peritoneal, or fallopian tube cancer (ROC).

Patients and Methods.—Patients with platinum-sensitive ROC (recurrence ≥ 6 months after front-line platinum-based therapy) and measurable disease were randomly assigned to GC plus either BV or placebo (PL) for six to 10 cycles. BV or PL, respectively, was then continued until disease progression. The primary end point was progression-free survival (PFS) by RECIST; secondary end points were objective response rate, duration of response (DOR), overall survival, and safety.

Results.—Overall, 484 patients were randomly assigned. PFS for the BV arm was superior to that for the PL arm (hazard ratio [HR], 0.484; 95% CI, 0.388 to 0.605; log-rank $P < .0001$); median PFS was 12.4 *v* 8.4 months, respectively. The objective response rate (78.5% *v* 57.4%; $P < .0001$) and DOR (10.4 *v* 7.4 months; HR, 0.534; 95% CI, 0.408 to 0.698) were significantly improved with the addition of BV. No new safety concerns were noted. Grade 3 or higher hypertension (17.4% *v* <1%) and proteinuria (8.5% *v* <1%) occurred more frequently in the BV arm. The rates of neutropenia and febrile neutropenia were similar in both arms. Two patients in the BV arm experienced GI perforation after study treatment discontinuation.

Conclusion.—GC plus BV followed by BV until progression resulted in a statistically significant improvement in PFS compared with GC plus PL in platinum-sensitive ROC.

► This article reports the results of a third phase III randomized trial evaluating bevacizumab in combination with chemotherapy in ovarian carcinoma. This study randomized patients with platinum-sensitive recurrent ovarian carcinoma to gemcitabine/carboplatin bevacizumab for 6 cycles followed by bevacizumab maintenance in the regimen containing bevacizumab. The primary endpoint of the trial was progression-free survival. Just as in the 2 frontline trials (Gynecologic Oncology Group study GOG218 and Gynecologic Cancer InterGroup study ICON7), the results show that the addition of bevacizumab followed by bevacizumab maintenance achieved a statistically significantly improved progression-free survival (hazard ratio = 0.484). This result is absolutely consistent with the results of the 2 frontline trials, which each showed an improved progression-free survival. None of the 3 trials show, as of yet, any improvement in overall survival. This is not surprising when one considers the large number of additional lines of therapy these patients receive when they relapse. In 2012 the American Society of Clinical Oncology initiated a fourth trial (Aurelia), this one in the platinum-resistant setting, also showing exactly the same thing: an improved progression-free survival with the addition of bevacizumab in the absence of an improved overall survival. We thus have 4 studies involving a total of over 4200 patients with ovarian carcinoma showing a consistent clinical benefit in the form of an improved progression-free survival with chemo/bevacizumab followed by maintenance bevacizumab. These data should be consistent to prompt the inclusion of bevacizumab in the treatment of these patients.

J. T. Thigpen, MD

Olaparib Maintenance Therapy in Platinum-Sensitive Relapsed Ovarian Cancer

Ledermann J, Harter P, Gourley C, et al (Univ College London, UK; Kliniken Essen Mitte, Germany; Univ of Edinburgh Cancer Res U.K. Centre; et al)

N Engl J Med 366:1382-1392, 2012

Background.—Olaparib (AZD2281) is an oral poly(adenosine diphosphate [ADP]–ribose) polymerase inhibitor that has shown antitumor activity in patients with high-grade serous ovarian cancer with or without *BRCA1* or *BRCA2* germline mutations.

Methods.—We conducted a randomized, double-blind, placebo-controlled, phase 2 study to evaluate maintenance treatment with olaparib in patients with platinum-sensitive, relapsed, high-grade serous ovarian cancer who had received two or more platinum-based regimens and had had a partial or complete response to their most recent platinum-based regimen. Patients were randomly assigned to receive olaparib, at a dose of 400 mg twice daily, or placebo. The primary end point was progression-free survival according to the Response Evaluation Criteria in Solid Tumors guidelines.

Results.—Of 265 patients who underwent randomization, 136 were assigned to the olaparib group and 129 to the placebo group. Progression-free survival was significantly longer with olaparib than with placebo (median, 8.4 months vs. 4.8 months from randomization on completion of chemotherapy; hazard ratio for progression or death, 0.35; 95% confidence interval [CI], 0.25 to 0.49; $P < 0.001$). Subgroup analyses of progression-free survival showed that, regardless of subgroup, patients in the olaparib group had a lower risk of progression. Adverse events more commonly reported in the olaparib group than in the placebo group (by more than 10% of patients) were nausea (68% vs. 35%), fatigue (49% vs. 38%), vomiting (32% vs. 14%), and anemia (17% vs. 5%); the majority of adverse events were grade 1 or 2. An interim analysis of overall survival (38% maturity, meaning that 38% of the patients had died) showed no significant difference between groups (hazard ratio with olaparib, 0.94; 95% CI, 0.63 to 1.39; $P = 0.75$).

Conclusions.—Olaparib as maintenance treatment significantly improved progression-free survival among patients with platinum-sensitive, relapsed, high-grade serous ovarian cancer. Interim analysis showed no overall survival benefit. The toxicity profile of olaparib in this population was consistent with that in previous studies. (Funded by Astra-Zeneca; ClinicalTrials.gov number, NCT00753545.)

▶ Repair of DNA damage in cancer cells usually takes place through homologous recombinant repair mechanisms. When these mechanisms are deficient, an alternate DNA repair pathway known as the PARP pathway becomes an important part of the cell's ability to repair DNA damage. One such population of patients among those with ovarian carcinomas is the population with BRCA1 or BRCA2 mutations. At least in ovarian carcinoma, many investigators believe that other patients also have deficiencies in homologous recombinant DNA repair and depend to a varying degree on the PARP pathway for DNA repair. In such patients, use of inhibitors of the PARP pathway can potentially be a successful approach to treating these cancers. This study evaluated 1 such agent, olaparib, as a maintenance therapy for patients with at least stable disease at the conclusion of initial chemotherapy. The study was a randomized phase II trial involving 265 patients with high-grade serous carcinoma of the ovary randomly assigned to either placebo or olaparib 400 mg twice daily by mouth. No substantial differences in toxicity were observed between the 2 arms. The olaparib arm showed a marked improvement in progression-free survival, the primary endpoint, with a hazard ratio of 0.35. This study was followed by a trial in newly diagnosed advanced ovarian carcinoma patients randomized to either paclitaxel/carboplatin for 6 cycles or paclitaxel/carboplatin/olaparib followed by olaparib maintenance, which showed a similar advantage for the patients receiving the olaparib. Again there was no substantial increase in toxicity with the addition of the olaparib. These data will need to be confirmed in a phase III trial, but the PARP inhibitors appear to be promising in ovarian carcinoma at least as maintenance agents.

J. T. Thigpen, MD

Ovarian low-grade serous carcinoma: A comprehensive update

Diaz-Padilla I, Malpica AL, Minig L, et al (Univ of Toronto, Ontario, Canada; The Univ of Texas M.D. Anderson Cancer Ctr, Houston; Hosp Universitario Madrid, Spain; et al)

Gynecol Oncol 126:279-285, 2012

Ovarian low-grade serous ovarian carcinoma (OvLGSCa) comprises a minority within the heterogeneous group of ovarian carcinomas. Despite biological differences with their high-grade serous counterparts, current treatment guidelines do not distinguish between these two entities. OvLGSCas are characterized by an indolent clinical course. They usually develop from serous tumors of low malignant potential, although they can also arise *de novo*. When compared with patients with ovarian high grade serous carcinoma (OvHGSCa) patients with OvLGSCa are younger and have better survival outcomes. Current clinical and treatment data available for OvLGSCa come from retrospective studies, suggesting that optimal cytoreductive surgery remains the cornerstone in treatment, whereas chemotherapy has a limited role. Molecular studies have revealed the preponderance of the RAS–RAF–MAPK signaling pathway in the pathogenesis of OvLGSCa, thereby representing an attractive therapeutic target for patients affected by this disease. Improved clinical trial designs and international collaboration are required to optimally address the unmet medical treatment needs of patients affected by this disease.

▶ This article is a further discussion of the now-in-place 2-tiered system for grading serous carcinomas of the ovary. The authors discuss the molecular difference between the 2 categories of serous carcinomas as a basis for future trials with targeted agents, particularly in the low-grade group of cancers for which there are few systemic therapeutic options that appear to be effective. Some of these trials are already under way within the Gynecologic Oncology Group and in intergroup settings in the Gynecologic Cancer Intergroup. Because the majority (> 80%) of ovarian cancers entered into Gynecologic Oncology Group trials are high-grade serous carcinomas, there should be sufficient numbers of patients available for study to permit continued phase III trials evaluating the standard of care for these more common lesions. The studies of low-grade serous carcinomas will of necessity be primarily phase II studies because this population of patients is too small to permit phase III trials, but will serve as a basis for a more rational approach to the management of these cancers than simply lumping them in with the high-grade serous cancers.

J. T. Thigpen, MD

Phase II, Open-Label, Randomized, Multicenter Study Comparing the Efficacy and Safety of Olaparib, a Poly (ADP-Ribose) Polymerase Inhibitor, and Pegylated Liposomal Doxorubicin in Patients With *BRCA1* or *BRCA2* Mutations and Recurrent Ovarian Cancer

Kaye SB, Lubinski J, Matulonis U, et al (The Royal Marsden Natl Health Service Foundation Trust and The Inst of Cancer Res, Sutton, Surrey, UK; International Hereditary Cancer Ctr, Szczecin, Poland; Dana-Farber Cancer Inst, Boston, MA; et al)

J Clin Oncol 30:372-379, 2012

Purpose.—Olaparib (AZD2281), an orally active poly (ADP-ribose) polymerase inhibitor that induces synthetic lethality in *BRCA1*- or *BRCA2*-deficient cells, has shown promising clinical efficacy in nonrandomized phase II trials in patients with ovarian cancer with *BRCA1* or *BRCA2* deficiency. We assessed the comparative efficacy and safety of olaparib and pegylated liposomal doxorubicin (PLD) in this patient population.

Patients and Methods.—In this multicenter, open-label, randomized, phase II study, patients with ovarian cancer that recurred within 12 months of prior platinum therapy and with confirmed germline *BRCA1* or *BRCA2* mutations were enrolled. Patients were assigned in a 1:1:1 ratio to olaparib 200 mg twice per day or 400 mg twice per day continuously or PLD 50 mg/m^2 intravenously every 28 days. The primary efficacy end point was Response Evaluation Criteria in Solid Tumors (RECIST)–assessed progression-free survival (PFS). Secondary end points included objective response rate (ORR) and safety.

Results.—Ninety-seven patients were randomly assigned. Median PFS was 6.5 months (95% CI, 5.5 to 10.1 months), 8.8 months (95% CI, 5.4 to 9.2 months), and 7.1 months (95% CI, 3.7 to 10.7 months) for the olaparib 200 mg, olaparib 400 mg, and PLD groups, respectively. There was no statistically significant difference in PFS (hazard ratio, 0.88; 95% CI, 0.51 to 1.56; P = .66) for combined olaparib doses versus PLD. RECIST-assessed ORRs were 25%, 31%, and 18% for olaparib 200 mg, olaparib 400 mg, and PLD, respectively; differences were not statistically significant. Tolerability of both treatments was as expected based on previous trials.

Conclusion.—The efficacy of olaparib was consistent with previous studies. However, the efficacy of PLD was greater than expected. Olaparib 400 mg twice per day is a suitable dose to explore in further studies in this patient population.

► Poly adenosine diphosphate ribose polymerase (PARP) inhibitors are agents that inhibit the activity of an alternate DNA repair pathway. When these agents are used in patients with ovarian cancers who are deficient in other mechanisms of DNA repair, there is evidence of efficacy in early observations. The classic group of patients with such deficiencies in DNA repair are those patients with *BRCA1* and *BRCA2* mutations. This phase II trial randomized such patients with recurrent ovarian carcinoma to either pegylated liposomal doxorubicin or 1 of 2 doses of the PARP inhibitor olaparib. The study shows efficacy for all 3 regimens with no significant difference among the 3 noted in terms of the primary endpoint, the Response Evaluation Criteria in Solid Tumors. Subsequent to the completion of this trial, olaparib had been assessed in randomized phase II trials as a maintenance therapy and as a regimen of chemotherapy with olaparib followed by olaparib maintenance in a mix of patients with *BRCA* mutations and those without such mutations. Both studies suggest that olaparib is effective and adds substantially to progression-free survival. This leaves 2 major questions unanswered: First, the efficacy of olaparib as a maintenance therapy needs to be validated in a phase III trial. Second, we need to better define the patient population that is most likely to benefit from PARP inhibition. As of yet, none of these agents have been approved for use in ovarian carcinoma

J. T. Thigpen, MD

Randomized, Double-Blind, Placebo-Controlled Phase II Study of AMG 386 Combined With Weekly Paclitaxel in Patients With Recurrent Ovarian Cancer

Karlan BY, Oza AM, Richardson GE, et al (Cedars-Sinai Med Ctr, Los Angeles, CA; Princess Margaret Hosp, Toronto, Ontario, Canada; Cabrini Hosp, Melbourne, Victoria, Australia; et al)

J Clin Oncol 30:362-371, 2012

Purpose.—To estimate the efficacy and toxicity of AMG 386, an investigational peptide-Fc fusion protein that neutralizes the interaction between the Tie2 receptor and angiopoietin-1/2, plus weekly paclitaxel in patients with recurrent ovarian cancer.

Patients and Methods.—Patients with recurrent epithelial ovarian, fallopian tube, or primary peritoneal cancer were randomly assigned 1:1:1 to receive paclitaxel (80 mg/m^2 once weekly [QW], 3 weeks on/1 week off) plus intravenous AMG 386 10 mg/kg QW (arm A), AMG 386 3 mg/kg QW (arm B), or placebo QW (arm C). The primary end point was progression-free survival (PFS). Secondary end points included overall survival, objective response, CA-125 response, safety, and pharmacokinetics.

Results.—One hundred sixty-one patients were randomly assigned. Median PFS was 7.2 months (95% CI, 5.3 to 8.1 months) in arm A, 5.7 months (95% CI, 4.6 to 8.0 months) in arm B, and 4.6 months (95% CI, 1.9 to 6.7 months) in arm C. The hazard ratio for arms A and B combined versus arm C was 0.76 (95% CI, 0.52 to 1.12; $P = .165$). Further analyses suggested an exploratory dose-response effect for PFS across arms (Tarone's test, $P = .037$). Objective response rates for arms A, B, and C were 37%, 19%, and 27%, respectively. The incidence of grade ≥3 adverse events (AEs) in arms A, B, and C was 65%, 55%, and 64%, respectively. Frequent AEs included hypertension (8%, 6%, and 5% in arms A, B, and C, respectively), peripheral edema (71%, 51%, and 22% in arms A, B, and C, respectively), and hypokalemia (21%, 15%, and 5% in arms A, B, and C, respectively). AMG 386 exhibited linear pharmacokinetic properties at the tested doses.

Conclusion.—AMG 386 combined with weekly paclitaxel was tolerable, with a manageable and distinct toxicity profile. The data suggest evidence of antitumor activity and a dose-response effect, warranting further studies in ovarian cancer.

▶ Ovarian carcinoma is characterized by genomic instability; therefore, the identification of drugable targets within the cancer cell itself has not been overly productive. The most promising efforts have focused on targeting the microenvironment, particularly in respect to angiogenesis. The agent under study in this article is a peptide-Fc fusion protein that neutralizes the interaction between the Tie2 receptor and angiopoietin-1/2 (an angiopoietin inhibitor). Dubbed AMG 386, this agent was tested in combination with weekly paclitaxel in a mix of platinum-sensitive and platinum-resistant patients with recurrent ovarian cancer and up to 3 prior chemotherapeutic regimens. The study was a randomized phase II assigning patients to either placebo or 1 of 2 dose levels of AMG 386. The results show definite trends toward improved progression-free survival, time to progression, and response rate with evidence of a dose-response relationship favoring the higher dose of AMG 386. These results have led to the activation of phase III trials in both recurrent and front-line settings combining AMG 386 with chemotherapy. The trial in the United States is GOG 3001, which randomizes newly diagnosed patients with advanced disease to paclitaxel/carboplatin AMG 386. The ultimate role of this agent in ovarian carcinoma will be determined by the outcome of these studies.

J. T. Thigpen, MD

Reclassification of Serous Ovarian Carcinoma by a 2-Tier System: A Gynecologic Oncology Group Study

Bodurka DC, Deavers MT, Tian C, et al (The Univ of Texas MD Anderson Cancer Ctr, Houston; Roswell Park Cancer Inst, Buffalo, NY; et al)
Cancer 118:3087-3094, 2012

Background.—A study was undertaken to use the 2-tier system to reclassify the grade of serous ovarian tumors previously classified using the International Federation of Gynecology and Obstetrics (FIGO) 3-tier system and determine the progression-free survival (PFS) and overall survival (OS) of patients treated on Gynecologic Oncology Group (GOG) Protocol 158.

Methods.—The authors retrospectively reviewed demographic, pathologic, and survival data of 290 patients with stage III serous ovarian carcinoma treated with surgery and chemotherapy on GOG Protocol 158, a cooperative multicenter group trial. A blinded pathology review was performed by a panel of 6 gynecologic pathologists to verify histology and regrade tumors using the 2-tier system. The association of tumor grade with PFS and OS was assessed.

Results.—Of 241 cases, both systems demonstrated substantial agreement when combining FIGO grades 2 and 3 (overall agreement, 95%; kappa statistic, 0.68). By using the 2-tier system, patients with low-grade versus high-grade tumors had significantly longer PFS (45.0 vs 19.8 months, respectively; $P = .01$). By using FIGO criteria, median PFS for patients with grade 1, 2, and 3 tumors was 37.5, 19.8, and 20.1 months, respectively ($P = .07$). There was no difference in clinical outcome in patients with grade 2 or 3 tumors in multivariate analysis. Woman with high grade versus low-grade tumors demonstrated significantly higher risk of death (hazard ratio, 2.43; 95% confidence interval, 1.17-5.04; $P = .02$).

Conclusions.—Women with high-grade versus low-grade serous carcinoma of the ovary are 2 distinct patient populations. Adoption of the 2-tier grading system provides a simple yet precise framework for predicting clinical outcomes.

► Serous ovarian carcinoma is by far the most common histology of epithelial ovarian carcinomas. These lesions account for more than 80% of patients entered into Gynecologic Oncology Group studies. The vast majority of these serous cancers are, under the current grading system, grade 2 or grade 3, with a small minority being classified as grade 1 lesions. The current report evaluates 241 cases of advanced stage serous carcinoma. Pertinent findings include the fact that only 6% were classified as grade 1, that these cases demonstrated a markedly superior progression-free survival, and that grade 2 and grade 3 cancers showed no difference in outcome. The investigators recommend that, based on these observations, patients with serous ovarian carcinomas be classified into a 2-tiered system of low-grade and high-grade cancers. Because the prognosis and the response to therapy differ substantially for the low-grade cancers, these should be studied in separate trials from the high-grade lesions. The Gynecologic Oncology Group has already acted on these recommendations and now pursues separate trials for the 2 groups.

J. T. Thigpen, MD

Vignette-Based Study of Ovarian Cancer Screening: Do U.S. Physicians Report Adhering to Evidence-Based Recommendations?

Baldwin L-M, Trivers KF, Matthews B, et al (Univ of Washington, Seattle; Ctrs for Disease Control and Prevention, Atlanta, GA; Dana-Farber Cancer Inst, Boston, MA)

Ann Intern Med 156:182-194, 2012

Background.—No professional society or group recommends routine ovarian cancer screening, yet physicians' enthusiasm for several cancer screening tests before benefit has been proven suggests that some women may be exposed to potential harms.

Objective.—To provide nationally representative estimates of physicians' reported nonadherence to recommendations against ovarian cancer screening.

Design.—Cross-sectional survey of physicians offering women's primary care. The 12-page questionnaire contained a woman's annual examination vignette and questions about offers or orders for transvaginal ultrasonography (TVU) and cancer antigen 125 (CA-125).

Setting.—United States.

Participants.—3200 physicians randomly sampled equally from the 2008 American Medical Association Physician Masterfile lists of family physicians, general internists, and obstetrician-gynecologists; 61.7% responded. After exclusions, 1088 respondents were included; their responses were weighted to represent the specialty distribution of practicing U.S. physicians nationally.

Measurements.—Reported nonadherence to screening recommendations (defined as sometimes or almost always ordering screening TVU or CA-125 or both).

Results.—Twenty-eight percent (95% CI, 24.5% to 32.9%) of physicians reported nonadherence to screening recommendations for women at low risk for ovarian cancer; 65.4% (CI, 61.1% to 69.4%) did so for women at medium risk for ovarian cancer. Six percent (CI, 4.4% to 8.9%) reported routinely ordering or offering ovarian cancer screening for low-risk women, as did 24.0% (CI, 20.5% to 28.0%) for medium-risk women ($P \leq 0.001$). Thirty-three percent believed TVU or CA-125 was an effective screening test. In adjusted analysis, actual and physician-perceived patient risk, patient request for ovarian cancer screening, and physician belief that TVU or CA-125 was an effective screening test were the strongest predictors of physician-reported nonadherence to published recommendations.

Limitation.—The results are limited by their reliance on survey methods; there may be respondent-nonrespondent bias.

Conclusion.—One in 3 physicians believed that ovarian cancer screening was effective, despite evidence to the contrary. Substantial proportions of physicians reported routinely offering or ordering ovarian cancer screening, thereby exposing women to the documented risks of these tests.

Primary Funding Source.—Centers for Disease Control and Prevention and the National Cancer Institute.

▶ Ovarian cancer is the most common cause of death among gynecologic cancers. Unlike the other 2 common gynecologic cancers, endometrial and cervical cancers, there is no effective screening test for ovarian cancer. Most recently, 2 large studies of serial cancer antigen-125 (CA-125) and transvaginal sonography as a screening approach were reported. The ovarian component of the PLCO trial in the United States showed a positive predictive value of only 1.3%. In the UK study, a positive predictive value of 36% was reported with the use of an algorithm to analyze CA-125 data (Risk of Ovarian Cancer Algorithm). Neither study, however, has shown a reduction in mortality from the disease as a result of screening. The purpose of a screening test is to reduce mortality from the screened-for disease process. The reason that it is important not to use these screening approaches until and unless mortality reduction is shown is that screening for ovarian cancer has an important adverse effect. If the screening test is positive, that patient in all likelihood will undergo a major invasive procedure (either laparoscopy or, more likely, laparotomy) to look for ovarian cancer. Most studies of ovarian cancer screening show ratios of laparotomies to ovarian cancers diagnosed as high as 20 or 40 to 1. The bottom line is that screening for ovarian cancer with currently available approaches is inappropriate because the tests have not been shown to be effective and can have a substantial adverse impact on the patient.

J. T. Thigpen, MD

Cervix

A multi-institutional phase II trial of paclitaxel and carboplatin in the treatment of advanced or recurrent cervical cancer

Kitagawa R, Katsumata N, Ando M, et al (NTT Med Ctr Tokyo, Japan; Nippon Med School Musashikosugi Hosp, Kanagawa, Japan; Natl Cancer Ctr Hosp, Tokyo, Japan; et al)

Gynecol Oncol 125:307-311, 2012

Objective.—The aim of this prospective trial was to evaluate the efficacy and safety of the combination of paclitaxel and carboplatin (TC) in patients with metastatic or recurrent cervical cancer.

Methods.—This was a multicenter phase II trial of 3 weekly paclitaxel 175 mg/m^2 3-hour iv day 1 followed by carboplatin AUC5 1-hour iv day 1 for maximum of 6 cycles until disease progression or prohibitive toxicity. Eligible patients had squamous or adenocarcinoma of the cervix with measurable stage IVB or recurrent, aged 20–75 years, Eastern Cooperative Oncology Group performance status 0–2, prior platinum-containing regimen 0–1, and no prior taxane. The primary endpoint was overall response rate (ORR) by RECIST.

Results.—41 patients were enrolled, of which 39 were evaluable for analysis. 33 patients (84.6%) received prior radiotherapy. The confirmed ORR was 59% (95% CI, 43% to 75%); 5 patients (13%) achieved a complete response and median response duration was 5.2 months. The response rates for patients who had adenocarcinoma (n = 10) and prior platinum-based chemotherapy <6 months (n = 7) were 40.0% and 0%, respectively. The median progression-free survival and overall survival times were 5.3 and 9.6 months, respectively. The most frequent grade 3 or 4 adverse events were neutropenia (79%), anemia (46%), thrombocytopenia (15%), and fatigue (8%). No treatment-related death was seen.

Conclusions.—TC seemed to be feasible and effective similar to other cisplatin-based doublets for the treatment of metastatic or recurrent cervical cancer. Phase III trial is warranted to establish the clinical benefits of this combination.

▶ Thirty years ago, as the activity of cisplatin in cervical cancer was becoming apparent, efforts were made to assess the less toxic platinum agent carboplatin. Trials showed, however, that carboplatin produced a consistently lower response rate (cisplatin 23% across 815 patients as opposed to carboplatin 15% across 177 patients). From that point forward, cisplatin was regarded as the preferred platinum agent in cervical carcinoma. Subsequent studies of the Gynecologic Oncology Group (GOG 110, GOG 169, and GOG 179) have established the superiority of doublets of cisplatin plus 1 other agent and the ultimate superiority of paclitaxel/cisplatin over other doublets (GOG 204). This study attempts to resurrect the possibility of using paclitaxel/carboplatin instead because of its greater ease of administration and fewer adverse effects. Although the study does show that the doublet is feasible, its phase II nature makes it impossible to determine whether the earlier observations about the superiority of cisplatin were in error. At the 2012 meeting of the American Society of Oncology, however, a randomized comparison of paclitaxel/cisplatin versus paclitaxel/carboplatin was presented. Involving 253 patients, the study reported that there was no overall difference between the 2 doublets. The caveat was, however, that in those patients without prior to exposure to cisplatin paclitaxel/cisplatin was statistically significantly superior in terms of overall survival. In those with prior exposure to cisplatin as a radiation sensitizer (the majority of US patients), there was no difference in the 2 regimens with actually a trend favoring carboplatin. The bottom line is that, for most patients, paclitaxel/carboplatin can be used. For those with no prior cisplatin, however, paclitaxel/cisplatin continues to be the preferred regimen.

J. T. Thigpen, MD

Chemoradiation and adjuvant chemotherapy in advanced cervical adenocarcinoma

Tang J, Tang Y, Yang J, et al (Hunan Provincial Tumor Hosp, Changsha, P.R. China)

Gynecol Oncol 125:297-302, 2012

Purpose.—The optimal treatment of women with advanced adenocarcinoma of uterine cervix is still undefined. We compared concurrent chemoradiation (CCRT) and adjuvant cisplatin-based chemotherapy with CCRT alone for advanced cervical adenocarcinoma in a randomized trial at the Hunan Provincial Tumor Hospital in China.

Methods.—From 1998 to 2007, 880 patients with clinical FIGO stages IIB–IVA cervical adenocarcinoma were randomized to receive either CCRT or chemoradiation with one cycle of neo-adjuvant chemotherapy with Paclitaxel (135 mg/m^2) + Cisplatin (75 mg/m^2) before receiving radiation and two cycles of consolidation chemotherapy with the same drugs after radiotherapy in 3-week intervals. The disease control and survival rates were calculated using the Kaplan–Meier method.

Results.—All patients completed the treatment plan. 340 patients have relapsed, with a median follow-up duration of 60 months. Patients who received chemoradiation with adjuvant chemotherapy showed a significantly longer disease-free ($P < .05$), cumulative survival ($P < .05$) and long-term local tumor control ($P < .05$). Patients who received CCRT alone had significantly more distant metastasis and pelvic failure than those who received chemoradiation with adjuvant chemotherapy ($P < .05$).

Conclusion.—Incorporating neo-adjuvant and consolidation chemotherapy with Paclitaxel and Cisplatin into concomitant chemoradiation is highly effective, safe and may be a very promising treatment protocol for advanced cervical adenocarcinoma.

▶ Based on 6 comparisons in 5 large phase III trials all reported at about the same time in 1999 as a part of a National Cancer Institute (NCI) Clinical Alert, the standard of care for patients with locally advanced (stages IB2-IVA) carcinoma of the cervix has been concurrent chemoradiation with the preferred regimen being weekly cisplatin plus radiation (survival hazard ratios range from 0.49 to 0.76 across these 6 comparisons favoring concurrent chemoradiation). Most of the patients in these trials had squamous cell carcinoma of the cervix, although most have assumed that adenocarcinomas would respond as well. This phase II study seeks to extend the concurrent chemoradiation with not only a combination radiation sensitizing regimen of paclitaxel/cisplatin but also neoadjuvant and adjuvant chemotherapy with the same 2 drugs before and after the completion of the concurrent chemoradiation. Although the investigators describe the results as promising, the precise assessment of this approach awaits a phase III trial, which is underway minus the neoadjuvant part of the regimen. This is an intergroup study known as the OUTBACK trial. For now, the standard of care remains weekly cisplatin plus radiation given concurrently.

J. T. Thigpen, MD

Comparison of treatment outcomes between squamous cell carcinoma and adenocarcinoma in locally advanced cervical cancer

Katanyoo K, Sanguanrungsirikul S, Manusirivithaya S (Navamindradhiraj Univ, Bangkok, Thailand; Chulalongkorn Univ, Bangkok, Thailand)

Gynecol Oncol 125:292-296, 2012

Objective.—To compare the treatment outcomes between squamous cell carcinoma (SCC) and adenocarcinoma (ACA) in locally advanced cervical cancer patients.

Methods.—All medical records of stages IIB–IVA of cervical cancer patients who had completed treatment between 1995 and 2008 were reviewed. ACA 1 case was matched for SCC 2 cases with clinical stage, tumor size, treatment modalities (radiation therapy (RT) vs concurrent chemoradiation (CCRT)). Treatment outcomes including response to RT/CCRT, time to complete response (CR), patterns of treatment failure and survival outcomes were analyzed.

Results.—A total of 423 patients with stages IIB–IVA (141 ACA: 282 SCC) were included. Most of the patients (about 60%) had stage IIB. The overall complete responses (CR) between ACA and SCC were 86.5% and 94.7%, respectively ($p = 0.004$). Median time to clinical CR from RT/CCRT of ACA were 2 months (0–5 months) compared with 1 month (0–4 months) for SCC ($p = 0.001$). Pelvic recurrence and distant failure were found in 2.1% and 14.9% in ACA, and corresponding with 3.9% and 15.6% in SCC. The 5-year overall survival rates of ACA compared to SCC were 59.9% and 61.7% ($p = 0.191$), respectively. When all prognostic factors are adjusted, clinical staging was the only factor that influenced overall survival.

Conclusion.—ACA in locally advanced cervical cancer had poorer response rate from treatment and also used longer time to achieve CR than SCC. However, these effects were not determinants of survival outcomes.

▶ Studies of the treatment of carcinoma of the cervix generally include mostly patients with squamous cell carcinoma because this is by far the most common cell type. Almost all of these studies do include approximately 15% of patients with other cell types, predominantly adenocarcinomas. Based on these studies, treatment recommendations generally do not distinguish different cell types. There has always been a concern that perhaps patients with something other than squamous cell carcinoma might not fare as well with the recommended treatment. This study examines outcomes of 423 patients (141 adenocarcinomas and 282 squamous cell carcinomas) to determine whether patients with adenocarcinomas are adversely affected by this approach. The data show that, as feared, patients with adenocarcinomas experienced lower response rates and longer times to complete response, but the overall survival of the 2 groups is essentially identical. Until sufficient numbers of patients can be accrued to allow studies of these cell types in separate trials, the practice of lumping these patients together seems to be reasonable based on overall survival results.

J. T. Thigpen, MD

Consensus guidelines for delineation of clinical target volume for intensity-modulated pelvic radiotherapy for the definitive treatment of cervix cancer

Lim K, for the Gyn IMRT Consortium (Univ Health Network, Toronto, Ontario, Canada; et al)

Int J Radiat Oncol Biol Phys 79:348-355, 2011

Purpose.—Accurate target definition is vitally important for definitive treatment of cervix cancer with intensity modulated radiotherapy (IMRT), yet a definition of clinical target volume (CTV) remains variable within the literature. The aim of this study was to develop a consensus CTV definition in preparation for a Phase 2 clinical trial being planned by the Radiation Therapy Oncology Group.

Methods and Materials.—A guidelines consensus working group meeting was convened in June 2008 for the purposes of developing target definition guidelines for IMRT for the intact cervix. A draft document of recommendations for CTV definition was created and used to aid in contouring a clinical case. The clinical case was then analyzed for consistency and clarity of target delineation using an expectation maximization algorithm for simultaneous truth and performance level estimation (STAPLE), with kappa statistics as a measure of agreement between participants.

Results.—Nineteen experts in gynecological radiation oncology generated contours on axial magnetic resonance images of the pelvis. Substantial STAPLE agreement sensitivity and specificity values were seen for gross tumor volume (GTV) delineation (0.84 and 0.96, respectively) with a kappa statistic of 0.68 ($p < 0.0001$). Agreement for delineation of cervix, uterus, vagina, and parametria was moderate.

Conclusions.—This report provides guidelines for CTV definition in the definitive cervix cancer setting for the purposes of IMRT, building on previously published guidelines for IMRT in the postoperative setting.

▶ Radiation therapy has been used to treat cervix cancer for decades. During that time, advances have occurred in both the external beam portion and for appropriate patients, the brachytherapy portion.

From an external beam perspective, the advances have allowed for increase conformality, which can decrease dose to surrounding normal tissues, and therefore, decrease toxicity. The challenge we as oncologists face as we increase conformality is the threat of missing microscopic disease that was previously treated with less conformal techniques.

To use Intensity Modulated Radiation Therapy (IMRT) for increased treatment conformality and yet avoid missing disease, gynecologic radiation oncology experts have developed these consensus guidelines. The approach using simultaneous truth and performance level estimation (STAPLE) has been used successfully in other disease sites to develop consensus volumes. These guidelines should be adhered to for IMRT treatment of cervix cancer unless there are clear patient- or tumor-specific indications to the contrary.

C. Lawton, MD

Management of recurrent cervical cancer: A review of the literature

Peiretti M, Zapardiel I, Zanagnolo V, et al (European Inst of Oncology, Milan, Italy; La Paz Univ Hosp, Madrid, Spain; et al)

Surg Oncol 21:e59-e66, 2012

Objective.—The aim of this narrative review is to update the current knowledge on the treatment of recurrent cervical cancer based on a literature review.

Material and Methods.—A web based search in Medline and CancerLit databases has been carried out on recurrent cervical cancer management and treatment. All relevant information has been collected and analyzed, prioritizing randomized clinical trials.

Results.—Cervical cancer still represents a significant problem for public health with an annual incidence of about half a million new cases worldwide. Percentages of pelvic recurrences fluctuate from 10% to 74% depending on different risk factors. Accordingly to the literature, it is suggested that chemoradiation treatment (containing cisplatin and/or taxanes) could represent the treatment of choice for locoregional recurrences of cervical cancer after radical surgery. Pelvic exenteration is usually indicated for selected cases of central recurrence of cervical cancer after primary or adjuvant radiation and chemotherapy with bladder and/or rectum infiltration neither extended to the pelvic side walls nor showing any signs of extrapelvic spread of disease. Laterally extended endopelvic resection (LEER) for the treatment of those patients with a locally advanced disease or with a recurrence affecting the pelvic wall has been described.

Conclusions.—The treatment of recurrences of cervical carcinoma consists of surgery, and of radiation and chemotherapy, or the combination of different modalities taking into consideration the type of primary therapy, the site of recurrence, the disease-free interval, the patient symptoms, performance status, and the degree to which any given treatment might be beneficial.

► Carcinoma of the cervix is the third most common gynecologic malignancy in the United States. In developed countries with widespread Pap smear screening programs, the frequency of deaths has declined remarkably since the 1950s. In less developed countries, however, this disease remains a major killer. This article reviews in detail the management of recurrent carcinoma of the cervix. In particular, the article reviews studies of systemic therapy for disseminated recurrence and points out that a taxane/platinum regimen appears to be the optimal regimen currently available for the treatment of the disease. More recent information suggests that paclitaxel/carboplatin is an acceptable regimen in those patients who have previously received cisplatin in the setting of concurrent chemoradiation for locally advanced disease, but in those patients who have not been previously exposed to cisplatin, it remains the platinum agent of choice to combine with a taxane. The article is worth reading in detail for the discussion of the role of surgery and radiation in patients with recurrent carcinoma of the cervix.

J. T. Thigpen, MD

Endometrial

Association of number of positive nodes and cervical stroma invasion with outcome of advanced endometrial cancer treated with chemotherapy or whole abdominal irradiation: A Gynecologic Oncology Group study

Tewari KS, Filiaci VL, Spirtos NM, et al (Univ of California Med Ctr, Irvine; GOG Statistical and Data Ctr, Buffalo, NY; Women's Cancer Ctr of Nevada, Las Vegas; et al)

Gynecol Oncol 125:87-93, 2012

Objective.—To determine whether the number of positive pelvic nodes (PPN), cervical stromal involvement (CSI), and/or lymphovascular space involvement (LVSI) were prognostic factors among women with advanced endometrial carcinoma treated with adriamycin plus cisplatin (AP) or whole abdominal irradiation (WAI).

Methods.—Data were abstracted from records of patients treated with adjuvant WAI or AP in a GOG randomized trial. Cox proportional hazards models were used to estimate the association of CSI and PPN with differences in PFS and OS while adjusting for treatment and previously studied factors.

Results.—WAI was randomly allocated to 202 and AP to 194 eligible patients. CSI (n = 93 total) was associated with a 44% increase in risk of progression and a 33% increase in risk of death. There was a trend for increasing number of PPN being associated with a 7% per positive node increase in risk of progression/death. For CSI, the estimated unadjusted treatment hazard ratios (HRs) were: PFS 0.85 (0.53, 1.38); OS 0.81 (0.50, 1.33). For metastatic disease limited to a single PPN (n = 25), the unadjusted HRs were: PFS 0.96 (0.34, 2.74); OS 0.73 (0.24, 2.18). The test of homogeneity of treatment effect (ie., AP vs WAI) across subgroups (CSI, number of positive pelvic nodes) was not statistically significant for either endpoint, thus supporting the superiority of chemotherapy as reported in the original manuscript.

Conclusions.—The presence of CSI and increasing number of PPN were associated with poor prognosis. On average, patients with CSI experienced improved PFS and OS when treated with AP relative to WAI.

▶ Prior to 2003, chemotherapy had no well-defined role in the management of endometrial carcinoma. That year marked the reporting of 2 Gynecologic Oncology Group (GOG) trials that essentially changed the paradigm for treating patients with advanced or recurrent disease. GOG 122 involved patients with stage III-IV disease. These patients were optimally debulked and then randomized to receive either whole abdominal radiation (the standard of care at the time) or chemotherapy consisting of doxorubicin/cisplatin. Those receiving chemotherapy demonstrated a superior progression-free (hazard ratio [HR] = 0.70) and overall (HR = 0.66) survival. At the same time, a trial in disseminated recurrent disease (GOG 177) showed an advantage in terms of response, complete response, progression-free survival, and overall survival for a 3-drug combination (paclitaxel/doxorubicin/cisplatin) as compared with the 2-drug combination (doxorubicin/cisplatin). Since the publication of these 2 trials, chemotherapy has generally been considered to be the preferred treatment for both patients with locally advanced disease and patients with disseminated disease. Studies now are seeking to determine whether chemotherapy should be a part of the management of even earlier-stage disease. As a result, it is crucial to determine accurately what constitutes high-risk early disease. This study of the GOG evaluated patients entered onto GOG 122 to determine those factors that increased risk of recurrence and death. Factors evaluated and found to indicate high risk included the number of positive pelvic nodes and involvement of the cervical stroma. Both factors were also associated with an enhanced outcome with the use of chemotherapy as opposed to whole abdominal radiation.

J. T. Thigpen, MD

Metformin potentiates the effects of paclitaxel in endometrial cancer cells through inhibition of cell proliferation and modulation of the mTOR pathway

Hanna RK, Zhou C, Malloy KM, et al (Univ of North Carolina, Chapel Hill; et al)
Gynecol Oncol 125:458-469, 2012

Objectives.—To examine the effects of combination therapy with metformin and paclitaxel in endometrial cancer cell lines.

Methods.—ECC-1 and Ishikawa endometrial cancer cell lines were used. Cell proliferation was assessed after exposure to paclitaxel and metformin. Cell cycle progression was assessed by flow cytometry. hTERT expression was determined by real-time RT-PCR. Western immunoblotting was performed to determine the effect of metformin/paclitaxel on the mTOR pathway.

Results.—Paclitaxel inhibited proliferation in a dose-dependent manner in both cell lines with IC_{50} values of 1–5 nM and 5–10 nM for Ishikawa and ECC-1 cells, respectively. Simultaneous exposure of cells to various doses of paclitaxel in combination with metformin (0.5 mM) resulted in a significant synergistic anti-proliferative effect in both cell lines (Combination Index <1). Metformin induced G1 arrest in both cell lines. Paclitaxel alone or in combination with metformin resulted in predominantly G2 arrest. Metformin decreased hTERT mRNA expression while paclitaxel alone had no effect on telomerase activity. Metformin stimulated AMPK phosphorylation and decreased phosphorylation of the S6 protein. In contrast, paclitaxel inhibited AMPK phosphorylation in the ECC-1 cell line and induced phosphorylation of S6 in both cell lines. Treatment with metformin and paclitaxel resulted in decreased phosphorylation of S6 in both cell lines but only had an additive effect on AMPK phosphorylation in the ECC-1 cell line.

Conclusions.—Metformin potentiates the effects of paclitaxel in endometrial cancer cells through inhibition of cell proliferation and modulation of the mTOR pathway. This combination may be a promising targeted therapy for endometrial cancer.

▶ Endometrial carcinoma is the most common invasive malignancy of the female genital tract. What is often overlooked is the fact that it is the second leading cause of death from gynecologic cancers and accounts for over 8000 deaths per year in the United States. Since 2003, systemic therapy with chemotherapy has assumed an increasing role in the management of recurrent or disseminated disease as well as locally advanced disease. Active agents include paclitaxel, the platinum compounds, and the anthracyclines. The most commonly used regimen in clinical practice is paclitaxel/carboplatin. Targeted agents are being evaluated, but none as yet have a defined role. This particular study evaluates the ability of a diabetic agent, metformin, to enhance the cytotoxicity of paclitaxel through modulation of the mTOR pathway. The results suggest that metformin may well improve results with taxane-based combinations. The result has been that the Gynecologic Oncology Group plans to conduct a phase III trial of paclitaxel/carboplatin metformin. Until this trial is performed, metformin's role in endometrial carcinoma remains as a treatment for diabetes, which many of these patients have.

J. T. Thigpen, MD

Recurrence and Survival After Random Assignment to Laparoscopy Versus Laparotomy for Comprehensive Surgical Staging of Uterine Cancer: Gynecologic Oncology Group LAP2 Study

Walker JL, Piedmonte MR, Spirtos NM, et al (Univ of Oklahoma Health Science Ctr; Roswell Park Cancer Inst, Buffalo, NY; Women's Cancer Ctr of Nevada, Las Vegas; et al)

J Clin Oncol 30:695-700, 2012

Purpose.—The primary objective was to establish noninferiority of laparoscopy compared with laparotomy for recurrence after surgical staging of uterine cancer.

Patients and Methods.—Patients with clinical stages I to IIA disease were randomly allocated (two to one) to laparoscopy (n = 1,696) versus laparotomy (n = 920) for hysterectomy, salpingo-oophorectomy, pelvic cytology, and pelvic and para-aortic lymphadenectomy. The primary study end point was noninferiority of recurrence-free interval defined as no more than a 40% increase in the risk of recurrence with laparoscopy compared with laparotomy.

Results.—With a median follow-up time of 59 months for 2,181 patients still alive, there were 309 recurrences (210 laparoscopy; 99 laparotomy) and 350 deaths (229 laparoscopy; 121 laparotomy). The estimated hazard ratio for laparoscopy relative to laparotomy was 1.14 (90% lower bound, 0.92; 95% upper bound, 1.46), falling short of the protocol-specified definition of noninferiority. However, the actual recurrence rates were substantially lower than anticipated, resulting in an estimated 3-year recurrence rate of 11.4% with laparoscopy and 10.2% with laparotomy, or a difference of 1.14% (90% lower bound, −1.28; 95% upper bound, 4.0). The estimated 5-year overall survival was almost identical in both arms at 89.8%.

Conclusion.—This study previously reported that laparoscopic surgical management of uterine cancer is superior for short-term safety and length-of-stay end points. The potential for increased risk of cancer recurrence with laparoscopy versus laparotomy was quantified and found to be small, providing accurate information for decision making for women with uterine cancer.

▶ This study of the Gynecologic Oncology Group undertook to determine whether laparoscopy offered a reasonable alternative to laparotomy for the surgical staging and treatment of patients with clinical stage I or IIA endometrial carcinoma. The study included over 2100 patients randomized 2 to 1 to laparoscopy or laparotomy. The primary endpoint was recurrence rate, and the intent of the study was to demonstrate noninferiority of laparoscopy. The study actually showed that laparoscopy resulted in a shorter hospital stay, fewer complications, less pain, and faster recovery with no difference in overall survival and an absolute 1.14% difference in recurrence rate. All of these observations support the use of laparoscopy as a valid alternative to laparotomy for the surgical staging and treatment of endometrial carcinoma regardless of histologic type. However, it must also be noted that the study did not meet its primary endpoint of noninferiority of recurrence rate, although all other parameters indicate essentially equivalence. This probably relates to the fact that recurrence was lower than expected in both arms of the trial. On balance, the conclusion of the authors that the study supports laparoscopy as a valid and probably preferred alternative for surgical staging and management of early-stage endometrial carcinoma seems reasonable and appropriate.

J. T. Thigpen, MD

The role of lymphadenectomy in endometrial cancer: Was the ASTEC trial doomed by design and are we destined to repeat that mistake?

Naumann RW (The Blumenthal Cancer Ctr at Carolinas Med Ctr, Charlotte, NC)

Gynecol Oncol 126:5-11, 2012

Objective.—This study examines the design of previous and future trials of lymph node dissection in endometrial cancer.

Methods.—Data from previous trials were used to construct a decision analysis modeling the risk of lymphatic spread and the effects of treatment on patients with endometrial cancer. This model was then applied to previous trials as well as other future trial designs that might be used to address this subject.

Results.—Comparing the predicted and actual results in the ASTEC trial, the model closely mimics the survival results with and without lymph node dissection for the low and high risk groups. The model suggests a survival difference of less than 2% between the experimental and control arms of the ASTEC trial under all circumstances. Sensitivity analyses reveal that these conclusions are robust. Future trial designs were also modeled with hysterectomy only, hysterectomy with radiation in intermediate risk patients, and staging with radiation only with node positive patients. Predicted outcomes for these approaches yield survival rates of 88%, 90%, and 93% in clinical stage I patients who have a risk of pelvic node involvement of approximately 7%. These estimates were 78%, 82%, and 89% in intermediate risk patients who have a risk of nodal spread of approximately 15%.

Conclusions.—This model accurately predicts the outcome of previous trials and demonstrates that even if lymph node dissection was therapeutic, these trials would have been negative due to study design. Furthermore, future trial designs that are being considered would need to be conducted in high-intermediate risk patients to detect any difference.

▶ The overall survival of patients with endometrial carcinoma is excellent because most patients are stage I, grade 1, with a very high cure rate with hysterectomy. Of concern, however, are the approximately 20% to 25% of patients who recur after surgery and die of their cancer. Studies have identified prognostic factors associated with ultimate recurrence and death; these include myometrial invasion, involvement of the cervical stroma, and extrauterine spread to sites such as pelvic and para-aortic lymph nodes. Careful surgical staging to determine as accurately as possible the extent of disease in each patient is considered in the United States to be standard of care. One of the ongoing controversies about surgical staging is whether patients should undergo pelvic and para-aortic lymphadenectomy as a part of staging. Those who favor lymph node dissection cite not only perhaps some potential therapeutic effect of the lymphadenectomy, but also information that leads to different therapeutic approaches if there is clinically unsuspected involvement of nodes. Two recent randomized trials in Europe claim results that indicate no benefit from lymph node dissection. This article discusses these 2 studies in detail and points out that 1 trial was underpowered to the point that it could not have detected what is, if it exists, almost certainly a very small therapeutic advantage. The other is criticized for failure to control for the use of postoperative therapy. The bottom line is that neither European trial answers the question as to whether lymph node dissection offers patient benefit and that the answer remains unknown. Any further study of this issue must meet 2 particular criteria before it is undertaken. First, the trial should be adequately powered to detect any expected advantage for lymph node dissection. This means it would have to include a huge number of patients or else focus on a very high risk subset of patients. Second, the trial must specify or randomize the postoperative therapy so that any effect of node dissection can be identified and quantitated. Until such a trial has been done, lymph node dissection should be carried out only if the physician plans to use the findings to determine further management because a direct therapeutic benefit of the dissection itself seems unlikely.

J. T. Thigpen, MD

Miscellaneous

A phase II trial of radiation therapy and weekly cisplatin chemotherapy for the treatment of locally-advanced squamous cell carcinoma of the vulva: A gynecologic oncology group study

Moore DH, Ali S, Koh W-J, et al (Gynecologic Oncology of Indiana, Indianapolis; GOG Statistical & Data Ctr, Buffalo, NY; Fred Hutchinson Cancer Res Ctr, Seattle, WA; et al)
Gynecol Oncol 124:529-533, 2012

Objectives.—To determine the efficacy and toxicity of radiation therapy and concurrent weekly cisplatin chemotherapy in achieving a complete clinical and pathologic response when used for the primary treatment of locally-advanced vulvar carcinoma.

Methods.—Patients with locally-advanced (T3 or T4 tumors not amenable to surgical resection via radical vulvectomy), previously untreated squamous cell carcinoma of the vulva were treated with radiation (1.8 Gy daily $\times$ 32 fractions = 57.6 Gy) plus weekly cisplatin (40 mg/m^2) followed by surgical resection of residual tumor (or biopsy to confirm complete clinical response). Management of the groin lymph nodes was standardized and was not a statistical endpoint. Primary endpoints were complete clinical and pathologic response rates of the primary vulvar tumor.

Results.—A planned interim analysis indicated sufficient activity to reopen the study to a second stage of accrual. Among 58 evaluable patients, there were 40 (69%) who completed study treatment. Reasons for prematurely discontinuing treatment included: patient refusal ($N = 4$), toxicity ($N = 9$), death ($N = 2$), other ($N = 3$). There were 37 patients with a complete clinical response (37/58; 64%). Among these women there were 34 who underwent surgical biopsy and 29 (78%) who also had a complete pathological response. Common adverse effects included leukopenia, pain, radiation dermatitis, pain, or metabolic changes.

Conclusions.—This combination of radiation therapy plus weekly cisplatin successfully yielded high complete clinical and pathologic response rates with acceptable toxicity.

▶ Vulvar carcinoma is a relatively uncommon cancer. Because of this, there is little information on the management of these lesions from well-done prospective trials. It is rational to extrapolate from the treatment of cervix carcinoma because both are squamous cell carcinomas for the most part, but we need prospective trials to validate these approaches. This study undertook to assess the standard treatment for locally advanced cervix cancer, a concurrent combination of weekly cisplatin plus radiation with pathological and clinical complete response as the primary endpoints. The approach was associated with increased toxicity because 13 of the 58 patients either refused to continue or experienced toxicity that prompted cessation of therapy. There were, however, very high pathologic and clinical complete response rates. This strongly suggests that such an approach is an effective treatment for patients with vulvar carcinoma. It is therefore reasonable to conclude that vulvar cancers that are not resectable should be treated with a concurrent chemoradiation in a fashion similar to that used for cervix cancers.

J. T. Thigpen, MD

8 Gastrointestinal

Screening and Detection

Association Between Lymph Node Evaluation for Colon Cancer and Node Positivity Over the Past 20 Years

Parsons HM, Tuttle TM, Kuntz KM, et al (Natl Cancer Inst, Bethesda, Maryland; Univ of Minnesota, Minneapolis)

JAMA 306:1089-1097, 2011

Context.—Among patients surgically treated for colon cancer, better survival has been demonstrated in those with more lymph nodes evaluated. The presumed mechanism behind this association suggests that a more extensive lymph node evaluation reduces the risk of understaging, leading to improved survival.

Objective.—To further evaluate the mechanism behind lymph node evaluation and survival by examining the association between more extensive lymph node evaluation, identification of lymph node–positive cancers, and hazard of death.

Design.—Observational cohort study.

Setting.—Surveillance, Epidemiology, and End Results (SEER) program data from 1988 through 2008.

Patients.—86 394 patients surgically treated for colon cancer.

Main Outcome Measure.—We examined the relationship between lymph node evaluation and node positivity using Cochran-Armitage tests and multivariate logistic regression. The association between lymph node evaluation and hazard of death was evaluated using Cox proportional hazards modeling.

Results.—The number of lymph nodes evaluated increased from 1988 to 2008 but did not result in a significant overall increase in lymph node positivity. During 1988-1990, 34.6% of patients (3875/11,200) had 12 or more lymph nodes evaluated, increasing to 73.6% (9798/13,310) during 2006-2008 ($P < .001$); however, the proportion of node-positive cancers did not change with time (40% in 1988-1990, 42% in 2006-2008, $P = .53$). Although patients with high levels of lymph node evaluation were only slightly more likely to be node positive (adjusted odds ratio for 30-39 nodes vs 1-8 nodes, 1.11; 95% CI, 1.02-1.20), these patients experienced significantly lower hazard of death compared with those with fewer nodes evaluated (adjusted hazard ratio for 30-39 nodes vs 1-8 nodes, 0.66; 95% CI, 0.62-0.71; unadjusted 5-year mortality, 35.3%).

Conclusion.—The number of lymph nodes evaluated for colon cancer has markedly increased in the past 2 decades but was not associated with an overall shift toward higher-staged cancers, questioning the upstaging mechanism as the primary basis for improved survival in patients with more lymph nodes evaluated.

▶ Colon cancer remains a serious malignant disease for which improvements in diagnosis and staging are very important. Screening colonoscopy has markedly improved the diagnosis of earlier stages of disease for which cure is possible for many patients. Yet once the diagnosis has been made, the next step is surgery. Clearly, as with all oncologic surgeries, the extent of the surgery is important with regard to accurate staging and treatment. But it is also important with regard to postoperative complications. Thus, it is important to do the best operation with the fewest complications. The extent of lymph node dissection during surgery for colon cancer patients is important from both of these perspectives. These data suggest that the more extensive lymph node dissection did not result in more patients with positive lymph nodes. Therefore, one might question the need for these extensive lymph node dissections with their associated morbidity.

Likely only a randomized trial to study the extent of lymph node dissection will answer this question. Perhaps it needs to be asked.

C. Lawton, MD

Esophagus, Stomach

Adjuvant capecitabine and oxaliplatin for gastric cancer after D2 gastrectomy (CLASSIC): a phase 3 open-label, randomised controlled trial

Bang Y-J, for the CLASSIC trial investigators (Seoul Natl Univ College of Medicine, South Korea; et al)

Lancet 379:315-321, 2012

Background.—D2 gastrectomy is recommended in US and European guidelines, and is preferred in east Asia, for patients with resectable gastric cancer. Adjuvant chemotherapy improves patient outcomes after surgery, but the benefits after a D2 resection have not been extensively investigated in large-scale trials. We investigated the effect on disease-free survival of adjuvant chemotherapy with capecitabine plus oxaliplatin after D2 gastrectomy compared with D2 gastrectomy only in patients with stage II–IIIB gastric cancer.

Methods.—The capecitabine and oxaliplatin adjuvant study in stomach cancer (CLASSIC) study was an open-label, parallel-group, phase 3, randomised controlled trial undertaken in 37 centres in South Korea, China, and Taiwan. Patients with stage II–IIIB gastric cancer who had had curative D2 gastrectomy were randomly assigned to receive adjuvant chemotherapy of eight 3-week cycles of oral capecitabine (1000 mg/m^2 twice daily on days 1 to 14 of each cycle) plus intravenous oxaliplatin (130 mg/m^2 on day 1 of each cycle) for 6 months or surgery only. Block randomisation was done by a central interactive computerised system, stratified by country and disease stage. Patients, and investigators giving interventions, assessing outcomes, and analysing data were not masked. The primary endpoint was 3 year disease-free survival, analysed by intention to treat. This study reports a pre-specified interim efficacy analysis, after which the trial was stopped after a recommendation by the data monitoring committee. The trial is registered at ClinicalTrials.gov (NCT00411229).

Findings.—1035 patients were randomised (520 to receive chemotherapy and surgery, 515 surgery only). Median follow-up was 34·2 months (25·4–41·7) in the chemotherapy and surgery group and 34·3 months (25·6–41·9) in the surgery only group. 3 year disease-free survival was 74% (95% CI 69–79) in the chemotherapy and surgery group and 59% (53–64) in the surgery only group (hazard ratio 0·56, 95% CI 0·44–0·72; $p < 0{\cdot}0001$). Grade 3 or 4 adverse events were reported in 279 of 496 patients (56%) in the chemotherapy and surgery group and in 30 of 478 patients (6%) in the surgery only group. The most common adverse events in the intervention group were nausea (n = 326), neutropenia (n = 300), and decreased appetite (n = 294).

Interpretation.—Adjuvant capecitabine plus oxaliplatin treatment after curative D2 gastrectomy should be considered as a treatment option for patients with operable gastric cancer.

▶ Gastric cancer manifests high recurrence rates of 40% to 80% after surgical resection. The Intergroup (INT-0116) and the British Medical Research Council Adjuvant Gastric Infusional Chemotherapy (MAGIC) randomized phase III trials demonstrated significant survival benefit by using either postoperative 5-fluorouracil (5-FU) chemotherapy and 5-FU–based chemoradiation, or perioperative epirubicin, cisplatin, and 5-FU (ECF), respectively. In the INT-0116 trial, the median survival rates with 5-FU–based chemoradiotherapy were 36 months versus 27 months in the surgery alone arm, while the MAGIC trial noted median survival rates of 24 months with ECF versus 20 months in the surgery alone group. None of these trials required an optimal D2 lymph node dissection, and only 10% of patients in the INT-0116 trial and 41% of patients in the MAGIC trial underwent D2 gastrectomy. It is appropriately thought that a D2 dissection will significantly increase the odds of long-term disease-free survival (DFS) and overall survival (OS).

D2 dissection is considered standard of care in Asia, and the overall superior long-term outcomes for resected gastric cancer in Asian patients were in part attributed to a more successful surgery. The Capecitabine and Oxaliplatin Adjuvant Study in Stomach Cancer (CLASSIC) randomized phase III trial studied the role of 6 months of adjuvant capecitabine plus oxaliplatin (XELOX) after surgery compared to surgery alone, with the primary endpoint being 3-year DFS.

With a median follow-up of 34 months, the 3-year DFS was significantly better with XELOX versus surgery alone (74% vs 59%), irrespective of disease staging. Although the OS data are not yet mature, prior meta-analyses noted a good correlation between 3-year DFS and 5-year OS benefit.

In comparison with the INT-0116 trial, where the 3-year DFS rates were 48% (study arm) versus 31% (control), and the MAGIC trial with 3-year DFS rates of 40% (study arm) versus 25% (control), it is clear that adjuvant chemotherapy with XELOX sustains benefit following D2 gastrectomy. This is highly relevant for the current adjuvant treatment of gastric cancer patients worldwide, particularly with the adoption of D2 gastrectomy as standard of care in Europe and the United States.

E. G. Chiorean, MD

Bevacizumab in Combination With Chemotherapy As First-Line Therapy in Advanced Gastric Cancer: A Randomized, Double-Blind, Placebo-Controlled Phase III Study

Ohtsu A, Shah MA, Van Cutsem E, et al (Natl Cancer Ctr Hosp East, Kashiwa, Chiba; Memorial Sloan-Kettering Cancer Ctr, NY; Univ Hosp Gasthuisberg, Leuven, Belgium; et al)

J Clin Oncol 29:3968-3976, 2011

Purpose.—The Avastin in Gastric Cancer (AVAGAST) trial was a multinational, randomized, placebo-controlled trial designed to evaluate the efficacy of adding bevacizumab to capecitabine-cisplatin in the first-line treatment of advanced gastric cancer.

Patients and Methods.—Patients received bevacizumab 7.5 mg/kg or placebo followed by cisplatin 80 mg/m^2 on day 1 plus capecitabine 1,000 mg/m^2 twice daily for 14 days every 3 weeks. Fluorouracil was permitted in patients unable to take oral medications. Cisplatin was given for six cycles; capecitabine and bevacizumab were administered until disease progression or unacceptable toxicity. The primary end point was overall survival (OS). Log-rank test was used to test the OS difference.

Results.—In all, 774 patients were enrolled; 387 were assigned to each treatment group (intention-to-treat population), and 517 deaths were observed. Median OS was 12.1 months with bevacizumab plus fluoropyrimidine-cisplatin and 10.1 months with placebo plus fluoropyrimidine-cisplatin (hazard ratio 0.87; 95% CI, 0.73 to 1.03; $P = .1002$). Both median progression-free survival (6.7 *v* 5.3 months; hazard ratio, 0.80; 95% CI, 0.68 to 0.93; $P = .0037$) and overall response rate (46.0% *v* 37.4%; $P = .0315$) were significantly improved with bevacizumab versus placebo. Preplanned subgroup analyses revealed regional differences in efficacy outcomes. The most common grade 3 to 5 adverse events were neutropenia (35%, bevacizumab plus fluoropyrimidine-cisplatin; 37%, placebo plus fluoropyrimidine-cisplatin), anemia (10% *v* 14%), and decreased appetite (8% *v* 11%). No new bevacizumab-related safety signals were identified.

Conclusion.—Although AVAGAST did not reach its primary objective, adding bevacizumab to chemotherapy was associated with significant increases in progression-free survival and overall response rate in the first-line treatment of advanced gastric cancer.

▶ Gastric cancer accounts for more than 700 000 deaths worldwide, and while less prevalent in the United States, it is an extremely aggressive malignancy mostly diagnosed in advanced stages in the Western world. Overall survival rates average less than 1 year when the disease is metastatic, even with the use of chemotherapy. New biological targets, such as HER2, EGFR, and cMET, have been identified for gastroesophageal malignancies, and the anti-HER2 monoclonal antibody trastuzumab has already shown significant survival improvement for HER2-positive tumors.

Increased angiogenesis has been linked to poor prognosis in gastric and gastroesophageal cancer, and preliminary phase II studies showed encouraging activity of chemotherapy plus the anti–vascular endothelial growth factor (VEGF) antibody, bevacizumab (Avastin).

The Avastin in Gastric Cancer Study (AVAGAST) was a randomized, double-blind, placebo-controlled phase III trial of a fluoropyrimidine (94% capecitabine and 6% 5-fluorouracil) plus cisplatin chemotherapy with or without bevacizumab in the first-line treatment of metastatic (96%) or locally advanced (4%) gastric or GE junction carcinomas. The primary endpoint was overall survival, with the aim of obtaining a 22% increase with the addition of bevacizumab. Approximately 50% of the patients were accrued in Asia and 50% in Europe and South and North America, combined.

The overall survival for the intent-to-treat population was 12.1 versus 10.1 months in favor of the bevacizumab-treated arm but without statistical significance (HR = 0.87, $P = .1$). Interestingly, prior gastric cancer studies suggested superior survival rates in general for Asian patients compared with those from the Western world. In a preplanned subgroup analysis in this trial, the control group treated with chemotherapy alone showed survival rates of 12 months in Asia, 8.6 months in Europe, and only 6.8 months in the Pan-America group. Interestingly, it seemed that the advantage conferred by bevacizumab was differential based on the geographic region, such that there was a significant survival benefit for the Pan-America patients: 11.5 months versus 6.8 months (hazard ratio [HR], 0.63, 95% confidence interval [CI], 0.43–0.94) but not for the Asian patients (13.9 vs 12.1 months, HR 0.97), with an intermediate effect for European patients (11.1 vs 8.6 months, HR 0.85, 95% CI 0.63–1.14). The addition of bevacizumab was associated with significantly improved response rates and an absolute increase in progression-free survival of 1.4 months ($P = .003$). Nevertheless, bevacizumab did not achieve its preplanned objective of increasing median overall survival from 10 to 12.8 months and a HR of 0.78.

With this caveat, one needs to recognize that gastric cancer is not a uniform disease, and the potential benefit observed by adding bevacizumab to fluoropyrimidine and cisplatin chemotherapy in the Pan-America patients should prompt future studies in this patient population. Analysis of angiogenesis-related biomarkers, which was conducted in this study, may further guide the use of anti-VEGF agents in gastric and gastroesophageal malignancies.

E. G. Chiorean, MD

Salvage Chemotherapy for Pretreated Gastric Cancer: A Randomized Phase III Trial Comparing Chemotherapy Plus Best Supportive Care With Best Supportive Care Alone

Kang JH, Lee SI, Lim DH, et al (Gyeongsang Natl Univ Hosp, Jinju, Korea; Dankook Univ Hosp, Cheonan, South Korea; et al)

J Clin Oncol 30:1513-1518, 2012

Purpose.—When designing this trial, there was no evidence that salvage chemotherapy (SLC) in advanced gastric cancer (AGC) resulted in substantial prolongation of survival when compared with best supportive care (BSC). However, SLC is often offered to pretreated patients with AGC for anecdotal reasons.

Patients and Methods.—Patients with AGC with one or two prior chemotherapy regimens involving both fluoropyrimidines and platinum and with an Eastern Cooperative Oncology Group performance status (PS) 0 or 1 were randomly assigned in a ratio of 2:1 to SLC plus BSC or BSC alone. Choice of SLC—either docetaxel 60 mg/m^2 every 3 weeks or irinotecan 150 mg/m^2 every 2 weeks—was left to the discretion of investigators. Primary end point was overall survival (OS).

Results.—Median OS was 5.3 months among 133 patients in the SLC arm and 3.8 months among 69 patients in the BSC arm (hazard ratio, 0.657; 95% CI, 0.485 to 0.891; one-sided $P=.007$). OS benefit for SLC was consistent in most of the prospectively defined subgroups, including age, PS, number of prior treatments, metastatic sites, hemoglobin levels, and response to prior chemotherapy. SLC was generally well tolerated, and adverse events were similar in the SLC and BSC arms. We found no median OS difference between docetaxel and irinotecan (5.2 *v* 6.5 months; $P=.116$).

Conclusion.—To our knowledge, this is the largest phase III trial comparing SLC plus BSC with BSC alone in AGC. In pretreated patients, SLC is tolerated and significantly improves OS when added to BSC.

▶ This study assesses the efficacy of further chemotherapy after progression following initial 1 or 2 lines of systemic treatment. Although such treatment is commonly offered to patients, there is a lack of extensive supporting of such an approach. Patients were randomly assigned to either salvage chemotherapy with best supportive care or best supportive care alone in a 2:1 ratio. Investigators were allowed to choose the single-agent chemotherapy from between docetaxel (60 mg/m^2 every 3 weeks) and irinotecan (150 mg/m^2 every 2 weeks). Those who received salvage chemotherapy showed a statistically significant survival benefit (HR = 0.657) without evidence of an excess of toxicity compared with best supportive care. Although the choice of chemotherapy was not randomized, no difference between the 2 single agents could be discerned. This, along with another phase III trial, provides evidence to support the use of salvage chemotherapy for recurrent gastric cancer in the second- or third-line setting as a standard approach.

J. T. Thigpen, MD

Pancreas

Gemcitabine Alone Versus Gemcitabine Plus Radiotherapy in Patients With Locally Advanced Pancreatic Cancer: An Eastern Cooperative Oncology Group trial

Loehrer PJ Sr, Feng Y, Cardenes H, et al (Indiana Univ, Indianapolis; Dana Farber Cancer Inst, Boston, MA; et al)

J Clin Oncol 29:4105-4112, 2011

Purpose.—The purpose of this trial was to evaluate the role of radiation therapy with concurrent gemcitabine (GEM) compared with GEM alone in patients with localized unresectable pancreatic cancer.

Patients and Methods.—Patients with localized unresectable adenocarcinoma of the pancreas were randomly assigned to receive GEM alone (at 1,000 mg/m^2/wk for weeks 1 to 6, followed by 1 week rest, then for 3 of 4 weeks) or GEM (600 mg/m^2/wk for weeks 1 to 5, then 4 weeks later 1,000 mg/m^2 for 3 of 4 weeks) plus radiotherapy (starting on day 1, 1.8 Gy/Fx for total of 50.4 Gy). Measurement of quality of life using the Functional Assessment of Cancer Therapy—Hepatobiliary questionnaire was also performed.

Results.—Of 74 patients entered on trial and randomly assigned to receive GEM alone (arm A; n = 37) or GEM plus radiation (arm B; n = 34), patients in arm B had greater incidence of grades 4 and 5 toxicities (41% *v* 9%), but grades 3 and 4 toxicities combined were similar (77% in A *v* 79% in B). No statistical differences were seen in quality of life measurements at 6, 15 to 16, and 36 weeks. The primary end point was survival, which was 9.2 months (95% CI, 7.9 to 11.4 months) and 11.1 months (95% CI, 7.6 to 15.5 months) for arms A and B, respectively (one-sided P = .017 by stratified log-rank test).

Conclusion.—This trial demonstrates improved overall survival with the addition of radiation therapy to GEM in patients with localized unresectable pancreatic cancer, with acceptable toxicity.

▶ Locally advanced pancreatic cancer (LAPC) represents approximately 35% of all newly diagnosed pancreatic adenocarcinomas and is generally associated with survival rates of 8 to 12 months. Previously used treatment regimens for LAPC incorporated chemotherapy, mostly 5-fluorouracil (5-FU) or gemcitabine with or without 5-FU—based radiotherapy.[1-3] Gemcitabine has been studied in phase I and II trials as a radiosensitizer, but head-to-head studies comparing it with 5-FU have not declared a preferred regimen, despite some suggesting better tolerability versus 5-FU. The role of radiotherapy has been subject to much debate for both resectable and unresectable localized pancreatic cancer.

ECOG4201 has been designed as a prospectively randomized, controlled trial to test the efficacy (ie, overall survival as primary endpoint) of gemcitabine-based chemoradiotherapy (CRT) in addition to gemcitabine versus gemcitabine alone for LAPC. Among 316 patients intended for accrual, only 74 patients were enrolled. The poor accrual was likely due to preconceived physician expectations, such as always including, or not, radiotherapy in their patients' regimens. Nevertheless, the primary endpoint was met, with the gemcitabine-based CRT arm conferring a modest but significant survival benefit of 11.1 versus 9.2 months (1-sided $P = .017$) for gemcitabine alone. The fact that the progression-free survival rates of 6 months were equivalent in both groups makes the overall results harder to interpret and this justifies skepticism.

Many investigators, including European groups, have been incorporating induction chemotherapy regimens for 2 to 6 months prior to CRT for LAPC. Retrospective analyses of GERCOR phase II and III studies found a significant survival benefit (15 vs 11.7 months, $P = .0009$) for those patients exposed to CRT compared with those maintained on chemotherapy after an initial 3- to 6-month period of systemic treatment.[4] It is clear that exposure to effective systemic chemotherapy is essential to control metastatic cancer spread and helps select patients most likely to benefit from CRT.

ECOG4201, while designed with an initial CRT regimen, offers the background that there may be a role for CRT in LAPC and justifies future trials with effective and novel systemic therapies as well as the addition of biomarkers to help select those most likely to benefit.

E. G. Chiorean, MD

References

1. Moertel CG, Frytak S, Hahn RG, et al. Therapy of locally unresectable pancreatic carcinoma: a randomized comparison of high dose (6000 rads) radiation alone, moderate dose radiation (4000 rads +5-fluorouracil), and high dose radiation +5-fluorouracil: the Gastrointestinal Tumor Study Group. *Cancer.* 1981;48:1705-1710.
2. Cardenes HR, Moore AM, Johnson CS, et al. A phase II study of gemcitabine in combination with radiation therapy in patients with localized, unresectable pancreatic cancer: a Hoosier Oncology Group study. *Am J Clin Oncol.* 2011;34:460-465.
3. Cardenes H, Chiorean EG, Dewitt J, Schmidt M, Loehrer PJ. Locally advanced pancreatic cancer: current therapeutic approach. *Oncologist.* 2006;11:612-623.
4. Huguet F, André T, Hammel P, et al. Impact of chemoradiotherapy after disease control with chemotherapy in locally advanced pancreatic adenocarcinoma in GERCOR phase II and III studies. *J Clin Oncol.* 2007;25:326-331.

Rectal Carcinoma

A Phase II Trial of Neoadjuvant Chemoradiation and Local Excision for T2N0 Rectal Cancer: Preliminary Results of the ACOSOG Z6041 Trial

Garcia-Aguilar J, Shi Q, Thomas CR Jr, et al (Dept of Surgery, City of Hope, Duarte; Mayo Clinic, Rochester, MN; Oregon Health and Science Univ, Portland; et al)
Ann Surg Oncol 19:384-391, 2012

Purpose.—We designed American College of Surgeons Oncology Group (ACOSOG) Z6041, a prospective, multicenter, single-arm, phase II trial to assess the efficacy and safety of neoadjuvant chemoradiation (CRT) and local excision (LE) for T2N0 rectal cancer. Here, we report tumor response, CRT-related toxicity, and perioperative complications (PCs).

Methods.—Clinically staged T2N0 rectal cancer patients were treated with capecitabine and oxaliplatin during radiation followed by LE. Because of toxicity, capecitabine and radiation doses were reduced. LE was performed 6 weeks after CRT. Patients were evaluated for clinical and pathologic response. CRT-related complications and PCs were recorded.

Results.—Ninety patients were accrued; 6 received nonprotocol treatment. The remaining 84 were 65% male; median age 63 years; 83% Eastern Cooperative Oncology Group performance score 0; 92% white; mean tumor size 2.9 cm; and average distance from anal verge 5.1 cm. Five patients were considered ineligible. Therapy was completed per protocol in 79 patients, but two patients did not undergo LE. Among 77 eligible patients who underwent LE, 34 patients achieved a pathologic complete response (44%) and 49 (64%) tumors were downstaged (ypT0−1), but 4 patients (5%) had ypT3 tumors. Five LE specimens contained lymph nodes; one T3 tumor had a positive node. All but one patient had negative margins. Thirty-three (39%) of 84 patients developed CRT-related grade ≥3 complications. Rectal pain was the most common PC.

Conclusions.—CRT before LE for T2N0 tumors results in a high pathologic complete response rate and negative resection margins. However, complications during CRT and after LE are high. The true efficacy of this approach will ultimately be assessed by the long-term oncologic outcomes.

▶ Total mesorectal excision (TME) is the standard surgical treatment for localized rectal cancer, with the main caveat of resulting in permanent colostomy for distal tumors. Neoadjuvant chemoradiotherapy is an established means of reducing the odds of local recurrence for patients with T3-4 or node-positive rectal cancers.[1] In contrast, patients with clinical T1 tumors can be treated safely with transanal local excisions (LE), but T2 rectal cancers have traditionally been treated with TME. LE alone in small rectal cancers confers a higher risk of local recurrences.[2] Several small studies have already found that neoadjuvant chemoradiation followed by local excision may be as effective as TME in terms of local control, but they are limited by mostly retrospective methodology, diverse eligibility criteria, and treatment regimens.[3,4]

ACOSOG Z6041 is a large prospective phase II trial that tested the safety and efficacy of neoadjuvant chemoradiotherapy followed by LE for T2N0 rectal cancers. Ninety patients were enrolled, and 84 received study treatment. The chemotherapy used was capecitabine plus oxaliplatin.

Even though the pathological complete response (pCR) rate was 44%, the surgical specimens of locally excised tumors rarely contained any lymph nodes; thus, the possibility of overestimating pCR is high. Only 1 patient had positive margins and required TME. This regimen was associated with substantial toxicity, mainly gastrointestinal and dermatologic (41% grade 3 and 4). Perioperative complications (rectal pain, hemorrhage, infections) were common in 16% of patients.

While this regimen resulted in a high pCR rate, toxicity was significant, and long-term results regarding local and distant relapse are needed before considering this approach as standard for early stage T2N0 rectal cancer.

E. G. Chiorean, MD

References

1. Sauer R, Becker H, Hohenberger W, et al. Preoperative versus postoperative chemoradiotherapy for rectal cancer. *N Engl J Med.* 2004;351:1731-1740.
2. Bleday R, Breen E, Jessup JM, et al. Prospective evaluation of local excision for small rectal cancers. *Dis Colon Rectum.* 1997;40:388-392.
3. Lezoche G, Baldarelli M, Guerrieri M, et al. A prospective randomized study with a 5-year minimum follow-up evaluation of transanal endoscopic microsurgery versus laparoscopic total mesorectal excision after neoadjuvant therapy. *Surg Endosc.* 2008;22:352-358.
4. Borschitz T, Wachtlin D, Mohler M, et al. Neoadjuvant chemoradiation and local excision for T2-3 rectal cancer. *Ann Surg Oncol.* 2008;15:712-720.

Primary Tumor Response to Preoperative Chemoradiation With or Without Oxaliplatin in Locally Advanced Rectal Cancer: Pathologic Results of the STAR-01 Randomized Phase III Trial

Aschele C, Cionini L, Lonardi S, et al (Istituto Nazionale per la Ricerca sul Cancro, Genova, Italy; Centro Oncologico Fiorentino Villanova, Sesto Fiorentino, Italy; Istituto Oncologico Veneto, Padova, Italy; et al)

J Clin Oncol 29:2773-2780, 2011

Purpose.—To investigate oxaliplatin combined with fluorouracil-based chemoradiotherapy as preoperative treatment for locally advanced rectal cancer.

Patients and Methods.—Seven hundred forty-seven patients with resectable, locally advanced (cT3-4 and/or cN1-2) adenocarcinoma of the mid-low rectum were randomly assigned to receive pelvic radiation (50.4 Gy in 28 daily fractions) and concomitant infused fluorouracil (225 mg/m^2/d) either alone (arm A, n = 379) or combined with oxaliplatin (60 mg/m^2 weekly × 6; arm B, n = 368). Overall survival is the primary end point. A protocol-planned analysis of response to preoperative treatment is reported here.

Results.—Grade 3 to 4 adverse events during preoperative treatment were more frequent with oxaliplatin plus fluorouracil and radiation than with radiation and fluorouracil alone (24% *v* 8% of treated patients; $P < .001$). In arm B, 83% of the patients treated with oxaliplatin had five or more weekly administrations. Ninety-one percent, compared with 97% in the control arm, received ≥45 Gy ($P < .001$). Ninety-six percent versus 95% of patients underwent surgery with similar rates of abdominoperineal resections (20% v 18%, arm A v arm B). The rate of pathologic complete responses was 16% in both arms (odds ratio = 0.98; 95% CI, 0.66 to 1.44; $P = .904$). Twenty-six percent versus 29% of patients had pathologically positive lymph nodes (arm A *v* arm B; $P = .447$), 46% versus 44% had tumor infiltration beyond the muscularis propria ($P = .701$), and 7% versus 4% had positive circumferential resection margins ($P = .239$). Intra-abdominal metastases were found at surgery in 2.9% versus 0.5% of patients (arm A *v* arm B; $P = .014$).

Conclusion.—Adding oxaliplatin to fluorouracil-based preoperative chemoradiotherapy significantly increases toxicity without affecting primary tumor response. Longer follow-up is needed to assess the impact on efficacy end points.

▶ Locally advanced rectal cancer is a devastating condition for afflicted patients for 2 reasons. The first is that it often results in the need for colostomy, which is a significant change in quality of life. The second reason is that it can cause the development of distant metastasis and result in mortality for these patients.

The use of preoperative chemotherapy and radiation to decrease the risk of the need for colostomy has been a standard option for years. Fluorouracil is the chemotherapy of choice used in combination with radiation. It has been shown to decrease the tumor size compared with radiation alone. Yet patients still have significant problems with distant metastasis.

This trial randomly assigned these locally advanced rectal cancer patients to fluorouracil and radiation plus or minus oxaliplatin to test the potential benefit of oxaliplatin in the prevention of distant metastasis. Unfortunately, the results showed no significant benefit to oxaliplatin in prevention of distant metastasis and unfortunately also showed an increase in toxicity. Therefore, oxaliplatin should not be used in this setting, and we need to look to other chemotherapeutic agents to help prevent distant metastasis.

C. Lawton, MD

Colorectal Cancer

Long-term risk of colorectal cancer after negative colonoscopy

Brenner H, Chang-Claude J, Seilor CM, et al (German Cancer Res Ctr, Heidelberg, Germany)

J Clin Oncol 29:3761-3767, 2011

Purpose.—Colonoscopy is thought to be a powerful and cost-effective tool to reduce colorectal cancer (CRC) incidence and mortality. Empirical evidence for overall and risk group-specific definition of screening intervals is sparse. We aimed to assess the risk of CRC according to time since negative colonoscopy, overall, and by sex, smoking, and family history of CRC, in a large population-based case-control study.

Patients and Methods.—In all, 1,945 patients with CRC and 2,399 population controls were recruited in 22 hospitals and through population registers in the Rhine-Neckar region of Germany from 2003 to 2007. Data on history of colonoscopy and important covariates were obtained by personal interviews and from medical records.

Results.—Compared with people who had never undergone colonoscopy, people with a previous negative colonoscopy had a strongly reduced risk of CRC. Adjusted odds ratios for time windows of 1 to 2, 3 to 4, 5 to 9, 10 to 19, and 20+ years after negative colonoscopy were 0.14 (95% CI, 0.10 to 0.20), 0.12 (95% CI, 0.08 to 0.19), 0.26 (95% CI, 0.18 to 0.39), 0.28 (95% CI, 0.17 to 0.45), and 0.40 (95% CI, 0.24 to 0.66), respectively. Low risks even beyond 10 years after negative colonoscopy were observed for both left- and right-sided CRC and in all risk groups assessed except current smokers, who had a risk similar to that of never smokers with no previous colonoscopy 10 or more years after a negative colonoscopy.

Conclusion.—These results support suggestions that screening intervals for CRC screening by colonoscopy could be longer than the commonly recommended 10 years in most cases, perhaps even among men and people with a family history of CRC, but probably not among current smokers.

▶ The use of screening colonoscopy has become a very important tool to decrease the incidence and mortality associated with colorectal cancer. Few patients, physicians, and even insurers question the need for this screening examination. Yet once a patient has a colonoscopy and the results are negative, what is the next appropriate interval for subsequent ones? The answer to this question is not known with certainty and is very important from a cost, patient convenience, and colorectal cancer risk perspective.

We know as physicians that the current answer to the question of timing of subsequent screening colonoscopies after an initial negative one has been 10 years. The data to verify that 10 years is the correct timeframe are lacking. These authors have attempted to answer the question through the use of population-based registries in Germany. Based on their data, especially in nonsmokers, the interval could be every 20 years. These results need to be evaluated in a larger cohort of patients, but they do provide tantalizing data to encourage us to pursue this important question.

C. Lawton, MD

9 Hematologic Malignancies

Leukemia and Myelodysplastic Syndrome

Clonal origins of relapse in *ETV6-RUNX1* acute lymphoblastic leukemia

van Delft FW, Horsley S, Colman S, et al (Inst of Cancer Res, Sutton, UK; et al)

Blood 117:6247-6254, 2011

B-cell precursor childhood acute lymphoblastic leukemia with *ETV6-RUNX1 (TEL-AML1)* fusion has an overall good prognosis, but relapses occur, usually after cessation of treatment and occasionally many years later. We have investigated the clonal origins of relapse by comparing the profiles of genomewide copy number alterations at presentation in 21 patients with those in matched relapse (12-119 months). We identified, in total, 159 copy number alterations at presentation and 231 at relapse (excluding Ig/TCR). Deletions of *CDKN2A/B or CCNC* (6q16.2-3) or both increased from 38% at presentation to 76% in relapse, suggesting that cell-cycle deregulation contributed to emergence of relapse. A novel observation was recurrent gain of chromosome 16 (2 patients at presentation, 4 at relapse) and deletion of plasmocytoma variant translocation 1 in 3 patients. The data indicate that, irrespective of time to relapse, the relapse clone was derived from either a major or minor clone at presentation. Backtracking analysis by FISH identified a minor subclone at diagnosis whose genotype matched that observed in relapse ~ 10 years later. These data indicate subclonal diversity at diagnosis, providing a variable basis for intraclonal origins of relapse and extended periods (years) of dormancy, possibly by quiescence, for stem cells in *ETV6-RUNX1*$^+$ acute lymphoblastic leukemia.

▶ Charles Darwin and Alfred Russel Wallace made important insights into the evolution of species. The belief is that all species of life descended over time from common ancestors, which in turn retained traceable, common traits. The concepts of evolution and survival of the fittest have also been applied to the development of cancer and the resistance of cancer to treatment through selective pressure-mediated molecular changes. However, the re-emergence of cancer many years after a patient has been presumed cured has remained a mystery. Van Delft et al demonstrate that specific molecular changes are shared between newly diagnosed samples and very late relapses in B-cell precursor childhood acute lymphoblastic leukemia (ALL) characterized by the *ETV6-RUNX1* translocation. Specifically, they examined genomewide copy number changes between matched diagnosis and relapsed samples. They indicated that certain changes, such as deletions at chromosome position 6q16.2-3, involving *CDKN2A/B* or *CCNC*, are seen in 38% of diagnostic and 76% of relapse samples. Other changes are seen in quite small numbers of patients, such as recurrent gain of chromosome 16 in 2 patients at presentation and 4 at relapse. Detailed mapping at the nucleotide level was not done, raising the possibility that quite different clones (maybe even completely new) developed to contribute to relapse but still involved selective, critical regions that contribute to leukemogenesis. Another issue that is unanswered by such studies is how a cell stays dormant for so long if it is indeed such a cell that contributes to relapse in contrast to the de novo development of a new leukemia.

R. J. Arceci, MD, PhD

Radiation therapy for leukemia cutis

Bakst R, Yahalom J (Memorial Sloan-Kettering Cancer Ctr, NY)

Pract Radiat Oncol 1:182-187, 2011

Purpose.—Leukemia cutis (LC) is the infiltration of the epidermis, dermis, or subcutis by neoplastic leukocytes, resulting in clinically identifiable cutaneous lesions. Electron-based radiation therapy (RT) is often used in the treatment of LC; however, modern studies of RT are lacking. We reviewed our experience to analyze treatment response, disease control, and toxicity associated with RT in order to develop treatment recommendations for patients with LC.

Methods and Materials.—Fifteen patients who underwent treatment for LC at our institution from November 1994 to August 2009 were identified and their medical records were reviewed and analyzed.

Results.—LC presented after a median of 2 (range 0-24) months from acute myeloid leukemia diagnosis. Median survival from time of LC presentation was 23 months (range 0.5-137 months). Thirteen courses of radiation were administered to 12 patients: 9 total skin electron beam (TSEB) therapy and 4 focal treatments. Of patients receiving TSEB, 89% had diffuse LC involvement and 67% were in marrow remission. By contrast, only 25% of patients receiving focal therapy had diffuse LC involvement and only 25% were in marrow remission. Median TSEB dose was 1600 (range 600-2400) cGy. Fifty percent of patients had a complete response to RT but 1-year local control was only 33%. All patients who developed a skin relapse either had active marrow disease at the time of RT or marrow recurrence shortly thereafter. Median survival since RT was 5 (range 0.5-136) months. RT was well tolerated without significant acute effects; however, 1 patient receiving chemotherapy developed radiation recall 1 month after RT.

Conclusions.—Patients with LC have aggressive disease with few long-term survivors. Definitive treatment with TSEB should be utilized only in cases of marrow remission with focal electron therapy reserved for palliation of symptomatic lesions. Long-term prognosis and durable cutaneous remission is dependent on systemic disease control.

▶ Leukemia cutis is a relatively rare entity but can occur in patients with acute or chronic leukemia. It is usually associated with systemic leukemia and portends a poor outcome.

The primary treatment for leukemia cutis, regardless of whether it stems from acute or chronic leukemia, is systemic chemotherapy. Yet for symptomatic lesions or lesions that are chemotherapy resistant, radiation therapy can play an important role.

This review article is an excellent overview of the disease process, diagnosis, and treatment. A few points are worth underscoring:

1. The first is the need for a biopsy of any lesion thought to be leukemia cutis. Patients with leukemia can have many other reasons for abnormal skin lesions, and a biopsy, especially prior to local treatment, should be done to validate the diagnosis.
2. The second point is that chemotherapy is the mainstay of treatment, but radiation therapy can play a role. If lesions are diffuse then total skin electron beam therapy is appropriate with a fractionated course and a total dose of 18 to 20 Gy. For localized symptomatic lesions, the total dose is similar to 20 Gy fractionated.

C. Lawton, MD

The genetic basis of early T—cell precursor acute lymphoblastic leukaemia

Zhang J, Ding L, Holmfeldt L, et al (St Jude Children's Res Hosp, Memphis, TN; The Genome Inst at Washington Univ, St Louis, MO; et al)

Nature 481:157-163, 2012

Early T—cell precursor acute lymphoblastic leukaemia (ETP ALL) is an aggressive malignancy of unknown genetic basis. We performed whole—genome sequencing of 12 ETP ALL cases and assessed the frequency of the identified somatic mutations in 94 T—cell acute lymphoblastic leukaemia cases. ETP ALL was characterized by activating mutations in genes regulating cytokine receptor and RAS signalling (67% of cases; *NRAS, KRAS, FLT3, IL7R, JAK3, JAK1, SH2B3* and *BRAF*), inactivating lesions disrupting haematopoietic development (58%; *GATA3, ETV6, RUNX1, IKZF1* and *EP300*) and histone—modifying genes (48%; *EZH2, EED, SUZ12, SETD2* and *EP300*). We also identified new targets of recurrent mutation including *DNM2, ECT2L* and *RELN*. The mutational spectrum is similar to myeloid tumours, and moreover, the global transcriptional profile of ETP ALL was similar to that of normal and myeloid leukaemia haematopoietic stem cells. These findings suggest that addition of myeloid–directed therapies might improve the poor outcome of ETP ALL.

▶ There is always an immense sense of satisfaction in medicine and science when an enigmatic disease with a poor outcome is understood in a new light that in turn can be used to test a new approach to treatment. Early T-cell precursor acute lymphoblastic leukemia (ALL) was defined primarily by its immunophenotypic antigen expression pattern and poor outcome with conventional ALL-directed therapy. Using genomic approaches to better under this acute leukemia, these authors identify a group of activating mutations in genes that are primarily involved in normal and malignant hematopoietic myeloid development. They observe mutations in genes such as *NRAS*, *KRAS*, *FLT3*, *JAK3*, *SH2B3*, and *BRAF* as well as *GATA3*, *ETV6*, *RUNX1*, *IKZF1*, and *EP300*. In addition, mutations in chromatin remodeling enzymes such as EZH2, EED, SUZ12, SETD2, and EP300 are identified. Taken together, the mutational pattern resembles that of acute myelocytic leukemia (AML) rather than ALL, suggesting that AML-directed chemotherapeutic regimens might be more effective in this distinct leukemia. The clinical testing will be especially interesting to watch develop.

R. J. Arceci, MD, PhD

TP53 **alterations in acute myeloid leukemia with complex karyotype correlate with specific copy number alterations, monosomal karyotype, and dismal outcome**

Rücker FG, Schlenk RF, Bullinger L, et al (Univ Hosp of Ulm, Germany; et al)
Blood 119:2114-2121, 2012

To assess the frequency of *TP53* alterations and their correlation with other genetic changes and outcome in acute myeloid leukemia with complex karyotype (CK-AML), we performed integrative analysis using *TP53* mutational screening and array-based genomic profiling in 234 CKAMLs. *TP53* mutations were found in 141 of 234 (60%) and *TP53* losses were identified in 94 of 234 (40%) CK-AMLs; in total, 164 of 234 (70%) cases had *TP53* alterations. *TP53*-altered CK-AML were characterized by a higher degree of genomic complexity (aberrations per case, 14.30 vs 6.16; $P < .0001$) and by a higher frequency of specific copy number alterations, such as −5/5q−,−7/7q−,−16/16q−, −18/18q−, +1/+1p, and +11/+11q/ amp11q13∼25; among CK-AMLs, *TP53*-altered more frequently exhibited a monosomal karyotype (MK). Patients with *TP53* alterations were older and had significantly lower complete remission rates, inferior event-free, relapse-free, and overall survival. In multivariable analysis for overall survival, *TP53* alterations, white blood cell counts, and age were the only significant factors. In conclusion, *TP53* is the most frequently known altered gene in CK-AML. *TP53* alterations are associated with older age, genomic complexity, specific DNA copy number alterations, MK, and dismal outcome. In multivariable analysis, *TP53* alteration is the most important prognostic factor in CK-AML, outweighing all other variables, including the MK category.

▶ One of the first findings that arose from The Cancer Genome Project was that the most common mutation observed was not surprisingly that involving the tumor suppressor *TP53*, which has major roles in DNA damage responses and cell cycle control. Initial estimates showed less than 30% mutation frequency of *TP53* in acute myeloid leukemia (AML). However, a more detailed examination, as reported by Rucker et al, has refined this mutational frequency and which subtype of AML is most affected. Using mutational screening and array-based approaches, they identified *TP53* mutations and *TP53* losses in 60% and 40%, respectively, of AML characterized by a complex karyotype. Of further importance is that age, white blood cell count, and *TP53* status were all independent variables in predicting a poor prognosis. It remains unclear how alterations in *TP53* are directly linked to this subclass of AML. In addition, as Goethe has written, "Knowing is not enough ... we must do." Unfortunately, in this instance, knowing about the *TP53* status does not lead one to a selective therapeutic approach. Targeting *TP53* dysfunction therapeutically has been more difficult than identifying its alterations.

R. J. Arceci, MD, PhD

A phase 1/2 study of chemosensitization with the CXCR4 antagonist plerixafor in relapsed or refractory acute myeloid leukemia

Uy GL, Rettig MP, Motabi IH, et al (Washington Univ School of Medicine, St Louis, MO)

Blood 119:3917-3924, 2012

The interaction of acute myeloid leukemia (AML) blasts with the leukemic microenvironment is postulated to be an important mediator of resistance to chemotherapy and disease relapse. We hypothesized that inhibition of the CXCR4/CXCL12 axis by the small molecule inhibitor, plerixafor, would disrupt the interaction of leukemic blasts with the environment and increase the sensitivity of AML blasts to chemotherapy. In this phase 1/2 study, 52 patients with relapsed or refractory AML were treated with plerixafor in combination with mitoxantrone, etoposide, and cytarabine. In phase 1, plerixafor was escalated to a maximum of 0.24 mg/kg/d without any dose-limiting toxicities. In phase 2, 46 patients were treated with plerixafor 0.24 mg/kg/d in combination with chemotherapy with an overall complete remission and complete remission with incomplete blood count recovery rate (CR + CRi) of 46%. Correlative studies demonstrated a 2-fold mobilization in leukemic blasts into the peripheral circulation. No evidence of symptomatic hyperleukocytosis or delayed count recovery was observed with the addition of plerixafor. We conclude that the addition of plerixafor to cytotoxic chemotherapy is feasible in AML, and results in encouraging rates of remission with correlative studies demonstrating in vivo evidence of disruption of the CXCR4/CXCL12 axis. This study was registered at www.clinicaltrials.gov, no. NCT00512252.

▶ The importance of the microenvironment in the progression of cancers or their resistance to chemotherapy is becoming increasingly evident through a large number of experimental systems. Some of these data are now also being tested in clinical trials. The report by Uy et al represents one such attempt by describing the use of the CXCR4 (a chemokine receptor) antagonist, plerixafor, to mobilize acute myelogenous leukemia (AML) blasts from the bone marrow to the peripheral blood where they might be more sensitive to chemotherapy than when in the bone marrow and partially protected by that microenvironmental niche. CXCR4 is one of several key receptors that mediate adhesion of leukemic blasts to bone marrow stromal cells; preclinical data have shown that the inhibition of the interaction of CXCR4 with its ligand, CXCL12, induces release of stem cells from the bone marrow as well as generates a pro-apoptotic effect. Of note, plerixafor has been approved by the US Food and Drug Administration in combination with granulocyte colony-stimulating factor to mobilize hematopoietic stem cells for autologous, hematopoietic stem cell harvesting. The results of the phase I portion of the Uy et al report show that a maximum of 0.24 mg/kg/d of plerixafor in combination with chemotherapy resulted in no dose-limiting toxicities. Although this maximum dose tested was the dose established in phase III studies of stem cell mobilization, it is unfortunate that in this phase I trial, more of an attempt was not made to optimize the dose for leukemic cell mobilization, even with the observed variation among different patients. The phase II part of the trial then tested this dose of plerixafor in combination with chemotherapy in 52 patients with relapsed or refractory AML. A 46% complete remission or complete remission without full hematopoietic recovery was observed along with approximately a 2-fold mobilization in leukemic blasts into the peripheral circulation. Is this a result that might have been achieved with chemotherapy alone? Unfortunately, the opportunity to perform even a "pick the winner" randomized phase II trial was not done. In an era of decreasing funding and increasing needs, all efforts should be directed toward obtaining as much information as possible from early-phase clinical trials. Conventional single-arm phase II trials are certainly useful, but opportunities for squeezing more information from them should be a growing expectation.

R. J. Arceci, MD, PhD

Acute leukemia incidence and patient survival among children and adults in the United States, 2001-2007

Dores GM, Devesa SS, Curtis RE, et al (Dept of Veterans Affairs Med Ctr, OK; Natl Cancer Inst, Bethesda, MD)

Blood 119:34-43, 2012

Since 2001, the World Health Organization classification for hematopoietic and lymphoid neoplasms has provided a framework for defining acute leukemia (AL) subtypes, although few population-based studies have assessed incidence patterns and patient survival accordingly. We assessed

AL incidence rates (IRs), IR ratios (IRRs), and relative survival in the United States (2001-2007) in one of the first population-based, comprehensive assessments. Most subtypes of acute myeloid leukemia (AML) and acute lymphoblastic leukemia/lymphoma (ALL/L) predominated among males, from twice higher incidence of T-cell ALL/L among males than among females (IRR = 2.20) to nearly equal IRs of acute promyelocytic leukemia (APL; IRR = 1.08). Compared with non-Hispanic whites, Hispanics had significantly higher incidence of B-cell ALL/L (IRR = 1.64) and APL (IRR = 1.28); blacks had lower IRs of nearly all AL subtypes. All ALL/L but only some AML subtypes were associated with a bimodal age pattern. Among AML subtypes, survival was highest for APL and AML with inv(16). B-cell ALL/L had more favorable survival than T-cell ALL/L among the young; the converse occurred at older ages. Limitations of cancer registry data must be acknowledged, but the distinct AL incidence and survival patterns based on the World Health Organization classification support biologic diversity that should facilitate etiologic discovery, prognostication, and treatment advances.

▶ Although reporting outcomes for patients with cancer based on clinical trials suffers from the bias and lack of acknowledgment of what happens to patients not treated in those trials, population-based registries should provide a more global view of outcomes for patients with a particular cancer type. To this end, these authors report on the incidence and survival of children and adults with acute leukemia in the United States from 2001 to 2007. Consistent with the report (reviewed in this edition) by Hunger et al[1] on the outcomes of patients treated in Children's Oncology Group trials, the population-based study shows an overall inferior outcome for infants with acute lymphoblastic leukemia (ALL). However, unlike reports from pediatric cooperative groups or other consortia trials, these authors report that patients with B-cell ALL had a more favorable outcome than those with T-cell ALL. Does this reflect those patients who are not treated in such clinical trials? Other key points of this analysis are that Hispanics had a higher incidence of B-cell ALL and acute promyelocytic leukemia. Why is this? Such survey or epidemiological reports suffer profoundly from their lack of disease mechanism insights, but they surely can shine a spotlight on the questions that others can try to unravel biologically.

R. J. Arceci, MD, PhD

Reference

1. Hunger SP, Lu X, Devidas M, et al. Improved survival for children and adolescents with acute lymphoblastic leukemia between 1990 and 2005: a report from the children's oncology group. *J Clin Oncol.* 2012;30:1663-1669.

Age-Related Prognostic Impact of Different Types of *DNMT3A* Mutations in Adults With Primary Cytogenetically Normal Acute Myeloid Leukemia

Marcucci G, Metzeler KH, Schwind S, et al (The Ohio State Univ Comprehensive Cancer Ctr, Columbus; et al)

J Clin Oncol 30:742-750, 2012

Purpose.—To determine the frequency of *DNMT3A* mutations, their associations with clinical and molecular characteristics and outcome, and the associated gene- and microRNA-expression signatures in primary cytogenetically normal acute myeloid leukemia (CN-AML).

Patients and Methods.—Four hundred fifteen previously untreated adults were analyzed for *DNMT3A* mutations and established prognostic gene mutations and expression markers. Gene- and microRNA-expression profiles were derived using microarrays.

Results.—Younger (< 60 years; n = 181) and older (≥ 60 years; n = 234) patients had similar frequencies of DNMT3A mutations (35.3% *v* 33.3%). Missense mutations affecting arginine codon 882 (R882-*DNMT3A*) were more common (n = 92; 62%) than those affecting other codons (non–R882-*DNMT3A*). *DNMT3A*-mutated patients did not differ regarding complete remission rate, but had shorter disease-free survival (DFS; *P* =.03) and, by trend, overall survival (OS; *P* =.07) than *DNMT3A*–wild-type patients. In multivariable analyses, *DNMT3A* mutations remained associated with shorter DFS (*P* =.01), but not with shorter OS. When analyzed separately, the two *DNMT3A* mutation types had different significance by age group. Younger patients with non–R882-*DNMT3A* mutations had shorter DFS (*P* =.002) and OS (*P* =.02), whereas older patients with R882-*DNMT3A* mutations had shorter DFS (*P* =.005) and OS (*P* =.002) after adjustment for other clinical and molecular prognosticators. Gene- and microRNA-expression signatures did not accurately predict *DNMT3A* mutational status.

Conclusion.—*DNMT3A* mutations are frequent in CN-AML, and their clinical significance seems to be age dependent. *DNMT3A*-R882 mutations are associated with adverse prognosis in older patients, and non–R882-*DNMT3A* mutations are associated with adverse prognosis in younger patients. Low accuracy of gene- and microRNA-expression signatures in predicting *DNMT3A* mutation status suggested that the role of these mutations in AML remains to be elucidated.

▶ As Juliet appealed to Romeo in Shakespeare's immortal play "What's in a name? That which we call a rose by any other name would smell as sweet," the same may not necessarily be true of gene mutations. Numerous examples are emerging in which specific sites of mutations within the same gene manifest important differences in function and impact on clinical outcomes. Although this may not be surprising to the biochemist, to the clinician and patient, such information can be exceedingly important. These authors thus examine different types of mutations in *DMNT3A* in adults with acute myeloid leukemia and assess their association with outcome. They show that *R882-DN MT3A* mutations are associated with a longer disease-free survival (DFS) in younger patients, whereas they are associated with a shorter DFS in older patients. Gene and microRNA expression patterns did not predict *DNMT3A* mutational status. Unfortunately, no explanation is provided for such potentially interesting results. Alternatively, without validation in separate cohorts, one might also conclude that such information is too preliminary to base future functional studies or modeling.

R. J. Arceci, MD, PhD

Assessment of *BCR-ABL1* Transcript Levels at 3 Months Is the Only Requirement for Predicting Outcome for Patients With Chronic Myeloid Leukemia Treated With Tyrosine Kinase Inhibitors

Marin D, Ibrahim AR, Lucas C, et al (Hammersmith Hosp, London, UK; Royal Liverpool Univ Hosp, UK)

J Clin Oncol 30:232-238, 2012

Purpose.—We studied *BCR-ABL1* transcript levels in patients with chronic myeloid leukemia in chronic phase (CML-CP) at 3, 6, and 12 months after starting imatinib to identify molecular milestones that would predict for overall survival (OS) and other outcomes more reliably than serial marrow cytogenetics.

Patients and Methods.—We analyzed 282 patients with CML-CP who received imatinib 400 mg/d as first-line therapy followed by dasatinib or nilotinib if treatment with imatinib failed. We used a receiver operating characteristic curve to identify the cutoffs in transcript levels at 3, 6, and 12 months that would best predict patient outcome. We validated our findings in an independent cohort of 95 patients treated elsewhere.

Results.—Patients with transcript levels of more than 9.84% (n = 68) at 3 months had significantly lower 8-year probabilities of OS (56.9% *v* 93.3%; *P* < .001), progression-free survival, cumulative incidence of complete cytogenetic response, and complete molecular response than those with higher transcript levels. Similarly, transcript levels of more than 1.67% (n = 87) at 6 months and more than 0.53% (n = 93) at 12 months identified high-risk patients. However, transcript levels at 3 months were the most strongly predictive for the various outcomes. When we compared OS for the groups defined molecularly at 6 and 12 months with the usual cytogenetic milestones, categorization by transcript numbers was the only independent predictor for OS (relative risk, 0.207; *P* < .001 and relative risk, 0.158; *P* < .001, respectively).

Conclusion.—A single measurement of *BCR-ABL1* transcripts performed at 3 months is the best way to identify patients destined to fare poorly, thereby allowing early clinical intervention.

▶ That early response to therapy is good in patients with cancer has often been an accepted mantra in oncology. It is of interest that other published models, however, would suggest the opposite in that slow responses might be expected if therapies were really targeting cancer stem cells. The truth may more likely lie somewhere in the middle, depending on the type of cancer. For chronic myeloid leukemia, several studies dating back more than 6 years ago have reported data that documents early molecular responses are predictive of long-term outcomes. So now Marin et al publish additional data that essentially confirm previous studies. Why another study? One aspect of their report is that they used a standardized polymerase chain reaction assessment of *BCR-ABL* fusion transcripts, determined a value of 9.84% fusion transcripts following 3 months of imatinib therapy is a key cutoff value that separates poor from good outcomes, and validated their cutoff in a smaller, but independent cohort. The 9.84% is clearly a statistically derived cutoff of data that are continuous in character. So if early response continues to be repetitively reported to be a good predictor of outcome, why have standards of practice not been changed? What should the oncologist do for patients who have a good or poor 3-month response? If this is the only measurement that matters, why are patients having additional monitoring done before 3 months? If other TK inhibitors produce more rapid responses in more patients, why would a patient be treated with imatinib? Unfortunately, the rate and frequency of publishing reports can sometimes predict inversely the rate of change regarding standards of practice.

R. J. Arceci, MD, PhD

Chronic myeloid leukemia stem cells are not dependent on Bcr-Abl kinase activity for their survival

Hamilton A, Helgason GV, Schemionek M, et al (Univ of Glasgow, UK; Univ of Münster, Germany; et al)

Blood 119:1501-1510, 2012

Recent evidence suggests chronic myeloid leukemia (CML) stem cells are insensitive to kinase inhibitors and responsible for minimal residual disease in treated patients. We investigated whether CML stem cells, in a transgenic mouse model of CML-like disease or derived from patients, are dependent on Bcr-Abl. In the transgenic model, after retransplantation, donor-derived CML stem cells in which Bcr-Abl expression had been induced and subsequently shut off were able to persist in vivo and reinitiate leukemia in secondary recipients on Bcr-Abl reexpression. Bcr-Abl knockdown in human CD34$^+$ CML cells cultured for 12 days in physiologic growth factors achieved partial inhibition of Bcr-Abl and downstream targets p-CrkL and p-STAT5, inhibition of proliferation and colony forming cells, but no reduction of input cells. The addition of dasatinib further inhibited p-CrkL and p-STAT5, yet only reduced input cells by 50%. Complete growth factor withdrawal plus dasatinib further reduced input cells to 10%; however, the surviving fraction was enriched for primitive leukemic cells capable of growth in a long-term culture-initiating cell assay and expansion on removal of dasatinib and addition of growth factors. Together, these data suggest that CML stem cell survival is Bcr-Abl kinase independent and suggest curative approaches in CML must focus on kinase-independent mechanisms of resistance.

▶ The potential differences between cancer stem cells compared with their offspring have been proposed as one of the primary reasons why many treatments for cancer ultimately fail. But this can be a tricky business because studying stem cells can be difficult based on their often low frequency as well as how best to define their biological characteristics. Thus, preclinical animal models might be useful in helping to better define this population of cells. Chronic myeloid leukemia (CML) has been the preeminent example of targeted therapy of a primal genetic lesion (ie, the BCR-ABL translocation that produces the characteristic fusion kinase). Nevertheless, it remains unclear whether the molecular remissions obtained with BCR-ABL kinase inhibitors result in cures. There is some evidence that a BCR-ABL—negative CML stem cell exists that avoids the inhibitor effects of targeted inhibitors. Hamilton et al thus use a mouse model of BCR-ABL—driven CML in which the expression of BCR-ABL can be turned off. Using this model, the authors demonstrate that the BCR-ABL—negative stem cells were capable of reinitiating CML. Extending the studies to human CML cells, they observed that treatment with BCR-ABL inhibitors (eg, dasatinib) along with growth factor depletion was able to significantly reduce the number of leukemic cells capable of subsequent long term culture-initiating expansion on removal of dasatinib and addition of growth factors demonstrated that the CML stem cells survive in the absence of BCR-ABL activity. Although one can certainly argue that such animal models and in vitro studies are artificial, they do raise the important issue that alternative treatment approaches other than kinase inhibition may be essential for eradicating CML without using hematopoietic stem cell transplantation.

R. J. Arceci, MD, PhD

***DNMT3A* mutations in acute myeloid leukemia: stability during disease evolution and clinical implications**

Hou H-A, Kuo Y-Y, Liu C-Y, et al (Natl Taiwan Univ Hosp, Taipei; Natl Taipei College of Nursing, Taiwan; et al)

Blood 119:559-568, 2012

DNMT3A mutations are associated with poor prognosis in acute myeloid leukemia (AML), but the stability of this mutation during the clinical course remains unclear. In the present study of 500 patients with de novo AML, *DNMT3A* mutations were identified in 14% of total patients and in 22.9% of AML patients with normal karyotype. *DNMT3A* mutations were positively associated with older age, higher WBC and platelet counts, intermediate-risk and normal cytogenetics, *FLT3* internal tandem duplication, and *NPM1*, *PTPN11*, and *IDH2* mutations, but were negatively associated with *CEBPA* mutations. Multivariate analysis demonstrated that the *DNMT3A* mutation was an independent poor prognostic factor for overall survival and relapse-free survival in total patients and also in normokaryotype group. A scoring system incorporating the *DNMT3A* mutation and 8 other prognostic factors, including age, WBC count, cytogenetics, and gene mutations, into survival analysis was very useful in stratifying AML patients into different prognostic groups (*P* < .001). Sequential study of 138 patients during the clinical course showed that *DNMT3A* mutations were stable during AML evolution. In conclusion, *DNMT3A* mutations are associated with distinct clinical and biologic features and poor prognosis in de novo AML patients. Furthermore, the *DNMT3A* mutation may be a potential biomarker for monitoring of minimal residual disease.

▶ Risk stratification in patients with acute myeloid leukemia (AML) has taken on increasing levels of scientific sophistication with the inclusion of molecular markers along with traditional clinical and cytogenetic characteristics. The initial identification of mutations involving DNMT3A opened up a new class of molecules that could be involved in AML pathogenesis and behavior. Subsequent to the initial reporting of DNMT3A mutations, a series of articles followed with conflicting data on the molecular consequences and clinical outcomes. Of note, DNMT3A mutations are extremely rare in children compared with adults. The report by Hou et al examines multiple conventional and molecular characteristics leading to the conclusion that DNMT3A mutations show increased frequency with age, are independent predictors of poor prognosis, and are persistent from diagnosis to relapse, making them potentially useful in the detection of minimal residual disease. Unfortunately, this report also fails to validate the key findings in an independent cohort, again leaving open the all too likely possibility that such data end up not being confirmed or never being incorporated into clinical practice. Finally, while such information helps to possibly refine risk stratification, the data do not directly lead to the definition of risk groups whose AML biology can be therapeutically targeted.

R. J. Arceci, MD, PhD

Frequency and prognostic impact of mutations in *SRSF2, U2AF1,* and *ZRSR2* in patients with myelodysplastic syndromes

Thol F, Kade S, Schlarmann C, et al (Hannover Med School, Germany; et al)

Blood 119:3578-3584, 2012

Mutations in genes of the splicing machinery have been described recently in myelodysplastic syndromes (MDS). In the present study, we examined a cohort of 193 MDS patients for mutations in *SRSF2, U2AF1* (synonym *U2AF35*), *ZRSR2*, and, as described previously, *SF3B1*, in the context of other molecular markers, including mutations in *ASXL1, RUNX1, NRAS, TP53, IDH1, IDH2, NPM1*, and *DNMT3A*. Mutations in *SRSF2, U2AF1, ZRSR2*, and *SF3B1* were found in 24 (12.4%), 14 (7.3%), 6 (3.1%), and 28 (14.5%) patients, respectively, corresponding to a total of 67 of 193 MDS patients (34.7%). *SRSF2* mutations were associated with *RUNX1* (*P* < .001) and IDH1 (*P* =.013) mutations, whereas *U2AF1* mutations were associated with *ASXL1* (*P* =.005) and *DNMT3A* (*P* =.004) mutations. In univariate analysis, mutated *SRSF2* predicted shorter overall survival and more frequent acute myeloid leukemia progression compared with wild type *SRSF2*, whereas mutated *U2AF1*, *ZRSR2*, and *SF3B1* had no impact on patient outcome. In multivariate analysis, *SRSF2* remained an independent poor risk marker for overall survival (hazard ratio = 2.3; 95% confidence interval, 1.28-4.13; $P = .017$) and acute myeloid leukemia progression (hazard ratio = 2.83; 95% confidence interval, 1.31-6.12; $P = .008$). These results show a negative prognostic impact of *SRSF2* mutations in MDS. *SRSF2* mutations may become useful for clinical risk stratification and treatment decisions in the future.

▶ A criticism often tossed at genomic sequencing projects is that they represent a large investment of resources but have not produced substantial additional gene mutations than were already known in various cancers. Dr Sidney Brenner has reputedly characterized such studies as "Low input, high throughput, no output." Nevertheless, some of the astonishing exceptions and successes have opened up entirely new areas of understanding of cancer and started to provide several novel therapeutic approaches. One such exception was the initial identification of mutations in spliceosome proteins in myelodysplastic syndromes (MDS) by several investigators. Aberrant splicing of precursor RNAs has been known for many years, but the identification of spliceosome machinery mutations began to potentially shed light on this mysterious phenomenon. In this article, data are presented that convincingly link mutations in splicing factor 3B subunit 1 (*SF3B1*) as an independent prognostic factor to outcome of patients with MDS as well as overall survival. Although mutations were observed in *U2AF1*, *ZRSR2*, and *SF3B1* splicing factors, they appeared to have an obvious impact on patient outcome. Nevertheless, the lack of influence on prognosis should not lead to the conclusion that such mutations do not have an impact on the biology of leukemia and still may represent important pathways for therapeutic targeting. A rewriting of the Brenner mantra might instead read: "Focused input, high throughput, surprising output."

R. J. Arceci, MD, PhD

Increased BMI correlates with higher risk of disease relapse and differentiation syndrome in patients with acute promyelocytic leukemia treated with the AIDA protocols

Breccia M, Mazzarella L, Bagnardi V, et al (Sapienza Univ, Rome, Italy; European Inst of Oncology, Milan, Italy; et al)

Blood 119:49-54, 2012

We investigated whether body mass index (BMI) correlates with distinct outcomes in newly diagnosed acute promyelocytic leukemia (APL). The study population included 144 patients with newly diagnosed and genetically confirmed APL consecutively treated at a single institution. All patients received All-*trans* retinoic acid and idarubicin according to the GIMEMA protocols AIDA-0493 and AIDA-2000. Outcome estimates according to the BMI were carried out together with multivariable analysis for the risk of relapse and differentiation syndrome. Fifty-four (37.5%) were under/normal weight (BMI < 25), whereas 90 (62.5%) patients were overweight/obese (BMI ≥ 25). An increased BMI was associated with older age ($P < .0001$) and male sex ($P = .02$). BMI was the most powerful predictor of differentiation syndrome in multivariable analysis (odds ratio = 7.24; 95% CI, 1.50-34; $P = .014$). After a median follow-up of 6 years, the estimated cumulative incidence of relapse at 5 years was 31.6% (95% CI, 22.7%-43.8%) in overweight/obese and 11.2% (95% CI, 5.3%-23.8%) in underweight/normal weight patients ($P = .029$). Multivariable analysis showed that BMI was an independent predictor of relapse (hazard ratio = 2.45, 95% CI, 1.00-5.99, in overweight/obese vs under/normal weight patients, $P = .049$). An increased BMI at diagnosis is associated with a higher risk of developing differentiation syndrome and disease relapse in APL patients treated with AIDA protocols.

▶ Obesity has been linked to increased risk of cardiovascular disease, diabetes, and more recently to cancer. The association of obesity in patients with cancer has been more controversial. In addition, very few data exist regarding the possible reasons for outcome differences when they are reported for obese patients with cancer. This article examines the issue of obesity in a cohort of patients with acute promyelocytic leukemia (APL) from a single institution and treated on 1 of 2 GIMEMA protocols. A significant increased frequency in differentiation syndrome associated with All-*trans* retinoic acid as well as an increased risk of relapse are shown to be independently predicted in the obese group of patients (ie, those with a body mass index greater than 25) (see Fig 2 in the original article). Although these are important associations, there are no biological studies included that would help us understand these associations or a clear path to addressing the consequences of being obese and having APL. Unfortunately, we live in an age of multiple publications rather than definitive narratives. However, these authors have defined a problem and we can hope another report will address the underlying reasons and solutions.

R. J. Arceci, MD, PhD

Outcomes after matched unrelated donor versus identical sibling hematopoietic cell transplantation in adults with acute myelogenous leukemia

Saber W, Opie S, Rizzo JD, et al (Ctr for International Blood and Marrow Transplant Res, Milwaukee, WI; Banner Blood and Marrow Transplant Program, Phoenix, AZ; et al)

Blood 119:3908-3916, 2012

Approximately one-third of patients with an indication for hematopoietic cell transplantation (HCT) have an HLA-matched related donor (MRD) available to them. For the remaining patients, a matched unrelated donor (MUD) is an alternative. Prior studies comparing MRD and MUD HCT provide conflicting results, and the relative efficacy of MRD and MUD transplantation is an area of active investigation. To address this issue, we analyzed outcomes of 2223 adult acute myelogenous leukemia patients who underwent allogeneic HCT between 2002 and 2006 (MRD, n = 624; 8/8 HLA locus matched MUD, n = 1193; 7/8 MUD, n = 406). The 100-day cumulative incidence of grades B-D acute GVHD was significantly lower in MRD HCT recipients than in 8/8 MUD and 7/8 MUD HCT recipients (33%, 51%, and 53%, respectively; $P < .001$). In multivariate analysis, 8/8 MUD HCT recipients had a similar survival rate compared with MRD HCT recipients (relative risk [RR], 1.03; $P = .62$). 7/8 MUD HCT recipients had higher early mortality than MRD HCT recipients (RR, 1.40; $P < .001$), but beyond 6 months after HCT, their survival rates were similar (RR, 0.88; $P = .30$). These results suggest that transplantation from MUD and MRD donors results in similar survival times for patients with acute myelogenous leukemia.

▶ Although there is little question that hematopoietic stem cell transplantation has saved many lives, this area of study remains clouded by the lack of randomized, prospective trials. All doctors think they're the best, but what is possibly less appreciated is that every transplant doctor knows the approach he or she uses to transplant is the best. Thus, few definitive, prospective, randomized trials have been performed. Instead, we are left with often retrospective registry studies or single or multiple institutional surveys of outcomes. These authors present 1 of the latter-type studies with the intent to compare outcomes of matched unrelated donor versus identical sibling hematopoietic transplants for adults with acute myelogenous leukemia. They conclude that while the frequency of graft-versus-host disease (GVHD) is more common in the matched unrelated donor (MUD) compared to HLA-matched related donor (MRD), overall survival percentages were similar. Not surprising, single mismatched MUD transplants had a higher early mortality than MRD recipients. It is also worth noting that the MRD, fully matched, unrelated donor cohorts and single mismatched, unrelated donor cohorts have significant differences in the distribution of various characteristics, including acute myelogenous leukemia of different flavors (ie, primary refractory, those in complete remission 1, or complete remission 2, or first relapse or with missing information). One does have to ask the question as to why such reports continue to be published and whether they have an impact on current standards of care. In fact, the field of transplantation has moved on from these types of transplants to a variety of other types of donors, including haploidentical or cord blood (single or double) as well as alternative preparative regimens and GVHD prophylaxis. Although not addressed in this article, the authors do make an important point in that with higher morbidity associated with GVHD linked to MUD transplants, there may be critical cost and societal consequences that should be considered. Information on that issue would have made the article potentially novel.

R. J. Arceci, MD, PhD

Pediatric-inspired intensified therapy of adult T-ALL reveals the favorable outcome of *NOTCH1/FBXW7* mutations, but not of low *ERG/BAALC* expression: a GRAALL study

Ben Abdelali R, for the Group for Research on Adult Acute Lymphoblastic Leukemia (Université Paris 5 Descartes, France; et al)

Blood 118:5099-5107, 2011

Despite recent progress in the understanding of acute lymphoblastic leukemia (T-ALL) oncogenesis, few markers are sufficiently frequent in large subgroups to allow their use in therapeutic stratification. Low *ERG* and *BAALC* expression (*E/B*^{low}) and *NOTCH1/FBXW7 (N/F)* mutations have been proposed as powerful prognostic markers in large cohorts of adult T-ALL. We therefore compared the predictive prognostic value of *N/F* mutations versus *E/B*^{low} in 232 adult T-ALLs enrolled in the LALA-94 and Group for Research on Adult Acute Lymphoblastic Leukemia (GRAALL) protocols. The outcome of T-ALLs treated in the pediatric-inspired GRAALL trials was significantly superior to the LALA-94 trial. Overall, 43% and 69% of adult T-ALL patients were classified as *E/B*^{low} and *N/F* mutated, respectively. Strikingly, the good prognosis of *N/F* mutated patients was stronger in more intensively treated, pediatric-inspired GRAALL patients. The *E/B* expression level did not influence the prognosis in any subgroup. *N/F* mutation status and the GRAALL trial were the only 2 independent factors that correlated with longer overall survival by multivariate analysis. This study demonstrates that the *N/F* mutational status and treatment protocol are major outcome determinants for adults with T-ALL, the benefit of pediatric inspired protocols being essentially restricted to the *N/F* mutated subgroup.

▶ A debate, not always data driven, as to whether pediatric-directed versus adult-directed trials for hematological malignancies are more effective has slowly been resolving with increased numbers of comparative trials, although few are prospective or randomized. The reluctance to simply apply pediatric trials to adults with acute myeloid leukemia or acute lymphoblastic leukemia (ALL) has in part been due to legitimate concerns that the often more intensive pediatric-directed regimens might not be as well tolerated in older patients. These authors report a twist on this debate by examining outcomes of adult patients with T-ALL treated on the adult-inspired LALA-94 (Leucémie Aigüe Lymphoblastique de l'Adulte) trial versus the pediatric-inspired Group for Research on Adult Acute Lymphoblastic Leukemia (GRAALL) trials. They ask the additional question as to whether different molecularly defined T-ALL subtypes show differential responses to the 2 types of therapeutic approaches. They show that the GRAALL treatment regimens result in a significantly improved outcome only for patients with *NOTCH1/FBXW7* mutations, but not with low *ERG* and *BAALC* expression (see Fig 3 in the original article). Thus, not surprisingly, one size does not fit all, especially when important biological heterogeneity exists. Despite the possible critique that there were more high-risk patients (ie, those with significantly higher presenting white blood cell counts) in the LALA-treated cohort, these results demonstrate the important conclusion that retrospective, subgroup analysis can lead to potentially important outcome predictions. Whether the data presented in this article are sufficiently robust to change what oncologists do in practice remains to be seen.

R. J. Arceci, MD, PhD

Poor response to second-line kinase inhibitors in chronic myeloid leukemia patients with multiple low-level mutations, irrespective of their resistance profile

Parker WT, Ho M, Scott HS, et al (Centre for Cancer Biology, Adelaide, Australia; et al)

Blood 119:2234-2238, 2012

Specific imatinib-resistant *BCR-ABL1* mutations (Y253H, E255K/V, T315I, F317L, and F359V/C) predict failure of second-line nilotinib or dasatinib therapy in patients with chronic myeloid leukemia; however, such therapy also fails in approximately 40% of patients in the chronic phase of this disease who do not have these resistant mutations. We investigated whether sensitive mutation analysis could identify other poor-risk subgroups. Analysis was performed by direct sequencing and sensitive mass spectrometry on 220 imatinib-resistant patients before they began nilotinib or dasatinib therapy. Patients with resistant mutations by either method (n = 45) were excluded because inferior response was known. Of the remaining 175 patients, 19% had multiple mutations by mass spectrometry versus 9% by sequencing. Compared with 0 or 1 mutation, the presence of multiple mutations was associated with lower rates of complete cytogenetic response (50% vs 21%, $P = .003$) and major molecular response (31% vs 6%, $P = .005$) and a higher rate of new resistant mutations (25% vs 56%, $P = .0009$). Sensitive mutation analysis identified a poor-risk subgroup (15.5% of all patients) with multiple mutations not identified by standard screening.

▶ It is often said that the truth lies in the method. This could not be more accurate than the data presented by Parker et al. They compared a multiplex mass spectrophotometric approach to mutational analysis with traditional nucleic acid sequencing and were able to identify 15.5% of patients with chronic phase chronic myelogenous leukemia (CML) as having multiple mutations and an associated lower rate of complete cytogenetic (50% compared with 21%) and major molecular (31% vs 6%) response to specific tyrosine kinase inhibitors compared with 9% identified by conventional sequencing. These data also show a significant level of molecular heterogeneity in any particular patient's CML, even during chronic phase. If validated, this approach should potentially set a new standard for the de novo molecular diagnostics of patients with CML as well as help to direct which targeted therapy is more likely to be effective, thus reducing the risk of a more resistant clone emerging as well as saving time, money, and lives.

R. J. Arceci, MD, PhD

Prediction of Early Death After Induction Therapy for Newly Diagnosed Acute Myeloid Leukemia With Pretreatment Risk Scores: A Novel Paradigm for Treatment Assignment

Walter RB, Othus M, Borthakur G, et al (Fred Hutchinson Cancer Res Ctr, Seattle, WA; The Univ of Texas MD Anderson Cancer Ctr, Houston)
J Clin Oncol 29:4417-4423, 2011

Purpose.—Outcome in acute myeloid leukemia (AML) worsens with age, at least in part because of higher treatment-related mortality (TRM) in older patients. Eligibility for intensive AML treatment protocols is therefore typically based on age as the implied principal predictor of TRM, although other health- and disease-related factors modulate this age effect.

Patients and Methods.—We empirically defined TRM using estimated weekly hazard rates in 3,365 adults of all ages administered intensive chemotherapy for newly diagnosed AML. We used the area under the receiver operator characteristic curve (AUC) to quantify the relative effects of age and other covariates on TRM in a subset of 2,238 patients. In this approach, an AUC of 1.0 denotes perfect prediction, whereas an AUC of 0.5 is analogous to a coin flip.

Results.—Regardless of age, risk of death declined once 4 weeks had elapsed from treatment start, suggesting that patients who die during this time comprise a qualitatively distinct group. Performance status (PS) and age were the most important individual predictors of TRM (AUCs of 0.75 and 0.65, respectively). However, multicomponent models were significantly more accurate in predicting TRM (AUC of 0.83) than PS or age alone. Elimination of age from such multicomponent models only minimally affected their predictive accuracy (AUC of 0.82).

Conclusion.—These data suggest that age is primarily a surrogate for other covariates, which themselves add significantly to predictive accuracy, thus challenging the wisdom of using age as primary or sole basis for assignment of intensive, curative intent treatment in AML.

▶ Although it is against the law (at least in the United States) to discriminate against someone because of age, in practice this is well known to happen. Medicine appears to be no exception, as described in this article in which the authors report on the role of age along with other covariates in determining outcomes for adults with acute myeloid leukemia (AML). They compared 2 cohorts of patients—1 treated on Southwest Oncology Group (SWOG) protocols and the other on a variety of trials at MD Anderson Comprehensive Cancer Center (MDACCC). The median age was 57 (range 17 to 88) in the SWOG group and 61 years (range 14 to 89) in the MDACCC. Although their data for death in the first month of treatment from toxicities were associated with performance status and age, the omission of age from the multicomponent model only minimally affected the predictive accuracy for treatment-related mortality. The authors conclude that enrollment of patients should not be based on age alone (some clinical trials do in fact do this), but that the more complex model provides a more accurate predictive model for restricting enrollment. Nevertheless, the elephant in the room, as shown in Fig 1A of the original article, is that overall survival for older adults with AML remains dismal. Although age may not be the only answer, an alternative approach to this group of patients is sorely needed.

R. J. Arceci, MD, PhD

Prognostic and therapeutic implications of minimal residual disease detection in acute myeloid leukemia

Buccisano F, Maurillo L, Del Principe MI, et al (Fondazione Policlinico Tor Vergata, Rome, Italy; et al)

Blood 119:332-341, 2012

The choice of either induction or postremission therapy for adults with acute myeloid leukemia is still largely based on the "one size fits all" principle. Moreover, pretreatment prognostic parameters, especially chromosome and gene abnormalities, may fail in predicting individual patient outcome. Measurement of minimal residual disease (MRD) is nowadays recognized as a potential critical tool to assess the quality of response after chemotherapy and to plan postremission strategies that are, therefore, driven by the individual risk of relapse. PCR and multiparametric flow cytometry have become the most popular methods to investigate MRD because they have been established as sensitive and specific enough to allow MRD to be studied serially. In the present review, we examine the evidence supporting the appropriateness of incorporating MRD detection into the AML risk assessment process. A comprehensive prognostic algorithm, generated by combining pretreatment cytogenetics/genetics and posttreatment MRD determination, should promote advances in development of personalized therapeutic approaches.

▶ The role of minimal residual disease (MRD) and the "quality of remission" for predicting outcome in patients with leukemia has been a mantra for quite a few years. Certainly in childhood acute lymphocytic leukemia (ALL) as well as in acute promyelocytic leukemia (APL) in any age, MRD is being used to risk stratify patients and, in addition, direct post-remission therapy. What is less clear is how best to evaluate such interventions in any way other than comparing them to historical controls. Even "pick the winner" analytical approaches have not been rigorously tested to help determine the success of risk-stratified directed therapy. This leads one to ask why would one want to see another review on this subject rather than actually focusing on doing the experiment. Yet reviews such as the one by Buccisano et al continue to be written. At some level, it reminds one of when Peter Finch in the movie "Network" shouted the now infamous words: "I'm as mad as hell and I'm not gonna take this anymore." The review does clearly point out that having MRD after induction therapy for adults with acute myeloid leukemia (AML) is a poor prognostic factor predicting inferior outcomes, but even with the inclusion of other genetic and clinical information, the predictions of outcome are far from perfect in terms of any studied cohort and still unclear in terms of the predictability of outcome for any particular patient. The reference to the non-APL pediatric trial by Rubnitz et al[1] as "...a trial of prospective MRD-driven therapy has also been initiated in childhood non-M3 AML, demonstrating an improvement of outcome in high-risk patients," is again overly enthusiastic and a misinterpretation of the data in that report, which did not definitively test or show an improvement. In fact, the question needs to be "improvement compared to what?" Thus, Peter Finch's words continue to be prophetic. Let's stop talking about it and actually carry out some definitive clinical trials.

R. J. Arceci, MD, PhD

Reference

1. Rubnitz JE, Inaba H, Dahl G, et al. Minimal residual disease-directed therapy for childhood acute myeloid leukaemia: results of the AML02 multicentre trial. *Lancet Oncol.* 2010;11:543-552.

Prognostic Relevance of Integrated Genetic Profiling in Acute Myeloid Leukemia

Patel JP, Gönen M, Figueroa ME, et al (Memorial Sloan-Kettering Cancer Ctr, NY, Weill Cornell Med College, NY; et al)
N Engl J Med 366:1079-1089, 2012

Background.—Acute myeloid leukemia (AML) is a heterogeneous disease with respect to presentation and clinical outcome. The prognostic value of recently identified somatic mutations has not been systematically evaluated in a phase 3 trial of treatment for AML.

Methods.—We performed a mutational analysis of 18 genes in 398 patients younger than 60 years of age who had AML and who were randomly assigned to receive induction therapy with high-dose or standard-dose daunorubicin. We validated our prognostic findings in an independent set of 104 patients.

Results.—We identified at least one somatic alteration in 97.3% of the patients. We found that internal tandem duplication in *FLT3* (*FLT3*-ITD), partial tandem duplication in *MLL* (*MLL*-PTD), and mutations in *ASXL1* and *PHF6* were associated with reduced overall survival ($P = 0.001$ for *FLT3*-ITD, $P = 0.009$ for *MLL*-PTD, $P = 0.05$ for *ASXL1*, and $P = 0.006$ for *PHF6*); *CEBPA* and *IDH2* mutations were associated with improved overall survival ($P = 0.05$ for *CEBPA* and $P = 0.01$ for *IDH2*). The favorable effect of *NPM1* mutations was restricted to patients with co-occurring *NPM1* and *IDH1* or *IDH2* mutations. We identified genetic predictors of outcome that improved risk stratification among patients with AML, independently of age, white-cell count, induction dose, and post-remission therapy, and validated the significance of these predictors in an independent cohort. High-dose daunorubicin, as compared with standard-dose daunorubicin, improved the rate of survival among patients with *DNMT3A* or *NPM1* mutations or *MLL* translocations ($P = 0.001$) but not among patients with wild-type *DNMT3A*, *NPM1*, and *MLL* ($P = 0.67$).

Conclusions.—We found that *DNMT3A* and *NPM1* mutations and *MLL* translocations predicted an improved outcome with high-dose induction chemotherapy in patients with AML. These findings suggest that mutational profiling could potentially be used for risk stratification and to inform prognostic and therapeutic decisions regarding patients with AML. (Funded by the National Cancer Institute and others.)

► The current holy grail of cancer biology is to fully enumerate all molecular changes characterizing a patient's cancer and then direct effective therapy toward the integrated pathway analysis with specifically targeted agents. This may or may not be ever achieved. Nevertheless, the goal seems rational and potentially less phenomenological than the use of the same chemotherapeutic regimen for all patients, only some of whom are likely to respond. These authors have attempted to accomplish at least 1 aspect of this overall goal in their mutational analysis, although limited to only 18 genes, in patients younger than age 60 years with newly diagnosed acute myeloid leukemia (AML). They rediscover known associations of some mutations with outcomes and provide some new information on genes known to be mutated in AML but with less clear prognostic value. They also demonstrate that high-dose versus standard-dose chemotherapy results in an improved outcome in patients whose AML carries *DNMT3A* and *NPM1* mutations or *MLL* translocations. In this outcome measure, the probability values are large, but the difference in survival (approximately 44% vs 25%) remains dismal (see Fig 5 in the original article). The results are importantly validated in a separate, albeit smaller group, which is not compared in detail with the initial test group. Of course, with such a limited assessment of molecular profiling, one could argue that they are missing a great deal of critical information that could further influence their conclusions. Nevertheless, with further prospective validation, these data could turn out to be important. Time and more data will tell.

R. J. Arceci, MD, PhD

Lymphoma

Minimal Disseminated Disease in High-Risk Burkitt's Lymphoma Identifies Patients With Different Prognosis

Mussolin L, Pillon M, d'Amore ES, et al (Università di Padova, Italy; Ospedali Riuniti, Bergamo, Italy; Ospedale Regina Margherita, Torino, Italy; et al)

J Clin Oncol 29:1779-1784, 2011

Purpose.—To study minimal disseminated disease (MDD) in children with Burkitt's lymphoma (BL) and to determine its impact on prognosis.

Patients and Methods.—We established a simplified long-distance polymerase chain reaction (LD-PCR) assay that can amplify up to 15 to 20 Kb of DNA sequence, making it possible to detect the t(8;14) at the genomic level with sensitivity of 10^{-4}. We prospectively studied diagnostic biopsies and bone marrow aspirates from 134 patients affected by BL.

Results.—A specific LD-PCR product was detected in 96 (72%) of 134 BL biopsies. Among 84 patients with t(8;14) positivity on tumor biopsy and bone marrow (BM), 26 (31%) had LD-PCR–positive BM, and 15 (18%) were positive at standard morphologic analysis. Twenty (85%) of 26 MDD-positive patients belonged to the R4 risk group, according to Berlin-Frankfurt-Munster definition. The 3-year progression-free survival was 68% (SE, 10%) in MDD-positive patients in R4 compared with 93% (SE, 5%) in MDD-negative patients in R4 ($P = .03$). By multivariate analysis (including MDD, sex, lactate dehydrogenase, CNS involvement), only MDD was predictive of higher risk of failure (hazard ratio, 4.7; $P = .04$).

Conclusion.—MDD identifies a poor-prognosis subgroup among children with high-risk BL. To improve disease control in these patients, a more effective risk-adapted therapy, possibly including anti-CD20 monoclonal antibody, should be considered.

▶ The use of multiparameter flow immunophenotyping or molecular approaches to defining minimal residual disease in leukemia have been standards of practice in evaluating patients in terms of risk group stratification. Less information has been obtained in lymphomas, although those that have a propensity for dissemination, such as Burkitt lymphoma, are potentially important candidates for such studies. Mussolin et al report on the utilization of a polymerase chain reaction–based assessment of minimal residual, or as they define it, minimal disseminated disease (MDD), for patients with Burkitt lymphoma. Their data demonstrate that in a multivariate analysis, the presence of MDD in the bone marrow was predictive of a progression-free survival of 68% compared with 98% for those patients who did not have positive MDD in the bone marrow. Within patients with disseminated disease, the presence of MDD was a powerful adverse prognostic variable. However, a significant limitation of this study is the lack of a prospective or even retrospective validation group, which raises the question as to whether such studies should be published until additional validation is provided. Hopefully, a replication of these results can independently confirm their validity because of their potential important implications.

R. J. Arceci, MD, PhD

10 Thoracic Cancer

Biology

DNA Repair Capacity in Peripheral Lymphocytes Predicts Survival of Patients With Non–Small-Cell Lung Cancer Treated With First-Line Platinum-Based Chemotherapy

Wang L-E, Yin M, Dong Q, et al (The Univ of Texas MD Anderson Cancer Ctr, Houston)

J Clin Oncol 29:4121-4128, 2011

Purpose.—Platinum-based regimens are the standard chemotherapy for patients with advanced non–small-cell lung cancer (NSCLC). DNA repair capacity (DRC) in tumor cells plays an important role in resistance to platinum-based drugs. We have previously reported that efficient DRC, as assessed by an in vitro lymphocyte-based assay, was a determinant of poor survival in patients with NSCLC in a relatively small data set. In this larger independent study of 591 patients with NSCLC, we further evaluated whether DRC in peripheral lymphocytes predicts survival of patients with NSCLC who receive platinum based chemotherapy.

Patients and Methods.—All patients were recruited at The University of Texas MD Anderson Cancer Center and donated blood samples before the start of any chemotherapy. We measured DRC in cultured T lymphocytes by using the host-cell reactivation assay, and we assessed associations between DRC in peripheral lymphocytes and survival of patients with NSCLC who were treated with first-line platinum-based chemotherapy.

Results.—We found an inverse association between DRC in peripheral lymphocytes and patient survival. Compared with patients in the low tertile of DRC, patients with NSCLC in the high tertile of DRC had significantly worse overall and 3-year survival (adjusted hazard ratio [HR], 1.33; 95% CI, 1.04 to 1.71; P =.023; and HR, 1.35; 95% CI, 1.04 to 1.76; P =.025, respectively). This trend was more pronounced in patients with early-stage tumors, adenocarcinoma, or squamous cell carcinoma.

Conclusion.—We confirmed that DRC in peripheral lymphocytes is an independent predictor of survival for patients with NSCLC treated with platinum-based chemotherapy.

► DNA repair capacity in tumor cells has been studied heavily as a mechanism of resistance to the platinum agents in non–small-cell lung cancer (NSCLC).

This particular study sought to identify a predictive biomarker in patient blood samples and measured the DNA repair capacity in peripheral lymphocytes. In a large number (n = 591) of chemonaïve patients scheduled for platinum-based therapy, T lymphocytes were harvested and the DNA repair capacity measured using a host-cell reactivation assay. This assay was previously verified in a prior publication. Patients with the highest or most efficient DNA repair capacity in peripheral lymphocytes had a worse overall survival (hazard ratio, 1.35; *P* = .025). This is consistent with results from prior publications that reported high NSCLC tumor ERCC1 conferred resistance to platinum agents. This assay to assess peripheral lymphocyte DNA repair capacity is being developed further for potential clinical use. Overall, this trial and the body of literature support the role of DNA repair pathways, specifically nucleotide excision repair in platinum resistance.

A. S. Tsao, MD

Genetic Variations and Patient-Reported Quality of Life Among Patients With Lung Cancer

Sloan JA, de Andrade M, Decker P, et al (Mayo Clinic, Rochester, MN)
J Clin Oncol 30:1699-1704, 2012

Purpose.—Recent evidence has suggested a relationship between the baseline quality of life (QOL) self-reported by patients with cancer and genetic disposition. We report an analysis exploring relationships among baseline QOL assessments and candidate genetic variations in a large cohort of patients with lung cancer.

Patients and Methods.—QOL data were provided by 1,299 patients with non–small-cell lung cancer observed at the Mayo Clinic between 1997 and 2007. Overall QOL and subdomains were assessed by either Lung Cancer Symptom Scale or Linear Analog Self Assessment measures; scores were transformed to a scale of 0 to 10, with higher scores representing better status. Baseline QOL scores assessed within 1 year of diagnosis were dichotomized as clinically deficient (CD) or not. A total of 470 single nucleotide polymorphisms (SNPs) in 56 genes of three biologic pathways were assessed for association with QOL measures. Logistic regression with training/validation samples was used to test the association of SNPs with CD QOL.

Results.—Six SNPs on four genes were replicated using our split schemes. Three SNPs in the *MGMT* gene (adjusted analysis, rs3858300; unadjusted analysis, rs10741191 and rs3852507) from DNA repair pathway were associated with overall QOL. Two SNPs (rs2287396 [*GSTZ1*] and rs9524885 [*ABCC4*]) from glutathione metabolic pathway were associated with fatigue in unadjusted analysis. In adjusted analysis, two SNPs (rs2756109 [*ABCC2*] and rs9524885 [*ABCC4*]) from glutathione metabolic pathway were associated with pain.

Conclusion.—We identified three SNPs in three glutathione metabolic pathway genes and three SNPs in two DNA repair pathway genes associated with QOL measures in patients with non–small-cell lung cancer.

▶ Ultimately, everything comes down to genetics and gene expression. This interesting trial looked at baseline quality-of-life (QOL) assessments and correlated outcomes to genetic variations in lung cancer patients (n = 1299) treated at the Mayo Clinic. The QOL assays used were validated and single nucleotide polymorphisms (SNPs) from 3 main biologic pathways were tested. From the results, it seems rather nonspecific that 3 SNPs from the *MGMT* gene pathway (a DNA repair pathway) would be relevant for overall QOL. But a rational biologic reason for this escapes me. However, the association of glutathione metabolic SNPs to fatigue and pain perception is much more biologically sound. Certainly these results need to be validated in future studies, but their role may be significant in the future. Currently, the art of oncology is that a physician eyeballs a patient and decides treatment dosages on their perception of how robust the patient is. It may not be a stretch of the imagination that genetic polymorphisms may one day play a role in deciding the amount and which treatments a patient receives.

A. S. Tsao, MD

Non–Small-Cell: Early Stage and Adjuvant Therapy

Occult metastases in lymph nodes predict survival in resectable non–small-cell lung cancer: report of the ACOSOG Z0040 trial

Rusch VW, Hawes D, Decker PA, et al (Memorial Sloan-Kettering Cancer Ctr, NY)

J Clin Oncol 29:4313-4319, 2011

Purpose.—The survival of patients with non–small-cell lung cancer (NSCLC), even when resectable, remains poor. Several small studies suggest that occult metastases (OMs) in pleura, bone marrow (BM), or lymph nodes (LNs) are present in early-stage NSCLC and are associated with a poor outcome. We investigated the prevalence of OMs in resectable NSCLC and their relationship with survival.

Patients and Methods.—Eligible patients had previously untreated, potentially resectable NSCLC. Saline lavage of the pleural space, performed before and after pulmonary resection, was examined cytologically. Rib BM and all histologically negative LNs (N0) were examined for OM, diagnosed by cytokeratin immunohistochemistry (IHC). Survival probabilities were estimated using the Kaplan-Meier method. The log-rank test and Cox proportional hazards regression model were used to compare survival of groups of patients. $P < .05$ was considered significant.

Results.—From July 1999 to March 2004, 1,047 eligible patients (538 men and 509 women; median age, 67.2 years) were entered onto the study, of whom 50% had adenocarcinoma and 66% had stage I NSCLC. Pleural lavage was cytologically positive in only 29 patients. OMs were identified in 66 (8.0%) of 821 BM specimens and 130 (22.4%) of 580 LN specimens. In univariate and multivariable analyses OMs in LN but not BM were associated with significantly worse disease-free survival (hazard ratio [HR], 1.50; $P = .031$) and overall survival (HR, 1.58; $P = .009$).

Conclusion.—In early-stage NSCLC, LN OMs detected by IHC identify patients with a worse prognosis. Future clinical trials should test the role of IHC in identifying patients for adjuvant therapy.

▶ ACOSOG Z0040 trial was a prospective trial designed to look at the predictive and prognostic value of occult metastases (OMs) in stage I non–small-cell lung cancer (NSCLC) (n = 1047) patients. OMs are defined as microscopic NSCLC disease identified by immunohistochemistry in the pleura, bone marrow, or lymph nodes. This study is important, as prior small retrospective trials with various detection techniques have suggested that OMs have a worse outcome. This study was able to report an 8% bone marrow OM rate and 22.4% lymph node OM rate. There were not enough patients to report on pleural effusion OM rates. Patients who had bone marrow OMs did not have a difference in overall survival (OS) or disease-free survival (DFS). Lymph node OMs did have a worse DFS (hazard ratio [HR]. 1.51; $P = .031$) and OS (HR, 1.58; $P = .008$). This was especially pronounced in the stage IB patients and indicates that IB patients should be considered for adjuvant chemotherapy. This analysis was unfortunately flawed, as the authors did not obtain any adjuvant chemotherapy or radiation therapy information; this trial was designed prior to the knowledge that adjuvant chemotherapy trials improved survival in resected IB-IIIA patients. Also, there were small numbers of patients with pleural fluid positivity and bone marrow OMs, and this may have affected the data analysis. In terms of clinical practice, the conglomerate data from adjuvant chemotherapy trials (CALBG 9633, JBR.10, IALT, ANITA, LACE meta-analysis) suggest that patients with stage IA and IB (tumors < 4 cm size) NSCLC tumors do not gain benefit from adjuvant chemotherapy. However, it is known that stage I NSCLC patients have a 30% risk of recurrence after resection; finding a predictive marker that would potentially help determine which patients should receive surgery or adjuvant chemotherapy would optimize treatment. Despite its flaws, this study does indicate that lymph node occult metastasis in stage IB patients can adversely affect survival, and this population of patients would likely benefit from adjuvant chemotherapy.

A. S. Tsao, MD

Phase III Comparison of Prophylactic Cranial Irradiation Versus Observation in Patients With Locally Advanced Non–Small-Cell Lung Cancer: Primary Analysis of Radiation Therapy Oncology Group Study RTOG 0214

Gore EM, Bae K, Wong SJ, et al (Med College of Wisconsin, Milwaukee; Radiation Therapy Oncology Group, Philadelphia, PA; Thomas Jefferson Univ Hosp, Philadelphia, PA; et al)

J Clin Oncol 29:272-278, 2011

Purpose.—This study was conducted to determine if prophylactic cranial irradiation (PCI) improves survival in locally advanced non–small-cell lung cancer (LA-NSCLC).

Patients and Methods.—Patients with stage III NSCLC without disease progression after treatment with surgery and/or radiation therapy (RT) with or without chemotherapy were eligible. Participants were stratified by stage (IIIA *v* IIIB), histology (nonsquamous *v* squamous), and therapy (surgery *v* none) and were randomly assigned to PCI or observation. PCI was delivered to 30 Gy in 15 fractions. The primary end point of the study was overall survival (OS). Secondary end points were disease-free survival (DFS), neurocognitive function (NCF), and quality of life (QoL). Kaplan-Meier and log-rank analyses were used for OS and DFS. The incidence of brain metastasis (BM) was evaluated with the logistic regression model.

Results.—Overall, 356 patients were accrued of the targeted 1,058. The study was closed early because of slow accrual; 340 of the 356 patients were eligible. The 1-year OS ($P = .86$; 75.6% *v* 76.9% for PCI *v* observation) and 1-year DFS ($P = .11$; 56.4% *v* 51.2% for PCI *v* observation) were not significantly different. The hazard ratio for observation versus PCI was 1.03 (95% CI, 0.77 to 1.36). The 1-year rates of BM were significantly different ($P = .004$; 7.7% *v* 18.0% for PCI *v* observation). Patients in the observation arm were 2.52 times more likely to develop BM than those in the PCI arm (unadjusted odds ratio, 2.52; 95% CI, 1.32 to 4.80).

Conclusion.—In patients with stage III disease without progression of disease after therapy, PCI decreased the rate of BM but did not improve OS or DFS.

▶ Historically, locally advanced non–small-cell lung cancer was a devastating disease with dismal outcomes in terms of survival. Although we clearly need to advance the field of treatment for this disease, there have been improvements in surgery, radiation therapy, and chemotherapy that now result in median survivals of 3 years or more.

Surviving longer increases the risk of these patients for developing intracranial metastatic disease, which can be devastating to the patient's quality of life. Decreasing the risk of brain metastases, therefore, is an important endeavor for oncologists. To that end, the Radiation Therapy Oncology Group launched this trial in 2002 hoping to accrue over 1000 patients with stage III lung cancer without disease progression after surgery and/or radiation therapy chemotherapy. Patients were randomized to prophylactic radiation therapy to the whole brain versus observation.

Unfortunately, the study did not accrue well, but 356 patients did enter the trial, of which the 340 eligible patients showed that the addition of prophylactic cranial irradiation (PCI) decreased the incidence of brain metastases statistically. Yet this change did not affect overall survival or disease-free survival. Patients who did not receive PCI had a 2.52-fold increase in the development of brain metastases. It is hard to believe that with longer follow-up, this trial will not reveal a survival benefit given the differences in development of brain metastases. Until that time though, these data do not support PCI in these patients. We look forward to a future analysis with longer follow-up to see whether improvement in survival endpoint is achieved.

C. Lawton, MD

Randomized Phase III Study of Surgery Alone or Surgery Plus Preoperative Cisplatin and Gemcitabine in Stages IB to IIIA Non–Small-Cell Lung Cancer

Scagliotti GV, Pastorino U, Vansteenkiste JF, et al (Univ of Turin, Italy; Natl Cancer Inst of Milan, Italy; Univ Hosp Gasthuisberg, Leuven, Belgium; et al)
J Clin Oncol 30:172-178, 2011

Purpose.—This study aimed to determine whether three preoperative cycles of gemcitabine plus cisplatin followed by radical surgery provides a reduction in the risk of progression compared with surgery alone in patients with stages IB to IIIA non–small-cell lung cancer (NSCLC).

Patients and Methods.—Patients with chemotherapy-naive NSCLC (stages IB, II, or IIIA) were randomly assigned to receive either three cycles of gemcitabine 1,250 mg/m^2 days 1 and 8 every 3 weeks plus cisplatin 75 mg/m^2 day 1 every 3 weeks followed by surgery, or surgery alone. Randomization was stratified by center and disease stage (IB/IIA *v* IIB/IIIA). The primary end point was progression-free survival (PFS).

Results.—The study was prematurely closed after the random assignment of 270 patients: 129 to chemotherapy plus surgery and 141 to surgery alone. Median age was 61.8 years and 83.3% were male. Slightly more patients in the surgery alone arm had disease stage IB/IIA (55.3% *v* 48.8%). The chemotherapy response rate was 35.4%. The hazard ratios for PFS and overall survival were 0.70 (95% CI, 0.50 to 0.97; P=.003) and 0.63 (95% CI, 0.43 to 0.92; P=.02), respectively, both in favor of chemotherapy plus surgery. A statistically significant impact of preoperative chemotherapy on outcomes was observed in the stage IIB/IIIA subgroup (3-year PFS rate: 36.1% *v* 55.4%; P=.002). The most common grade 3 or 4 chemotherapy-related adverse events were neutropenia and thrombocytopenia. No treatment-by-histology interaction effect was apparent.

Conclusion.—Although the study was terminated early, preoperative gemcitabine plus cisplatin followed by radical surgery improved survival in patients with clinical stage IIB/IIIA NSCLC.

▶ This phase III trial, Chemotherapy for Early Stages Trial (CHEST), was designed to compare neoadjuvant cisplatin-gemcitabine followed by surgery versus surgery alone in stages IB to IIIA non—small-cell lung cancer (NSCLC). The trial was closed early after 270 patients were randomly assigned. Patients were stratified by stage. Not surprisingly, the progression-free survival (PFS) was improved with the addition of chemotherapy (hazard ratio [HR], 0.7; $P = .03$) for all patients and especially pronounced for patients with stage IIB/IIIA (HR, 0.51; $P = .002$). Overall survival was also improved with the addition of chemotherapy (HR, 0.63; $P = .02$) for all patients, and the greatest benefit was seen in the stage IIB/IIIA group (HR, 0.42; $P < .001$). This is not surprising. Taken together with the literature, neoadjuvant chemotherapy appears to provide similar survival benefits to adjuvant chemotherapy in resected NSCLC patients. The recently published NATCH trial prospectively compared neoadjuvant chemotherapy with adjuvant chemotherapy and found similar survival benefits for patients with local-regionally advanced disease. The authors also provided an updated meta-analysis (n = 2200) from 10 neoadjuvant trials, including this study, which yielded an HR of 0.89 ($P = .02$) favoring the addition of preoperative chemotherapy to surgery versus surgery alone. Patients with NSCLC with stage II or III disease should definitely be considered for multimodality therapy. It appears that either neoadjuvant or adjuvant chemotherapy given in these stages will provide survival. The timing choice of when to use chemotherapy should be made after careful assessment of patient performance status, likelihood of tumor downstaging, patient compliance, and patients' underlying comorbidities.

A. S. Tsao, MD

Randomized Phase III Study of Thoracic Radiation in Combination With Paclitaxel and Carboplatin With or Without Thalidomide in Patients With Stage III Non–Small-Cell Lung Cancer: The ECOG 3598 Study

Hoang T, Dahlberg SE, Schiller JH, et al (Wisconsin Inst for Med Res, Madison)

J Clin Oncol 30:616-622, 2012

Purpose.—The primary objective of this study was to compare the survival of patients with unresectable stage III non–small-cell lung cancer (NSCLC) treated with combined chemoradiotherapy with or without thalidomide.

Patients and Methods.—Patients were randomly assigned to the control arm (PC) involving two cycles of induction paclitaxel 225 mg/m^2 and carboplatin area under the curve (AUC) 6 followed by 60 Gy thoracic radiation administered concurrently with weekly paclitaxel 45 mg/m^2 and carboplatin AUC 2, or to the experimental arm (TPC), receiving the same treatment in combination with thalidomide at a starting dose of 200 mg daily. The protocol allowed an increase in thalidomide dose up to 1,000 mg daily based on patient tolerability.

Results.—A total of 546 patients were eligible, including 275 in the PC arm and 271 in the TPC arm. Median overall survival, progression-free survival, and overall response rate were 15.3 months, 7.4 months, and 35.0%, respectively, for patients in the PC arm, in comparison with

16.0 months ($P = .99$), 7.8 months ($P = .96$), and 38.2% ($P = .47$), respectively, for patients in the TPC arm. Overall, there was higher incidence of grade 3 toxicities in patients treated with thalidomide. Several grade 3 or higher events were observed more often in the TPC arm, including thromboembolism, fatigue, depressed consciousness, dizziness, sensory neuropathy, tremor, constipation, dyspnea, hypoxia, hypokalemia, rash, and edema. Low-dose aspirin did not reduce the thromboembolic rate.

Conclusion.—The addition of thalidomide to chemoradiotherapy increased toxicities but did not improve survival in patients with locally advanced NSCLC.

▶ Thalidomide is an oral agent with antiangiogenic properties. E3598 was a randomized phase III trial comparing stage III non–small-cell lung cancer (NSCLC) patients receiving neoadjuvant chemotherapy then chemoradiation ± thalidomide. Patients received neoadjuvant carboplatin (area under the curve [AUC] 6) and paclitaxel (225 mg/m^2) for 2 cycles followed by weekly carboplatin (AUC 2) + paclitaxel (45 mg/m^2) with radiation. Half the patients received thalidomide (200 mg daily that was titrated up to 1000 mg daily) added to the chemoradiation and as maintenance therapy for 2 years. This trial showed no difference in response rate, progression-free survival, or overall survival and was stopped at the third interim analysis for futility. Patients who were on the thalidomide arm had more toxicities, especially thromboembolic events; 3 deaths occurred from thromboembolism before an amendment for prophylactic aspirin was put into place. Although no further deaths occurred, there was still an increase in thromboembolic events in the thalidomide arm (11% vs 3%, $P < .001$). This study clearly demonstrated that thalidomide does not have a role in combined modality therapy for stage III NSCLC.

A. S. Tsao, MD

Reduced Lung-Cancer Mortality with Low-Dose Computed Tomographic Screening

The National Lung Screening Trial Research Team (Univ of California at Los Angeles; et al)

N Engl J Med 365:395-409, 2011

Background.—The aggressive and heterogeneous nature of lung cancer has thwarted efforts to reduce mortality from this cancer through the use of screening. The advent of low-dose helical computed tomography (CT) altered the landscape of lung-cancer screening, with studies indicating that low-dose CT detects many tumors at early stages. The National Lung Screening Trial (NLST) was conducted to determine whether screening with low-dose CT could reduce mortality from lung cancer.

Methods.—From August 2002 through April 2004, we enrolled 53,454 persons at high risk for lung cancer at 33 U.S. medical centers. Participants were randomly assigned to undergo three annual screenings with either low-dose CT (26,722 participants) or single-view posteroanterior chest radiography (26,732). Data were collected on cases of lung cancer and deaths from lung cancer that occurred through December 31, 2009.

Results.—The rate of adherence to screening was more than 90%. The rate of positive screening tests was 24.2% with low-dose CT and 6.9% with radiography over all three rounds. A total of 96.4% of the positive screening results in the low-dose CT group and 94.5% in the radiography group were false positive results. The incidence of lung cancer was 645 cases per 100,000 person-years (1060 cancers) in the low-dose CT group, as compared with 572 cases per 100,000 person-years (941 cancers) in the radiography group (rate ratio, 1.13; 95% confidence interval [CI], 1.03 to 1.23). There were 247 deaths from lung cancer per 100,000 person-years in the low-dose CT group and 309 deaths per 100,000 person-years in the radiography group, representing a relative reduction in mortality from lung cancer with low-dose CT screening of 20.0% (95% CI, 6.8 to 26.7; $P = 0.004$). The rate of death from any cause was reduced in the low-dose CT group, as compared with the radiography group, by 6.7% (95% CI, 1.2 to 13.6; $P = 0.02$).

Conclusions.—Screening with the use of low-dose CT reduces mortality from lung cancer. (Funded by the National Cancer Institute; National Lung Screening Trial ClinicalTrials.gov number, NCT00047385.)

▶ Ten of thousands of American lose their lives to lung cancer each year, yet to date we have no proven screening tools to detect it early like we do for breast and prostate cancer. The National Lung Screening Trial research team was charged with evaluating the potential use of low-dose CT scanning as a screening tool to help diagnosis of this deadly disease at early potentially curable stages.

This article on the screening of over 50 000 high-risk individuals is an exciting step toward finding these tumors at a stage where surgery or radiation can eradicate them. Unfortunately, we still have 2 large hurdles to address: The first is that despite the improvement in mortality from lung cancer of 20% as seen with the use of low-dose CT screening, there were still 96.4% of the low-dose CT findings that were false positive. That number has to decrease. The second hurdle is the cost of these scans. Is the best use of our health care dollars put toward early detection of these tumors or should we place a bigger emphasis on smoking cessation programs so as to influence the cause of the cancer? These are not easy questions to answer, but they have to be addressed in the face of shrinking dollars for health care.

C. Lawton, MD

First-Line Metastatic Non–Small-Cell Lung Cancer

First-SIGNAL: First-Line Single-Agent Iressa Versus Gemcitabine and Cisplatin Trial in Never-Smokers With Adenocarcinoma of the Lung

Han J-Y, Park K, Kim S-W, et al (Natl Cancer Ctr, Goyang, Republic of Korea; Samsung Med Ctr, Seoul, Republic of Korea; Asan Med Ctr, Seoul, Republic of Korea; et al)

J Clin Oncol 30:1122-1128, 2012

Purpose.—Gefitinib has shown high response rate and improved progression-free survival (PFS) in never-smokers with lung adenocarcinoma (NSLAs). We compared efficacy of gefitinib with gemcitabine and cisplatin (GP) chemotherapy in this group of patients as first-line therapy.

Patients and Methods.—In this randomized phase III trial, a total of 313 Korean never-smokers with stage IIIB or IV lung adenocarcinoma, Eastern Cooperative Oncology Group performance status 0 to 2, and adequate organ function were randomly assigned to receive either gefitinib (250 mg daily) or GP chemotherapy (gemcitabine 1,250 mg/m^2 on days 1 and 8; cisplatin 80 mg/m^2 on day 1 every 3 weeks, for up to nine courses). The primary objective was to demonstrate better overall survival (OS) for gefitinib compared with GP in chemotherapy-naive NSLAs.

Results.—Three hundred nine patients were analyzed per protocol (gefitinib arm, n = 159; GP arm, n = 150). Gefitinib did not show better OS compared with GP (hazard ratio [HR], 0.932; 95% CI, 0.716 to 1.213; *P* =.604; median OS, 22.3 *v* 22.9 months, respectively). The 1-year PFS rates were 16.7% with gefitinib and 2.8% with GP (HR, 1.198; 95% CI, 0.944 to 1.520). Response rates were 55% with gefitinib and 46% with GP (*P* =.101). Myelosuppression, renal insufficiency, and fatigue were more common in the GP arm, but skin toxicities and liver dysfunction were more common in the gefitinib arm. Two patients (1.3%) in the gefitinib arm developed interstitial lung disease and died.

Conclusion.—Gefitinib failed to demonstrate superior OS compared with GP as first-line therapy for NSLAs.

▶ This Korean study randomized 313 non–small-cell lung cancer never-smoking adenocarcinomas (not molecularly selected) to receive gefitinib or cisplatin-gemcitabine for front-line therapy. Taken as a whole, this trial still confirms the results from the Iressa Pan-Asia Study that patients with epidermal growth factor receptor (EGFR) mutations have improved relative risk and progression-free survival with frontline EGFR tyrosine kinase inhibitors (TKIs) and does not alter or change the current treatment recommendations. The lack of overall survival difference noted in this trial is not unusual given the trial limitations: (1) that their mutation assay for EGFR had a higher false-negative rate; (2) atypical prolonged chemo (up to 9 cycles were allowed); (3) high crossover rate postdisease progression on trial; (4) lack of molecular selection for EGFR mutation prospectively; and (5) lack of *EML 4ALK* testing. *EML 4ALK* patients (which would be a significant percentage of the never-smoking adenocarcinoma patients) are generally resistant to EGFR TKIs. What can be learned from this trial is that front-line use of targeted agents should be reserved until patients can have molecular testing done. Clinical selection of patients (without molecular confirmation) for front-line EGFR tyrosine kinase inhibition is not recommended.

A. S. Tsao, MD

Impact on disease-free survival of adjuvant erlotinib or gefitinib in patients with resected lung adenocarcinomas that harbor EGFR mutations

Janjigian YY, Park BJ, Zakowski MF, et al (Weill Med College of Cornell Univ, NY)

J Thorac Oncol 6:569-575, 2011

Background.—Patients with stage IV lung adenocarcinoma and epidermal growth factor receptor (EGFR) mutation derive clinical benefit from treatment with EGFR tyrosine kinase inhibitors (TKIs). Whether treatment with TKI improves outcomes in patients with resected lung adenocarcinoma and EGFR mutation is unknown.

Methods.—Data were analyzed from a surgical database of patients with resected lung adenocarcinoma harboring EGFR exon 19 or 21 mutations. In a multivariate analysis, we evaluated the impact of treatment with adjuvant TKI.

Results.—The cohort consists of 167 patients with completely resected stages I to III lung adenocarcinoma. Ninety-three patients (56%) had exon 19 del, 74 patients (44%) had exon 21 mutations, and 56 patients (33%) received perioperative TKI. In a multivariate analysis controlling for sex, stage, type of surgery, and adjuvant platinum chemotherapy, the 2-year disease-free survival (DFS) was 89% for patients treated with adjuvant TKI compared with 72% in control group (hazard ratio = 0.53; 95% confidence interval: 0.28-1.03; $p = 0.06$). The 2-year overall survival was 96% with adjuvant EGFR TKI and 90% in the group that did not receive TKI (hazard ratio: 0.62; 95% confidence interval: 0.26-1.51; $p = 0.296$).

Conclusions.—Compared with patients who did not receive adjuvant TKI, we observed a trend toward improvement in DFS among individuals with resected stages I to III lung adenocarcinomas harboring mutations in EGFR exon 19 or 21 who received these agents as adjuvant therapy. Based on these data, 320 patients are needed for a randomized trial to prospectively validate this DFS benefit.

▶ This retrospective study conducted by the Memorial Sloan-Kettering Cancer Center evaluated stages I to III non–small-cell lung cancer (NSCLC) patients who had epidermal growth factor receptor (EGFR) mutations and analyzed the survival outcomes of these patients after adjuvant erlotinib for 2 years. In this analysis, patients with EGFR mutations were more likely to have a higher stage (stage III) and they had a trend toward an improved progression-free survival (hazard ratio [HR] 0.53; $P = .06$). This stands in contrast to the prospective Canadian BR.19 trial, which reported a detrimental effect for disease-free survival (DFS) and overall survival (OS) for adjuvant gefitinib for 2 years. The Canadian BR.19 enrolled stage IB through stage IIIA NSCLC patients and randomized them after surgery to gefitinib versus placebo for 2 years (presented by American Society of Clinical Oncology 2010). Unfortunately, for the EGFR mutations patients, there was no benefit to receiving adjuvant gefitinib (HR 1.58) and a detrimental effect for DFS and OS was seen. This is consistent with the detrimental effect of adjuvant gefitinib after chemo-external radiation therapy on the Southwest Oncology Group's study SWOG-0023. There are 2 trials that are ongoing or pending analysis (SELECT and RADIANT), which are prospective studies with adjuvant erlotinib, and will hopefully clarify the role of adjuvant erlotinib in EGFR mutation patients. The Massachusetts General Hospital is conducting a phase II trial (SELECT) of 100 patients with EGFR mutation and determining the role of adjuvant erlotinib therapy. The RADIANT trial is for unselected NSCLC stages I through IIIA patients and gives them up to 2 years of erlotinib adjuvant therapy after resection with or without radiation therapy. This trial has completed accrual but has not released survival outcomes yet. For now, until further data are known, the clinical recommendation is to not give any adjuvant EGFR tyrosine kinase inhibitor in resected NSCLC patients who have EGFR mutations.

A. S. Tsao, MD

Ipilimumab in Combination With Paclitaxel and Carboplatin As First-Line Treatment in Stage IIIB/IV Non–Small-Cell Lung Cancer: Results From a Randomized, Double-Blind, Multicenter Phase II Study

Lynch TJ, Bondarenko I, Luft A, et al (Yale Cancer Ctr and Smilow Cancer Hosp, New Haven, CT; City Clinical Hosp, Dnipropetrovsk, Ukraine; Leningrad Regional Clinical Hosp, St Petersburg, Russia; et al)
J Clin Oncol 30:2046-2054, 2012

Purpose.—Ipilimumab, which is an anti–cytotoxic T-cell lymphocyte-4 monoclonal antibody, showed a survival benefit in melanoma with adverse events (AEs) managed by protocol-defined guidelines. A phase II study in lung cancer assessed the activity of ipilimumab plus paclitaxel and carboplatin.

Patients and Methods.—Patients (N = 204) with chemotherapy-naive non–small-cell lung cancer (NSCLC) were randomly assigned 1:1:1 to receive paclitaxel (175 mg/m^2) and carboplatin (area under the curve, 6) with either placebo (control) or ipilimumab in one of the following two regimens: concurrent ipilimumab (four doses of ipilimumab plus paclitaxel and carboplatin followed by two doses of placebo plus paclitaxel and carboplatin) or phased ipilimumab (two doses of placebo plus paclitaxel and carboplatin followed by four doses of ipilimumab plus paclitaxel and carboplatin). Treatment was administered intravenously every 3 weeks for ≤18 weeks (induction). Eligible patients continued ipilimumab or placebo every 12 weeks as maintenance therapy. Response was assessed by using immune-related response criteria and modified WHO criteria. The primary end point was immune-related progression-free survival (irPFS). Other end points were progression-free survival (PFS), best overall response rate (BORR), immune-related BORR (irBORR), overall survival (OS), and safety.

Results.—The study met its primary end point of improved irPFS for phased ipilimumab versus the control (hazard ratio [HR], 0.72; $P = .05$), but not for concurrent ipilimumab (HR, 0.81; $P = .13$). Phased ipilimumab also improved PFS according to modified WHO criteria (HR, 0.69; $P = .02$). Phased ipilimumab, concurrent ipilimumab, and control treatments were associated with a median irPFS of 5.7, 5.5, and 4.6 months, respectively, a median PFS of 5.1, 4.1, and 4.2 months, respectively, an irBORR of 32%, 21% and 18%, respectively, a BORR of 32%, 21% and 14%, respectively, and a median OS of 12.2, 9.7, and 8.3 months. Overall rates of grade 3 and 4 immune-related AEs were 15%, 20%, and 6% for phased ipilimumab, concurrent ipilimumab, and the control, respectively. Two patients (concurrent, one patient; control, one patient) died from treatment-related toxicity.

Conclusion.—Phased ipilimumab plus paclitaxel and carboplatin improved irPFS and PFS, which supports additional investigation of ipilimumab in NSCLC.

▶ This phase II trial evaluates a new class of drug in non—small-cell lung cancer (NSCLC), ipilimumab, a fully human monoclonal antibody that targets cytotoxic T-lymphocyte antigen-4 (CTLA-4) and thus negatively regulates T-cell activation. Ipilimumab blocks CTLA-4 from binding to its ligands (CD80/CD86) and augments T-cell activation, proliferation, and invasion into tumors with an antitumor effect. Ipilimumab has completed phase III trials in melanoma. This phase II trial in metastatic chemo-naive NSCLC had 3 arms: (1) concurrent arm (ipilimumab plus carbo, plus paclitaxel for 4 cycles then carbo plus paclitaxel alone for 2 cycles); (2) phased arm (carbo plus paclitaxel for 2 cycles followed by ipilimumab plus carbo plus paclitaxel for 4 cycles); and (3) control arm (carbo plus paclitaxel plus placebo for up to 6 cycles). All 3 arms continued maintenance ipilimumab or placebo intravenously every 12 weeks until disease progression. The primary endpoint was immune-related progression-free survival (irPFS), with secondary endpoints of response rate (RR), disease control rate (DCR), and overall survival (OS) based on the new immune-related response criteria (irRC) and modified World Health Organization (mWHO) criteria. In this trial, the patients in the phased arm had an improvement in best overall RR, progression-free survival, and DCR by both irRC and mWHO criteria. There were no improvements in clinical outcomes in the concurrent ipilimumab arm over the control and no difference in OS for any of the 3 arms. However, in the phased ipilimumab arm, squamous cell carcinoma (SCC) patients had an improvement in irPFS (hazard ratio [HR] 0.4; $P = .55$) and an HR of 0.48 for OS. Interestingly, non-SCC patients had a worse OS (HR 1.17) in the phased ipilimumab arm. This trial is significant because it demonstrates that irRC can be used and that immunotherapy may have a role in NSCLC treatments, especially SCC. Immunotherapy is a novel avenue of research in NSCLC, especially in light of the recent exciting data on programmed death cell-1. Ipilimumab is being developed further and may have a greater role in earlier stage NSCLC disease in specific histologies. Although the SCC patient population appears to be prime candidates for this type of therapy, the adverse OS results in the non-SCC group without an explanation are concerning.

A. S. Tsao, MD

Prospective Molecular Marker Analyses of *EGFR* and *KRAS* From a Randomized, Placebo-Controlled Study of Erlotinib Maintenance Therapy in Advanced Non–Small-Cell Lung Cancer

Brugger W, Triller N, Blasinska-Morawiec M, et al (Univ of Freiburg, Germany; Clinic for Respiratory and Allergic Diseases, Golnik, Slovenia, Europe; Copernicus Memorial Hosp, Lodz, Poland, Europe; et al)
J Clin Oncol 29:4113-4120, 2011

Purpose.—The phase III, randomized, placebo-controlled Sequential Tarceva in Unresectable NSCLC (SATURN; BO18192) study found that erlotinib maintenance therapy extended progression-free survival (PFS) and overall survival in patients with advanced non–small-cell lung cancer (NSCLC) who had nonprogressive disease following first-line platinum-doublet chemotherapy. This study included prospective analysis of the prognostic and predictive value of several biomarkers.

Patients and Methods.—Mandatory diagnostic tumor specimens were collected before initiating first-line chemotherapy and were tested for epidermal growth factor receptor (EGFR) protein expression by using immunohistochemistry (IHC), *EGFR* gene copy number by using fluorescent in situ hybridization (FISH), and *EGFR* and *KRAS* mutations by using DNA sequencing. An *EGFR* CA simple sequence repeat in intron 1 (CA-SSR1) polymorphism was evaluated in blood.

Results.—All 889 randomly assigned patients provided tumor samples. EGFR IHC, *EGFR* FISH, *KRAS* mutation, and *EGFR* CA-SSR1 repeat length status were not predictive for erlotinib efficacy. A profound predictive effect on PFS of erlotinib relative to placebo was observed in the EGFR mutation–positive subgroup (hazard ratio [HR], 0.10; $P < .001$). Significant PFS benefits were also observed with erlotinib in the wild-type EGFR subgroup (HR, 0.78; $P = .0185$). *KRAS* mutation status was a significant negative prognostic factor for PFS.

Conclusion.—This large prospective biomarker study found that patients with activating *EGFR* mutations derive the greatest PFS benefit from erlotinib maintenance therapy. No other biomarkers were predictive for outcomes with erlotinib, although the study was not powered for clinical outcomes in biomarker subgroups. EGFR IHC–positive *KRAS* mutations were prognostic for reduced PFS. The study demonstrated the feasibility of prospective tissue collection for biomarker analyses in NSCLC.

▶ The Sequential Tarceva in Unresectable Non–Small Cell-Lung Cancer (NSCLC) (SATURN) trial was a phase III study comparing maintenance erlotinib to placebo after chemo-naive NSCLC patients were treated with a platinum doublet. Patients went on to receive maintenance erlotinib or placebo only if they did not progress after front-line doublet therapy. All patients were required to have tumor tissue biopsies, and the following biomarkers were assessed: epidermal growth factor receptor (EGFR) immunohistochemistry, EGFR fluorescent in situ hybridization, *EGFR* mutation, *KRAS* mutation, and EGFR CA simple sequence repeat in intron 1. The only biomarker with predictive benefit to maintenance erlotinib was the *EGFR* mutation (hazard ratio [HR] 0.10; $P < .001$). *KRAS* mutation was not predictive in any way for erlotinib, but was a prognostic factor for a worse progression-free survival for the entire group (HR 1.5; $P = .02$). The important aspects of this analysis are first, that patients with *EGFR*-sensitive mutations derive significant benefits from early treatment with EGFR tyrosine kinase inhibitors (TKIs). It is highly recommended to give these patients EGFR TKIs either frontline or as maintenance therapy. For quality-of-life purposes, I recommend treating these patients in the front-line setting if their *EGFR* mutation status is known. Second, patients who have wild-type EGFR still gain benefit from maintenance erlotinib (HR 0.81; $P = .0088$). Although the benefit is not as dramatic as that seen in the *EGFR* mutant population, the survival benefit is still significant for EGFR wild-type patients. Lastly, patients with *KRAS* mutations did not have a detrimental effect with the use of erlotinib. Although it did not reach statistical significance, patients with *KRAS* mutations had an HR of 0.77 with the addition of erlotinib maintenance. Taken together, patients who are reasonable candidates for maintenance therapy (regardless of biomarker status or histology) can be considered for switch maintenance. If a patient has a known sensitive *EGFR* mutation, they should receive EGFR TKIs as early as possible in therapy.

A. S. Tsao, MD

Randomized Phase II Trial of Erlotinib Alone or With Carboplatin and Paclitaxel in Patients Who Were Never or Light Former Smokers With Advanced Lung Adenocarcinoma: CALGB 30406 Trial

Jänne PA, Wang X, Socinski MA, et al (Dana-Farber Cancer Inst and Brigham and Women's Hosp, Boston, MA; Duke Univ Med Ctr, Durham; Univ of North Carolina, Chapel Hill; et al)

J Clin Oncol 30:2063-2069, 2012

Purpose.—Erlotinib is clinically effective in patients with non–small-cell lung cancer (NSCLC) who have adenocarcinoma, are never or limited former smokers, or have *EGFR* mutant tumors. We investigated the efficacy of erlotinib alone or in combination with chemotherapy in patients with these characteristics.

Patients and Methods.—Patients with advanced NSCLC (adenocarcinoma) who were epidermal growth factor receptor tyrosine kinase inhibitor and chemotherapy naive never or light former smokers (smokers of >100 cigarettes and ≤10 pack years and quit ≥1 year ago) were randomly assigned to continuous erlotinib or in combination with carboplatin and paclitaxel (ECP) for six cycles followed by erlotinib alone. The primary end point was progression-free survival (PFS). Tissue collection was mandatory.

Results.—PFS was similar (5.0 *v* 6.6 months; $P = .1988$) in patients randomly assigned to erlotinib alone (arm A; n = 81) or to ECP (arm B; n = 100). *EGFR* mutation analysis was possible in 91% (164 of 181) of patients, and *EGFR* mutations were detected in 40% (51 of 128) of never smokers and in 42% (15 of 36) of light former smokers. In arm A, response rate (70% *v* 9%), PFS (14.1 *v* 2.6 months), and overall survival (OS; 31.3 *v* 18.1 month) favored *EGFR*-mutant patients. In arm B, response rate (73% *v* 30%), PFS (17.2 *v* 4.8 months), and OS (38.1 *v* 14.4 months) favored *EGFR*-mutant patients. Incidence of grades 3 to 4 hematologic (2% *v* 49%; $P < .001$) and nonhematologic (24% *v* 52%; $P < .001$) toxicity was greater in patients treated with ECP.

Conclusion.—Erlotinib and erlotinib plus chemotherapy have similar efficacy in clinically selected populations of patients with advanced NSCLC. *EGFR* mutations identify patients most likely to benefit.

▶ This Cancer and Leukemia Group B 30406 trial was not powered to compare the 2 treatment arms: arm A erlotinib alone versus arm B erlotinib-carboplatin-paclitaxel. This trial demonstrates that front-line non–small-cell lung cancer patients with epidermal growth factor receptor (EGFR) mutation treated with erlotinib or erlotinib-carboplatin-paclitaxel do much better than EGFR wild-type patients. The EGFR mutation patients appeared to have similar outcomes regardless of which treatment arm they were in. Although this trial was not designed to compare the 2 arms with each other for the EGFR mutant patients, it does provide continued evidence that EGFR mutation patients will do extremely well with front-line EGFR tyrosine kinase inhibitors (TKIs) and that there is no evidence to suggest that these patients should receive chemotherapy combined with erlotinib in the front-line setting. Although there is widespread agreement that combination chemo-erlotinib is not recommended, some critics argue that these patients could be treated with the sequential SATURN trial regimen (4 cycles platinum doublet followed by erlotinib) instead of erlotinib monotherapy. Although it would not be wrong to do this, in my current clinical practice, I treat sensitive EGFR mutation patients with erlotinib monotherapy first for issues of quality of life and reserve chemotherapy for a time when they develop disease progression. Studies are currently under way to determine the optimal timing and sequencing of EGFR TKIs and chemotherapeutics.

A. S. Tsao, MD

Randomized, Double-Blind, Placebo-Controlled Phase II Study of Single-Agent Oral Talactoferrin in Patients With Locally Advanced or Metastatic Non–Small-Cell Lung Cancer That Progressed After Chemotherapy

Parikh PM, Vaid A, Advani SH, et al (Tata Memorial Hosp, Mumbai, India; Rajiv Gandhi Cancer Inst and Res Centre, New Delhi, India; Jaslok Hosp and Res Centre, Mumbai, India; et al)

J Clin Oncol 29:4129-4136, 2011

Purpose.—To investigate the activity and safety of oral talactoferrin (TLF) in patients with stages IIIB to IV non–small-cell lung cancer (NSCLC) for whom one or two prior lines of systemic anticancer therapy had failed.

Patients and Methods.—Patients (n = 100) were randomly assigned to receive either oral TLF (1.5 g in 15 mL phosphate-based buffer) or placebo (15 mL phosphate-based buffer) twice per day in addition to supportive care. Oral TLF or placebo was administered for a maximum of three 14-week cycles with dosing for 12 consecutive weeks followed by 2 weeks off. The primary objective was overall survival (OS) in the intent-to-treat (ITT) patient population. Secondary objectives included progression-free survival (PFS), disease control rate (DCR), and safety.

Results.—TLF was associated with improvement in OS in the ITT patient population, meeting the protocol-specified level of significance of a one-tailed $P = .05$. Compared with the placebo group, median OS increased by 65% in the TLF group (3.7 to 6.1 months; hazard ratio, 0.68; 90% CI, 0.47 to 0.98; $P = .04$ with one-tailed log-rank test). Supportive trends were also observed for PFS and DCR. TLF was well tolerated and, generally, there were fewer adverse events (AEs) and grade ≥3 AEs reported in the TLF arm. AEs were consistent with those expected in late-stage NSCLC.

Conclusion.—TLF demonstrated an apparent improvement in OS in patients with stages IIIB to IV NSCLC for whom one or two prior lines of systemic anticancer therapy had failed and was well tolerated. These results should be confirmed in a global phase III trial.

▶ This randomized, multicenter (India) phase II trial compared talactoferrin with placebo in patients with non–small-cell lung cancer (NSCLC) (n = 100) who had progressed on 1 to 2 lines of prior therapy. Talactoferrin (recombinant human lactoferrin) is an oral recombinant glycoprotein and is presumed to have immune modulatory properties with dendritic cell maturation and subsequent antitumor properties. Talactoferrin improved the median overall survival (hazard ratio (HR), 0.68; $P = .04$) and progression-free survival (HR, 0.73; $P = .05$) but was not significant for disease control rate. Patients receiving talactoferrin reported a lower toxicity rate. This agent is currently being studied in 2 phase III trials: a global salvage NSCLC study comparing talactoferrin with placebo, and one in combination with carboplatin-paclitaxel with or without talactoferrin followed by maintenance talactoferrin or placebo. The initial results from the talactoferrin studies are interesting, and the outcomes from the phase III trials are eagerly awaited. This is a novel mechanism of action that is reliant on the ability to modulate the patients' immune systems to stimulate antitumor activity. In thoracic oncology, there is a movement toward developing strategies to harness the immune system to fight cancer. Talactoferrin is one of the agents that is furthest along.

A. S. Tsao, MD

Weekly *nab*-Paclitaxel in Combination With Carboplatin Versus Solvent-Based Paclitaxel Plus Carboplatin as First-Line Therapy in Patients With Advanced Non–Small-Cell Lung Cancer: Final Results of a Phase III Trial

Socinski MA, Bondarenko I, Karaseva NA, et al (Univ of North Carolina at Chapel Hill; City Hosp #4, Dnepropetrovsk, Ukraine; City Oncology Ctr, St Petersburg, Russia; et al)

J Clin Oncol 30:2055-2062, 2012

Purpose.—This phase III trial compared the efficacy and safety of albumin-bound paclitaxel (*nab*-paclitaxel) plus carboplatin with solvent-based paclitaxel (sb-paclitaxel) plus carboplatin in advanced non–small-cell lung cancer (NSCLC).

Patients and Methods.—In all, 1,052 untreated patients with stage IIIB to IV NSCLC were randomly assigned 1:1 to receive 100 mg/m^2 *nab*-paclitaxel weekly and carboplatin at area under the concentration-time curve (AUC) 6 once every 3 weeks (*nab*-PC) or 200 mg/m^2 sb-paclitaxel plus carboplatin AUC 6 once every 3 weeks (sb-PC). The primary end point was objective overall response rate (ORR).

Results.—On the basis of independent assessment, *nab*-PC demonstrated a significantly higher ORR than sb-PC (33% *v* 25%; response rate ratio, 1.313; 95% CI, 1.082 to 1.593; $P = .005$) and in patients with squamous histology (41% *v* 24%; response rate ratio, 1.680; 95% CI, 1.271 to 2.221; $P < .001$). *nab*-PC was as effective as sb-PC in patients with nonsquamous histology (ORR, 26% *v* 25%; $P = .808$). There was an approximately 10% improvement in progression-free survival (median, 6.3 *v* 5.8 months; hazard ratio [HR], 0.902; 95% CI, 0.767 to 1.060; $P = .214$) and overall survival (OS; median, 12.1 *v* 11.2 months; HR, 0.922; 95% CI, 0.797 to 1.066; $P = .271$) in the *nab*-PC arm versus the sb-PC arm, respectively. Patients ≥ 70 years old and those enrolled in North America showed a significantly increased OS with *nab*-PC versus sb-PC. Significantly less grade ≥ 3 neuropathy, neutropenia, arthralgia, and myalgia occurred in the *nab*-PC arm, and less thrombocytopenia and anemia occurred in the sb-PC arm.

Conclusion.—The administration of *nab*-PC as first-line therapy in patients with advanced NSCLC was efficacious and resulted in a significantly improved ORR versus sb-PC, achieving the primary end point. *nab*-PC produced less neuropathy than sb-PC.

▶ Albumin-bound (*nab*) paclitaxel is a 130 nanomolar formulation of paclitaxel that is presumed to have better efficacy than solvent-bound paclitaxel because of its small size and ability to be preferentially taken up by cancer cells via caveolae-mediated transcytosis. Early phase II trials suggested that patients with non–small-cell lung cancer may experience significant clinical benefit. This phase III trial has been long awaited, and although it did show an improvement in response rate in the *nab*-paclitaxel arm, it disappointingly did not reach statistical significance for progression-free or overall survival. However, before throwing this agent into the bin of failed drugs, this trial did demonstrate that patients in the *nab*-paclitaxel arm had less neuropathy, and that subgroups of patients (elderly and squamous cell carcinoma [SCC]) appeared to have improved clinical outcomes. For elderly patients, this benefit could be because they were able to get more paclitaxel because of the minimized toxicity. It remains unclear why SCC would show improvement. So there may ultimately be a role for *nab*-paclitaxel to play in lung cancer, but only in a limited group of patients.

A. S. Tsao, MD

Second-Line Metastatic Non–Small-Cell Lung Cancer

Sunitinib Plus Erlotinib Versus Placebo Plus Erlotinib in Patients With Previously Treated Advanced Non–Small-Cell Lung Cancer: A Phase III Trial

Scagliotti GV, Krzakowski M, Szczesna A, et al (Univ of Turin, Orbassano, Italy; Maria Sklodowska-Curie Memorial Inst of Oncology, Warsaw, Poland; Regional Lung Diseases Hosp, Otwock, Poland; et al)

J Clin Oncol 30:2070-2078, 2012

Purpose.—Sunitinib plus erlotinib may enhance antitumor activity compared with either agent alone in non–small-cell lung cancer (NSCLC), based on the importance of the signaling pathways involved in tumor growth, angiogenesis, and metastasis. This phase III trial investigated overall survival (OS) for sunitinib plus erlotinib versus placebo plus erlotinib in patients with refractory NSCLC.

Patients and Methods.—Patients previously treated with one to two chemotherapy regimens (including one platinum-based regimen) for recurrent NSCLC, and for whom erlotinib was indicated, were randomly assigned (1:1) to sunitinib 37.5 mg/d plus erlotinib 150 mg/d or to placebo plus erlotinib 150 mg/d, stratified by prior bevacizumab use, smoking history, and epidermal growth factor receptor expression. The primary end point was OS. Key secondary end points included progression-free survival (PFS), objective response rate (ORR), and safety.

Results.—In all, 960 patients were randomly assigned, and baseline characteristics were balanced. Median OS was 9.0 months for sunitinib plus erlotinib versus 8.5 months for erlotinib alone (hazard ratio [HR], 0.922; 95% CI, 0.797 to 1.067; one-sided stratified log-rank $P = .1388$). Median PFS was 3.6 months versus 2.0 months (HR, 0.807; 95% CI, 0.695 to 0.937; one-sided stratified log-rank $P = .0023$), and ORR was 10.6% versus 6.9% (two-sided stratified log-rank $P = .0471$), respectively. Treatment-related toxicities of grade 3 or higher, including rash/dermatitis, diarrhea, and asthenia/fatigue were more frequent in the sunitinib plus erlotinib arm.

Conclusion.—In patients with refractory NSCLC, sunitinib plus erlotinib did not improve OS compared with erlotinib alone, but the combination was associated with a statistically significantly longer PFS and greater ORR. The incidence of grade 3 or higher toxicities was greater with combination therapy.

▶ Sunitinib is an oral tyrosine kinase inhibitor that targets VEGFR1,2,3, PDGFR a,b, KIT, FLT3, CSF-1R, and RET. Preclinical studies suggested that the combination of sunitinib and erlotinib, Food and Drug Administration (FDA)-approved for use in salvage non–small-cell lung cancer (NSCLC), would enhance antitumor activity. This phase III trial compared the combination of erlotinib plus sunitinib to erlotinib alone in a 1:1 randomized trial of 960 pretreated NSCLC patients. The primary endpoint was overall survival (OS). The combination of sunitinib with erlotinib improved the objective response rate (ORR; 10.6% vs 6.9%; $P = .047$) and median progression-free survival (hazard ratio 0.807; $P = .0023$), but failed to improve OS or quality of life. Subgroup analysis suggested that men, Asians, and North Americans had an OS benefit to the combination. Sunitinib is already FDA-approved for use in pancreatic neuroendocrine tumors, renal cancer, and gastrointestinal stromal tumors. However, it is unlikely to obtain further FDA approval in NSCLC as it has consistently failed to show an OS benefit (monotherapy or in combination with other systemic agents) and no predictive biomarker has been identified to date. Until a predictive reliable biomarker can be found, it is unlikely that sunitinib will be used in the unselected NSCLC population.

A. S. Tsao, MD

Vandetanib Versus Placebo in Patients With Advanced Non–Small-Cell Lung Cancer After Prior Therapy With an Epidermal Growth Factor Receptor Tyrosine Kinase Inhibitor: A Randomized, Double-Blind Phase III Trial (ZEPHYR)

Lee JS, Hirsh V, Park K, et al (Natl Cancer Ctr, Goyang, South Korea; McGill Univ Health Centre, Montreal, Quebec, Canada; Sungkyunkwan Univ School of Medicine, Seoul, South Korea; et al)
J Clin Oncol 30:1114-1121, 2012

Purpose.—Vandetanib is a once-daily oral inhibitor of vascular endothelial growth factor receptor, epidermal growth factor receptor (EGFR), and RET signaling. This placebo-controlled trial assessed whether vandetanib conferred an overall survival benefit in patients with advanced non–small-cell lung cancer (NSCLC) after prior treatment with an EGFR tyrosine kinase inhibitor and one or two chemotherapy regimens.

Patients and Methods.—Eligible patients were randomly assigned 2:1 to receive vandetanib 300 mg/d or placebo until disease progression or unacceptable toxicity. The primary objective was to compare the outcomes between the two arms with respect to overall survival.

Results.—Overall, 924 patients received vandetanib (n = 617) or placebo (n = 307). No significant increase in overall survival was detected in the vandetanib cohort compared with placebo (hazard ratio = 0.95; 95.2% CI, 0.81 to 1.11; *P* = .527); median overall survival was 8.5 months versus 7.8 months for vandetanib and placebo patients, respectively. Statistically significant advantages favoring vandetanib were observed for progression-free survival (hazard ratio = 0.63; *P* < .001) and objective response rate (2.6% *v* 0.7%; *P* = .028). Postprogression therapy was balanced across the cohorts in both number and type. Adverse events were generally consistent with previous NSCLC studies of vandetanib 300 mg; common events occurring with a greater frequency in the vandetanib arm versus placebo included diarrhea (46% *v* 11%), rash (42% *v* 11%), and hypertension (26% *v* 3%).

Conclusion.—The study did not demonstrate an overall survival benefit for vandetanib versus placebo. There was a higher incidence of some adverse events with vandetanib.

▶ The ZEPHYR is a phase III trial that compares vandetanib (vascular endothelial growth factor receptor, epidermal growth factor receptor, RET tyrosine kinase inhibitor) to placebo in a 2:1 randomized trial of 924 salvage non–small-cell lung cancer (NSCLC) patients. The primary endpoint was overall survival (OS). Although vandetanib improved progression-free survival (PFS; hazard ratio [HR] 0.63; *P* < .001), the response rate was 2.6% and there was no improvement in either quality of life or OS. Subgroup analysis suggested a PFS benefit in women, East Asians, never-smokers, adenocarcinomas, and in patients treated with gefitinib instead of erlotinib. No subgroups had an OS benefit. Vandetanib is currently Food and Drug Administration–approved for use in medullary thyroid carcinoma via RET inhibition. However, prior trials in both front-line and salvage NSCLC for vandetanib monotherapy and vandetanib chemotherapy have all consistently failed to show an OS benefit. And no biomarker exists that can identify the NSCLC patients who would benefit from the agent. These factors make it unlikely that vandetanib will have a role in NSCLC therapy. Use of this agent remains investigational in NSCLC.

A. S. Tsao, MD

Small-Cell Lung Cancer

Carboplatin- or Cisplatin-Based Chemotherapy in First-Line Treatment of Small-Cell Lung Cancer: The COCIS Meta-Analysis of Individual Patient Data

Rossi A, Di Maio M, Chiodini P, et al (S.G. Moscati Hosp, Avellino, Italy; Natl Cancer Inst, Naples, Italy; Second Univ, Naples, Italy; et al)
J Clin Oncol 30:1692-1698, 2012

Purpose.—Since treatment efficacy of cisplatin- or carboplatin-based chemotherapy in the first-line treatment of small-cell lung cancer (SCLC) remains contentious, a meta-analysis of individual patient data was performed to compare the two treatments.

Patients and Methods.—A systematic review identified randomized trials comparing cisplatin with carboplatin in the first-line treatment of SCLC. Individual patient data were obtained from coordinating centers of all eligible trials. The primary end point was overall survival (OS). All statistical analyses were stratified by trial. Secondary end points were progression-free survival (PFS), objective response rate (ORR), and treatment toxicity. OS and PFS curves were compared by using the log-rank test. ORR was compared by using the Mantel-Haenszel test.

Results.—Four eligible trials with 663 patients (328 assigned to cisplatin and 335 to carboplatin) were included in the analysis. Median OS was 9.6 months for cisplatin and 9.4 months for carboplatin (hazard ratio [HR], 1.08; 95% CI, 0.92 to 1.27; $P = .37$). There was no evidence of treatment difference between the cisplatin and carboplatin arms according to sex, stage, performance status, or age. Median PFS was 5.5 and 5.3 months for cisplatin and carboplatin, respectively (HR, 1.10; 95% CI, 0.94 to 1.29; $P = .25$). ORR was 67.1% and 66.0%, respectively (relative risk, 0.98; 95% CI, 0.84 to 1.16; $P = .83$). Toxicity profile was significantly different for each of the arms: hematologic toxicity was higher with carboplatin, and nonhematologic toxicity was higher with cisplatin.

Conclusion.—Our meta-analysis of individual patient data suggests no differences in efficacy between cisplatin and carboplatin in the first-line treatment of SCLC, but there are differences in the toxicity profile.

▶ This study was designed to duplicate the CISCA (cisplatin vs carboplatin) meta-analysis in non–small cell lung cancer (NSCLC), which demonstrated that cisplatin had an improved response rate and trend toward improved survival over carboplatin. The CISCA meta-analysis led to the recommendation in early stage NSCLC to use cisplatin-based regimens for any curative intent adjuvant or neoadjuvant or combined modality therapy if tolerated. This meta-analysis in SCLC ($n = 663$) showed no difference in clinical outcome between carboplatin and cisplatin in all SCLC patients. The subgroup analysis interestingly showed that while the limited-stage SCLC (who all received concurrent thoracic radiotherapy) had no difference in overall survival (OS), the extensive-stage SCLC patients had a nonstatistically significant trend toward improved OS with cisplatin ($P = .17$). Younger patients (younger than age 70) had an improved progression-free survival with cisplatin ($P = .005$). However, while this meta-analysis was well conducted, it has several limitations: (1) different dosages of platinum agents; (2) different schedules of agents given; (3) mixed limited and extensive stage SCLC patients with the confounding factor of radiotherapy in the limited stage patients; and (4) the time frame (1987–2004) when these trials were conducted was not during the era of improved antiemetics. Also the numbers of limited-stage SCLC patients were small. So I would not change my clinical practice based on the results of this study; in limited-stage SCLC patients, I still prefer cisplatin-etoposide when proceeding with curative intent, and in extensive-stage SCLC, I choose the platinum agent based on comorbidities, performance status, and age but will still prefer cisplatin if it can be well tolerated.

A. S. Tsao, MD

Cisplatin, Irinotecan, and Bevacizumab for Untreated Extensive-Stage Small-Cell Lung Cancer: CALGB 30306, a Phase II Study

Ready NE, Dudek AZ, Pang HH, et al (Duke Univ Med Ctr, Durham, NC)

J Clin Oncol 29:4436-4441, 2011

Purpose.—The efficacy of cisplatin, irinotecan, and bevacizumab was evaluated in patients with extensive-stage small-cell lung cancer (ES-SCLC).

Patients and Methods.—Patients with ES-SCLC received cisplatin 30 mg/m^2 and irinotecan 65 mg/m^2 on days 1 and 8 plus bevacizumab 15 mg/kg on day 1 every 21 days for six cycles on this phase II study. The primary end point was to differentiate between 50% and 65% 12-month survival rates.

Results.—Seventy-two patients were enrolled between March 2005 and April 2006; four patients canceled, and four were ineligible. Grade 3 or 4 toxicities included neutropenia (25%), all electrolyte (23%), diarrhea (16%), thrombocytopenia (10%), fatigue (10%), nausea (10%), hypertension (9%), anemia (9%), infection (7%), vascular access thrombosis (2%), stroke (2%), and bowel perforation (1%). Three deaths (5%) occurred on therapy as a result of pneumonitis (n = 1), stroke (n = 1), and heart failure (n = 1). Complete response, partial response, and stable disease occurred in three (5%), 45 (70%), and 11 patients (17%), respectively. Progressive disease occurred in one patient (2%). Overall response rate was 75%. Median progression-free survival (PFS) was 7.0 months (95% CI, 6.4 to 8.4 months). Median overall survival (OS) was 11.6 months (95% CI, 10.5 to 15.1 months). Hypertension ≥ grade 1 was associated with improved OS after adjusting for performance status (PS) and age (hazard ratio [HR], 0.55; 95% CI, 0.31 to 0.97; P = .04). Lower vascular endothelial growth factor levels correlated with worse PFS after adjusting for age and PS (HR, 0.90; 95% CI, 0.83 to 0.99; P = .03).

Conclusion.—PFS and OS times were higher compared with US trials in ES-SCLC with the same chemotherapy. However, the primary end point of the trial was not met. Hypertension was associated with improved survival after adjusting for age and PS.

▶ This phase II trial (n = 72) evaluated the use of cisplatin-irinotecan with bevacizumab in untreated patients with extensive-stage small-cell lung cancer (ES-SCLC). Bevacizumab has previously been approved in metastatic non—small-cell lung cancer (NSCLC), and significant rationale existed to study this regimen in SCLC. CALGB 30306 had reasonable results with an objective response rate (ORR) of 75%, median progression-free survival (PFS) of 7 months, and median overall survival (OS) 11.6 months; however, this difference was not impressive when compared with platinum-irinotecan alone arms from the JCOG 9511 trial in Japanese patients (12.8 month OS) and S0124 conducted in North America (ORR, 59%; median PFS, 5.8 months; and OS, 9.9 months). From the subgroup analysis from CALGB 30306, lower serum vascular endothelial growth factor levels correlated with a worse PFS, whereas HTN was associated with an improved OS. There was a 5% treatment-related mortality (3 patients).

A prior front-line ES-SCLC study, SALUTE, compared platinum-etoposide-bevacizumab with platinum-etoposide and reported a clinical benefit in relative risk and PFS but not OS with the addition of bevacizumab. Taken together, it does not appear that the addition of bevacizumab to front-line platinum-based doublet therapy in unselected ES-SCLC provides significant benefit to these patients and is not recommended for clinical practice. The quest for a predictive biomarker to bevacizumab remains elusive.

A. S. Tsao, MD

Advanced Diseases

Randomized Phase II Study of Dulanermin in Combination With Paclitaxel, Carboplatin, and Bevacizumab in Advanced Non–Small-Cell Lung Cancer

Soria JC, Màrk Z, Zatloukal P, et al (South Paris Univ, Villejuif, France)
J Clin Oncol 29:4442-4451, 2011

Purpose.—To evaluate the efficacy and safety of dulanermin combined with paclitaxel and carboplatin (PC) and bevacizumab (PCB) as first-line treatment for advanced or recurrent non–small-cell lung cancer (NSCLC).

Patients and Methods.—Patients with squamous NSCLC and/or CNS metastases received PC every 3 weeks alone (arm 1) or with dulanermin 8 mg/kg for 5 days (arm 2). Patients with nonsquamous NSCLC received PCB alone (arm 3) or with dulanermin 8 mg/kg for 5 days (arm 4) or 20 mg/kg for 2 days (arm 5). The primary end point was the objective response rate (ORR).

Results.—Overall, 213 patients were randomly assigned (arm 1, n = 41; arm 2, n = 39; arm 3, n = 42; arm 4, n = 40; arm 5, n = 41). The ORR in arms 1 to 5 was 39% (95% CI, 24% to 56%), 38% (95% CI, 24% to 54%), 50% (95% CI, 35% to 65%), 40% (95% CI, 25% to 56%), and 40% (95% CI, 25% to 56%), respectively. The odds ratio for ORR was 1.04 ($P = 1.000$) for arm 1 versus arm 2, 1.53 ($P = .391$) for arm 3 and versus arm 4, and 1.53 ($P = .391$) for arm 3 versus arm 5. The most common grade ≥3 adverse events were neutropenia, asthenia, anemia, thrombocytopenia, and hemoptysis. Of 161 available serum samples, a trend toward increased caspase-cleaved cytokeratin-18 was observed after dulanermin treatment in cycles 1 and 2. Among 84 patients evaluated for GalNT14 expression, there was a trend toward favorable progression-free survival and overall survival with dulanermin treatment in those with high GalNT14 expression.

Conclusion.—The addition of dulanermin to PC and PCB did not improve outcomes in unselected patients with previously untreated advanced or recurrent NSCLC.

▶ Dulanermin (recombinant human Apo2L/TRAIL) is a proapoptotic receptor antagonist to death receptors 4 and 5. Peptidyl O-glycosyltransferase GalNT14 analyzed by immunohistochemistry is a potential biomarker of dulanermin activity. Patients with squamous cell carcinoma (SCC) non–small-cell lung cancer (NSCLC) or brain metastases received carbo-paclitaxel (CP) with or without dulanermin, whereas patients with non-SCC NSCLC received carbo-paclitaxel-bevacizumab (CPB) with or without dulanermin. Dulanermin did not add significant benefit to patients receiving CP or CPB. No significant differences in relative risk, progression-free survival (PFS), overall survival (OS), TTP, or duration of response were seen. Of concern, in arm 2 (SCC or brain metastatic NSCLC receiving CP + dulanermin), there were 4 deaths from hemoptysis, 2 of which were attributed to dulanermin. The subgroup analysis did not reveal a predictive biomarker or patient characteristic for benefit to dulanermin. The GalNT14 IHC analysis showed that GalNT14 high expressors had a worse PFS with chemotherapy alone but, if treated with dulanermin, had a trend toward better OS and PFS. In terms of clinical practice, it is unlikely that dulanermin will be studied further in unselected NSCLC patients. It remains unclear whether this agent has a higher risk of hemoptysis for SCC patients and whether this is a drug class effect.

A. S. Tsao, MD

Randomized Phase II Study of Erlotinib in Combination With Placebo or R1507, a Monoclonal Antibody to Insulin-Like Growth Factor-1 Receptor, for Advanced-Stage Non–Small-Cell Lung Cancer

Ramalingam SS, Spigel DR, Chen D, et al (Winship Cancer Inst of Emory Univ, Atlanta, GA)

J Clin Oncol 29:4574-4580, 2011

Purpose.—R1507 is a selective, fully human, recombinant monoclonal antibody (immunoglobulin G1 subclass) against insulin-like growth factor-1 receptor (IGF-1R). The strong preclinical evidence supporting coinhibition of IGF-1R and epidermal growth factor receptor (EGFR) as anticancer therapy prompted this study.

Patients and Methods.—Patients with advanced-stage non–small-cell lung cancer (NSCLC) with progression following one or two prior regimens, Eastern Cooperative Oncology Group (ECOG) performance status 0 to 2, and measurable disease were eligible. Patients were randomly assigned to receive erlotinib (150 mg orally once a day) in combination with either placebo, R1507 9 mg/kg weekly, or R1507 16 mg/kg intravenously once every 3 weeks. Treatment cycles were repeated every 3 weeks. The primary end point was comparison of the 12-week progression-free survival (PFS) rate.

Results.—In all, 172 patients were enrolled: median age, 61 years; female, 33%; never-smokers, 12%; and performance status 0 or 1, 88%. The median number of R1507 doses was six for the weekly arm and 3.5 for the every-3-weeks arm. Grades 3 to 4 adverse events occurred in 37%, 44%, and 48% of patients with placebo, R1507 weekly, and R1507 every 3 weeks, respectively. The 12-week PFS rates were 39%, 37%, and 44%, and the median overall survival was 8.1, 8.1, and 12.1 months for the three groups, respectively, with statistically nonsignificant hazard ratios.

The 12-week PFS rate in patients with KRAS mutation was 36% with R1507 compared with 0% with placebo.

Conclusion.—The combination of R1507 with erlotinib did not provide PFS or survival advantage over erlotinib alone in an unselected group of patients with advanced NSCLC. Predictive biomarkers are essential for further development of combined inhibition of IGF-1R and EGFR.

▶ R1507 is a fully recombinant monoclonal antibody (immunoglobulin G1 [IgG-1]) to insulin-like growth factor receptor-1 (IGF-1R). Preclinical studies have reported that coinhibition of IGF-1R and epidermal growth factor receptor (EGFR) have a synergistic antitumor effect. This randomized phase II trial had 2 sequential randomizations and compared erlotinib monotherapy to erlotinib plus R1507 (at 2 different doses). The combination regimens had more treatment discontinuation rates due to toxicities. The most common grade 3 or 4 toxicities were deep vein thrombosis and nausea. Six patients treated with R1507 had hyperglycemia. There was no difference in any arm for response rate, 12-week progression-free survival, or overall survival. This is not surprising, as prior studies with other IGF-1R inhibitors have similarly failed to demonstrate benefit; figitumumab (a different IGF-1R inhibitor) has been assessed in a phase III trial with chemotherapy in non–squamous cell carcinoma NSCLC and has failed to show a survival benefit. Also, a phase III trial of erlotinib plus figitumumab closed early due to a lack of benefit. Although the results from this phase II trial were resoundingly negative in the unselected NSCLC population, this study is important in showing that patients who had a *KRAS* mutation had an improvement in 12-week progression-free survival with the combination of erlotinib plus R1507 compared to erlotinib alone ($P = .039$). The hypothesis is that IGF-R1 inhibition may be important in *KRAS* mutants or IGF-1R-driven EGFR resistance. Future studies with targeted agents should focus on molecular selection and not be widely used in unselected patients.

A. S. Tsao, MD

Randomized, Placebo-Controlled Phase III Study of Docetaxel Plus Carboplatin With Celecoxib and Cyclooxygenase-2 Expression as a Biomarker for Patients With Advanced Non–Small-Cell Lung Cancer: the NVALT-4 Study

Groen HJ, Sietsma H, Vincent A, et al (Univ Med Ctr Groningen, the Netherlands)
J Clin Oncol 29:4320-4326, 2011

Purpose.—Cyclooxygenase-2 (COX-2) protein expression in patients with non–small-cell lung cancer (NSCLC) may be not only a prognostic marker but also predictive for COX-2 inhibition. We hypothesized that COX-2 expression is associated with shorter survival and that celecoxib, being a potent COX-2 inhibitor, increases tumor response and survival.

Patients and Methods.—A phase III study was performed in patients with stage IIIb/IV NSCLC who had pathologic confirmation, no prior chemotherapy, Eastern Cooperative Oncology Group performance status of 0 to 2, and adequate organ function. Treatment consisted of docetaxel and carboplatin every 3 weeks for five cycles. Patients were randomly assigned to receive celecoxib 400 mg or placebo twice daily. COX-2 expression on tumor cells was detected by immunohistochemistry. Primary end point was overall survival (OS).

Results.—From July 2003 to December 2007, 561 patients were randomly assigned. Toxicity was mild, and no increase in cardiovascular events was observed. Tumor response was 38% in the celecoxib arm and 30% in the placebo arm ($P = .08$). Median progression-free survival was 4.5 months (95% CI, 4.0 to 4.8) for the celecoxib arm and 4.0 months (95% CI, 3.6 to 4.9) for the placebo arm (hazard ratio [HR], 0.8; 95% CI, 0.6 to 1.1; $P = .25$). Median OS was 8.2 months (95% CI, 7.5 to 8.8) for both treatment arms (HR, 0.9; 95% CI, 0.6 to 1.2; $P = .32$). COX-2 expression did not independently predict survival. Benefit from celecoxib, restricted to patients with low COX-2 expression, was not significant when adjusted for prognostic factors.

Conclusion.—In advanced NSCLC, celecoxib does not improve survival. In this study, COX-2 expression was not a prognostic biomarker and had no predictive value when celecoxib was added to chemotherapy.

► The NVALT-4 trial (n = 377) compared chemonaïve metastatic non–small-cell lung cancer (NSCLC) patients in a phase III trial with carboplatin-docetaxel with or without celecoxib (400 mg twice a day). There was no significant difference in relative risk, progression-free survival, or overall survival between the 2 arms. Also, COX-2 immunohistochemical (IHC) expression was not prognostic or predictive for benefit to celecoxib. These results are in direct contrast to CALGB 30203 results, which reported that COX-2 expression was predictive for benefit from celecoxib with chemotherapy. Also, it contradicts Khuri et al,[1] who reported that COX-2 expression was a negative prognostic factor in stage I NSCLC. This was a large prospective study with an extensive analysis. The evidence to date suggests that COX-2 inhibition is not a viable strategy in metastatic NSCLC.

A. S. Tsao, MD

Reference

1. Khuri F, Lotan R, Kemp B, et al. Retinoic acid receptor-beta as a prognostic indicator in stage I non–small-cell lung cancer. *J Clin Oncol.* 2000;18:2798-2804.

Miscellaneous

Longitudinal Perceptions of Prognosis and Goals of Therapy in Patients With Metastatic Non–Small-Cell Lung Cancer: Results of a Randomized Study of Early Palliative Care

Temel JS, Greer JA, Admane S, et al (Massachusetts General Hosp Cancer Ctr, Boston, MA; State Univ of New York, Buffalo; Yale Cancer Ctr, New Haven, CT)

J Clin Oncol 29:2319-2326, 2011

Purpose.—Understanding of prognosis among terminally ill patients impacts medical decision making. The aims of this study were to explore perceptions of prognosis and goals of therapy in patients with metastatic non–small-cell lung cancer (NSCLC) and to examine the effect of early palliative care on these views over time.

Patients and Methods.—Patients with newly diagnosed metastatic NSCLC were randomly assigned to receive either early palliative care integrated with standard oncology care or standard oncology care alone. Participants completed baseline and longitudinal assessments of their perceptions of prognosis and the goals of cancer therapy over a 6-month period.

Results.—We enrolled 151 participants on the study. Despite having terminal cancer, one third of patients (46 of 145 patients) reported that their cancer was curable at baseline, and a majority (86 of 124 patients) endorsed getting rid of all of the cancer as a goal of therapy. Baseline perceptions of prognosis (ie, curability) and goals of therapy did not differ significantly between study arms. A greater percentage of patients assigned to early palliative care retained or developed an accurate assessment of their prognosis over time (82.5% *v* 59.6%; $P = .02$) compared with those receiving standard care. Patients receiving early palliative care who reported an accurate perception of their prognosis were less likely to receive intravenous chemotherapy near the end of life (9.4% *v* 50%; $P = .02$).

Conclusion.—Many patients with newly diagnosed metastatic NSCLC hold inaccurate perceptions of their prognoses. Early palliative care significantly improves patient understanding of prognosis over time, which may impact decision making about care near the end of life.

▶ This study provides important confirmation of what we all know in the clinic: patients are less likely to choose aggressive end-of-life chemotherapy and additional treatment if they are well educated and accepting of their situation. However, busy clinicians rarely have the time to provide extended counseling and education during a clinic visit. The new integration of palliative care specialists to work with patients on this specific issue is a luxury and arguably a valid financially sound investment into clinical oncology. End-of-life treatment decisions for more aggressive yet futile therapy are often the most significant financial burden for the patient and the patient's family and health care institutions alike. For terminal oncology patients, this trial clearly shows the benefit of early integration of palliative care. This trial is important as it is the first to document specific outcome measures and scientifically demonstrate that early palliative care can positively affect treatment decisions later.

A. S. Tsao, MD

ROS1 Rearrangements Define a Unique Molecular Class of Lung Cancers
Bergethon K, Shaw AT, Ou SH, et al (Massachusetts General Hosp, Boston)
J Clin Oncol 30:863-870, 2012

Purpose.—Chromosomal rearrangements involving the ROS1 receptor tyrosine kinase gene have recently been described in a subset of non–small-cell lung cancers (NSCLCs). Because little is known about these tumors, we examined the clinical characteristics and treatment outcomes of patients with NSCLC with ROS1 rearrangement.

Patients and Methods.—Using a ROS1 fluorescent in situ hybridization (FISH) assay, we screened 1,073 patients with NSCLC and correlated ROS1 rearrangement status with clinical characteristics, overall survival, and when available, ALK rearrangement status. In vitro studies assessed the responsiveness of cells with ROS1 rearrangement to the tyrosine kinase inhibitor crizotinib. The clinical response of one patient with ROS1-rearranged NSCLC to crizotinib was investigated as part of an expanded phase I cohort.

Results.—Of 1,073 tumors screened, 18 (1.7%) were ROS1 rearranged by FISH, and 31 (2.9%) were ALK rearranged. Compared with the ROS1-negative group, patients with ROS1 rearrangements were significantly younger and more likely to be never-smokers (each $P < .001$). All of the ROS1-positive tumors were adenocarcinomas, with a tendency toward higher grade. ROS1-positive and -negative groups showed no difference in overall survival. The HCC78 ROS1-rearranged NSCLC cell line and 293 cells transfected with CD74-ROS1 showed evidence of sensitivity to crizotinib. The patient treated with crizotinib showed tumor shrinkage, with a near complete response.

Conclusion.—ROS1 rearrangement defines a molecular subset of NSCLC with distinct clinical characteristics that are similar to those observed in patients with ALK-rearranged NSCLC. Crizotinib shows in vitro activity and early evidence of clinical activity in ROS1-rearranged NSCLC.

▶ ROS1 is a receptor tyrosine kinase of the insulin receptor family and has been identified recently in non–small-cell lung cancer (NSCLC) chromosome rearrangements. There is significant preclinical and clinical evidence indicating that patients with ROS1 rearrangements will benefit from crizotinib therapy. In this study, 1073 patients were screened for ROS1 rearrangement by fluorescent in situ hybridization analysis ($n = 18$) and clinical outcomes reviewed. Although only 1.7% of patients screened had a ROS1 rearrangement, these patients were younger ($P < .001$), more likely to be never-smokers ($P < .001$), and all had adenocarcinomas (with higher grade). Given the recent Lung Cancer Mutation Consortium data indicating that identifiable driver mutations can be found in more than 54% of adenocarcinomas, this recent information on ROS1 rearrangements is promising and identifies a new subgroup of never-smoking adenocarcinomas that can potentially benefit from crizotinib. Clinical trials using crizotinib focused on this group of ROS1-rearranged NSCLC patients is ongoing. It will only be a matter of time before screening panels for NSCLC adenocarcinoma should include epidermal growth factor receptor mutation, EML 4ALK, and ROS1 rearrangements.

A. S. Tsao, MD

11 Endocrine

Combination Chemotherapy in Advanced Adrenocortical Carcinoma

Fassnacht M, for the FIRM-ACT Study Group (Univ of Würzburg, Germany; et al)

N Engl J Med 366:2189-2197, 2012

Background.—Adrenocortical carcinoma is a rare cancer that has a poor response to cytotoxic treatment.

Methods.—We randomly assigned 304 patients with advanced adrenocortical carcinoma to receive mitotane plus either a combination of etoposide (100 mg per square meter of body-surface area on days 2 to 4), doxorubicin (40 mg per square meter on day 1), and cisplatin (40 mg per square meter on days 3 and 4) (EDP) every 4 weeks or streptozocin (streptozotocin) (1 g on days 1 to 5 in cycle 1; 2 g on day 1 in subsequent cycles) every 3 weeks. Patients with disease progression received the alternative regimen as second-line therapy. The primary end point was overall survival.

Results.—For first-line therapy, patients in the EDP–mitotane group had a significantly higher response rate than those in the streptozocin–mitotane group (23.2% vs. 9.2%, $P < 0.001$) and longer median progression-free survival (5.0 months vs. 2.1 months; hazard ratio, 0.55; 95% confidence interval [CI], 0.43 to 0.69; $P < 0.001$); there was no significant between-group difference in overall survival (14.8 months and 12.0 months, respectively; hazard ratio, 0.79; 95% CI, 0.61 to 1.02; $P = 0.07$). Among the 185 patients who received the alternative regimen as second-line therapy, the median duration of progression-free survival was 5.6 months in the EDP–mitotane group and 2.2 months in the streptozocin–mitotane group. Patients who did not receive the alternative second-line therapy had better overall survival with first-line EDP plus mitotane (17.1 months) than with streptozocin plus mitotane (4.7 months). Rates of serious adverse events did not differ significantly between treatments.

Conclusions.—Rates of response and progression-free survival were significantly better with EDP plus mitotane than with streptozocin plus mitotane as first-line therapy, with similar rates of toxic events, although there was no significant difference in overall survival. (Funded by the Swedish Research Council and others; FIRM-ACT ClinicalTrials.gov number, NCT00094497.)

▶ Relatively little of a definitive nature is known about the optimal management of advanced adrenocortical carcinoma. Most of the literature is anecdotal in nature. This study is an exceedingly rare randomized phase III trial comparing 2 different systemic therapy approaches to these cancers. A total of 304 patients were randomized to receive mitotane plus either streptozocin or a 3-drug chemotherapy regimen consisting of etoposide, doxorubicin, and cisplatin. Mitotane is a derivative of DDT designed specifically for the treatment of adrenocortical cancers. Essentially all patients crossed over to the opposite regimen upon progression, so overall survival would not be expected to differ much. The study showed a response rate and substantial progression-free survival advantage for the triplet regimen (hazard ratio = 0.55). This leads to the conclusion that the regimen containing the triplet combination chemotherapy should be the preferred treatment for patients with advanced adrenocortical cancers.

J. T. Thigpen, MD

12 Head and Neck

A Phase 2 Trial of Bortezomib Followed by the Addition of Doxorubicin at Progression in Patients With Recurrent or Metastatic Adenoid Cystic Carcinoma of the Head and Neck: A trial of the Eastern Cooperative Oncology Group (E1303)

Argiris A, Ghebremichael M, Burtness B, et al (Univ of Pittsburgh School of Medicine, PA; Harvard Univ and Dana Farber Cancer Inst, Boston, MA; Fox Chase Cancer Ctr, Philadelphia, PA; et al)

Cancer 117:3374-3382, 2011

Background.—Bortezomib, an inhibitor of the 26S proteasome and NF-κB, may have antitumor activity in adenoid cystic carcinoma (ACC). Preclinical studies have shown synergy between bortezomib and doxorubicin.

Methods.—Eligibility criteria included incurable ACC, any number of prior therapies but without an anthracycline, unidimensionally measurable disease, Eastern Cooperative Oncology Group performance status 0-2, and ejection fraction within normal limits. Patients with stable disease for ≥9 months were excluded. Patients received bortezomib 1.3 mg/m^2 by intravenous (IV) push on Days 1, 4, 8, and 11, every 21 days until progression. Doxorubicin 20 mg/m^2 IV on Days 1 and 8 was added at the time of progression.

Results.—Twenty-five patients were enrolled, of whom 24 were eligible; the most common distant metastatic sites were the lung (n = 22) and the liver (n = 7). There was no objective response with single-agent bortezomib; best response was stable disease in 15 (71%) of 21 evaluable patients. The median progression-free survival and overall survival were 6.4 months and 21 months, respectively. Of 10 evaluable patients who received bortezomib plus doxorubicin, 1 had a partial response, and 6 had stable disease. The most frequent toxicity with bortezomib was grade 3 sensory neuropathy (16%). With bortezomib plus doxorubicin, serious toxicities seen more than once were grade 3-4 neutropenia (n = 3) and grade 3 anorexia (n = 2).

Conclusions.—Bortezomib was well tolerated and resulted in disease stabilization in a high percentage of patients but no objective responses. The combination of bortezomib and doxorubicin was also well tolerated and may warrant further investigation in ACC.

▶ There are no standard treatments that have been proven to provide clinically meaningful benefit for patients with locally advanced or metastatic adenoid cystic carcinoma. Thus, identification of new agents for treatment of this uncommon tumor is needed. That being said, testing novel agents for efficacy in patients with metastatic adenoid cystic cancer poses significant challenges for clinical researchers. This tumor type tends to progress slowly over time and may be asymptomatic for years. Thus, patients are usually observed until they develop tumor-related symptoms or the tumor demonstrates meaningful growth. Once treatment is initiated, confirmed partial or complete responses are uncommon. More commonly, clinical researchers report the rate of stable disease, which can be difficult to interpret in this population of patients. Nonetheless, continued research with an emphasis on molelcular targets should be encouraged.

B. A. Murphy, MD

A prospective, comparative study on the early effects of local and remote radiation therapy on carotid intima–media thickness and vascular cellular adhesion molecule-1 in patients with head and neck and prostate tumors

Pereira Lima MN, Biolo A, Foppa M, et al (Federal Univ of Rio Grande do sul, Porto Alegre, Brazil)

Radiother Oncol 101:449-453, 2011

Background and Purpose.—To investigate early vascular changes related to carotid atherosclerotic injury post-radiation therapy (RT), we studied carotid intima–media thickness (IMT) and vascular cellular adhesion molecule (VCAM)-1 at two time-points after RT and compared local and remote irradiation effects in patients with head and neck (HNC) and prostate cancer (PC), respectively.

Material and Methods.—We prospectively studied patients beginning RT for HNC or PC, performing carotid ultrasound before RT, early after and six months after treatment to measure carotid IMT. Blood samples were simultaneously collected to study VCAM-1 by ELISA.

Results.—We studied 19 patients with HNC and 24 with PC. Patients with HNC were younger (55 ± 10 years) than PC patients (68 ± 8 years). *Early post-RT* only HNC patients had an increase in IMT compared to baseline measurements (0.73 ± 0.04 mm *vs.* 0.80 ± 0.05 mm, $p = 0.029$). On the other hand, VCAM-1 levels decreased in PC patients, remaining unchanged in HNC patients. *Late post-RT* (six months from previous assessment), neither IMT nor VCAM-1 values changed in both groups.

Conclusion.—Local and remote RT seem to exert differential early effects regarding vascular-related changes: (1) local RT seems to affect vascular structure and increase IMT and (2) RT for PC is associated with reduction in VCAM levels, suggesting systemic modulation of cancer-related factors.

▶ The number of head and neck cancer (HNC) patients who survive long term is increasing. This is partly because of improvements in treatment, such as the use of combined modality therapy. In addition, there has been an increased incidence of human papilloma virus (HPV)–positive oropharyngeal cancer, which is associated with an improved survival. Regardless, it is important to understand the late effects of therapy and how they can affect quality of life and survival. Cardiovascular complications of cancer therapy have garnered recent interest, as it is becoming increasingly apparent that cancer treatment can increase both their incidence and severity. It has long been recognized that radiation therapy (RT) can cause damage to both large and small blood vessels. This can lead to long-term development of atherosclerotic plaques with increased risk for stenosis and thromboembolism. HNC patients have been shown to have an increased relative risk of stroke post-radiation therapy at 10 and 15 years of 10.1% (95% confidence interval [CI], 4.4% to 20.0%) and 12.0% (95% CI, 6.5% to 21.4%), respectively.[1] However, the trajectory of RT-induced vascular damage remains speculative, because studies have failed to look at the acute vascular effects in this population. This answers an important question: Is RT-induced vascular damage evident in the early stages after completion of RT? The study demonstrates that the initial effects of RT on the carotid artery as measured by intima—media thickness can be noted 3 months posttreatment. Thus, prevention of carotid artery disease due to RT may require early and prolonged intervention.

B. A. Murphy, MD

Reference

1. Dorresteijn LD, Kappelle AC, Boogerd W, et al. Increased risk of ischemic stroke after radiotherapy on the neck in patients younger than 60 years. *J Clin Oncol.* 2002;20:282-288.

13 Pediatric Cancer

Leukemia

Anti–*Escherichia coli* asparaginase antibody levels determine the activity of second-line treatment with pegylated *E coli* asparaginase: a retrospective analysis within the ALL-BFM trials

Willer A, Gerß J, König T, et al (Univ Children's Hosp of Muenster, Germany; Univ of Muenster, Germany; medac GmbH, Hamburg, Germany; et al)
Blood 118:5774-5782, 2011

Hypersensitivity reactions limit the use of the antileukemic enzyme asparaginase (ASE). We evaluated Ab levels against *Escherichia coli* ASE and ASE activity in 1221 serum samples from 329 patients with acute lymphoblastic leukemia who had received ASE treatment according to the ALL-BFM 2000 or the ALL-REZ BFM 2002 protocol for primary or relapsed disease. ASE activity during first-line treatment with native *E coli* ASE and second-line treatment with pegylated *E coli* ASE was inversely related to anti–*E coli* ASE Ab levels ($P < .0001$; Spearman rank order correlation). An effect on ASE activity during second-line treatment with pegylated *E coli* ASE was, however, only observed when anti–*E coli* ASE Ab levels were high (> 200 AU/mL). In the presence of moderate or intermediate Ab levels (6.25-200 AU/mL) the switch from native to pegylated *E coli* ASE resulted in a significant increase of ASE activity above the threshold of 100 U/L ($P < .05$). *Erwinia chrysanthemi* ASE activity was not correlated with anti–*E coli* ASE Ab levels. *Erwinia* ASE was found to be the best ASE alternative if Ab levels against *E coli* ASE exceed 200 AU/mL. This retrospective analysis is the first to describe the relationship between the level of anti–*E coli* ASE Abs and serum activity of pegylated *E coli* ASE used second-line after native *E coli* ASE.

▶ The use of L-asparaginase in the treatment of patients with acute lymphoblastic leukemia has been established in several prospective clinical trials. Unfortunately, because L-asparaginase is a foreign protein to humans, being isolated from bacteria, it can illicit anywhere from mild to severe host immunological reactions. The development of such allergic responses may, however, have additional and important consequences for treatment outcomes because the antibody responses can diminish the antileukemic activity of L-asparaginase. There can also be the development of clinically silent antibodies that can nevertheless neutralize the effectiveness of L-asparaginase. This article presents a detailed, although retrospective, analysis of such antibody levels in terms of their titers and influence on L-asparaginase activity in 329 patients treated in acute lymphoblastic leukemia Berlin-Frankfurt-Münster (ALL-BFM) 2000 and acute lymphoblastic leukemia relapse (ALL-REZ) BFM 2002 protocols in terms of clinical outcomes. The authors report that a change to *Erwinia*-derived L-asparaginase from the usual *Escherichia coli*—derived form is important when antibody levels against the *E coli* asparaginase exceed 200 AU/mL. For patients with lower titers, a switch to a pegylated form of *E coli* asparaginase may be efficacious (see Fig 6 in the original article). In any case, this report stresses the important need to monitor for anti-L-asparaginase antibodies and asparaginase levels. Unfortunately, this is not currently a routine part of practice, but clearly needs to be made so.

R. J. Arceci, MD, PhD

Developmental origins and impact of *BCR-ABL1* fusion and *IKZF1* deletions in monozygotic twins with Ph⁺ acute lymphoblastic leukemia

Cazzaniga G, van Delft FW, Lo Nigro L, et al (Università di Milano-Bicocca, Ospedale San Gerardo, Monza, Italy; The Inst of Cancer Res, Surrey, UK; Azienda Policlinico—Ospedale Vittorio Emanuele, Catania, Italy; et al)
Blood 118:5559-5564, 2011

The timing and developmental sequence of events for *BCR-ABL1*⁺ acute lymphoblastic leukemia (ALL), usually associated with *IKAROS (IKZF1)* deletions, are unknown. We assessed the status of *BCRABL1* and *IKZF1* genes in 2 pairs of monozygotic twins, one pair concordant, the other discordant for Philadelphia chromosome positive (Ph⁺) ALL. The twin pair concordant for ALL shared identical *BCRABL1* genomic sequence indicative of monoclonal, in utero origin. One twin had *IKZF1* deletion and died after transplantation. The other twin had hyperdiploidy, no *IKZF1* deletion, and is still in remission 8 years after transplantation. In the twin pair discordant for ALL, neonatal blood spots from both twins harbored the same clonotypic *BCR-ABL1* sequence. Low level *BCR-ABL1*⁺ cells were present in the healthy co-twin but lacked the *IKZF1* deletion present in the other twin's leukemic cells. The twin with ALL relapsed and died after transplantation. The co-twin remains healthy and leukemia free. These data show that in childhood Ph⁺ ALL, *BCR-ABL1* gene fusion can be a prenatal and possibly initiating genetic event. In the absence of additional, secondary changes, the leukemic clone remains clinically silent. *IKZF1* is a secondary and probable postnatal mutation in these cases, and as a recurrent but alternative copy number change is associated with poor prognosis.

▶ The study of leukemia in identical twins has provided investigators with important clues in terms of risk of leukemia development as well as the molecular characteristics and evolution of disease. It has long been accepted that the development of leukemia in identical twins has an extremely high concordance believed to be due to the common circulation of shared leukemic cells prenatally;

in contrast, in nonidentical twins, who do not share a common circulation, the concordance is significantly lower. A twist to this story is reported by Cassaniga et al in which they report on 2 sets of identical twins. In one set, both share a *BCR-ABL1* fusion in their leukemia, while one of them acquires an *IKZF1* mutation; this twin ultimately dies from progressive disease, while the other twin appears to be a long-term survivor. The other set of twins also both had evidence of hematopoietic cells present that were characterized by the presence of a *BCR-ABL1* translocation. However, only the twin that acquired an *IKZF1* deletion developed acute lymphoblastic leukemia, while the other twin was without leukemia 28 months later and at the time of the report. These data strongly suggest that a precursor genetic change sets up a susceptible cellular environment that can then develop into an overt leukemia with the acquisition of another leukemia-promoting mutation. In this instance, the "cooperativity" of *BCR-ABL1* and *IFZF1* provides for important details in terms of both monitoring such patients and for possible molecular mechanisms of leukemogenesis.

R. J. Arceci, MD, PhD

Improved Survival for Children and Adolescents With Acute Lymphoblastic Leukemia Between 1990 and 2005: A Report From the Children's Oncology Group

Hunger SP, Lu X, Devidas M, et al (Univ of Colorado School of Medicine, Aurora; Univ of Florida, Gainesville; et al)

J Clin Oncol 30:1663-1669, 2012

Purpose.—To examine population-based improvements in survival and the impact of clinical covariates on outcome among children and adolescents with acute lymphoblastic leukemia (ALL) enrolled onto Children's Oncology Group (COG) clinical trials between 1990 and 2005.

Patients and Methods.—In total, 21,626 persons age 0 to 22 years were enrolled onto COG ALL clinical trials from 1990 to 2005, representing 55.8% of ALL cases estimated to occur among US persons younger than age 20 years during this period. This period was divided into three eras (1990-1994, 1995-1999, and 2000-2005) that included similar patient numbers to examine changes in 5- and 10-year survival over time and the relationship of those changes in survival to clinical covariates, with additional analyses of cause of death.

Results.—Five-year survival rates increased from 83.7% in 1990 1994 to 90.4% in 2000-2005 ($P < .001$). Survival improved significantly in all subgroups (except for infants age ≤ 1 year), including males and females; those age 1 to 9 years, 10+ years, or 15+ years; in whites, blacks, and other races; in Hispanics, non-Hispanics, and patients of unknown ethnicity; in those with B-cell or T-cell immunophenotype; and in those with National Cancer Institute (NCI) standard- or high-risk clinical features. Survival rates for infants changed little, but death following relapse/disease progression decreased and death related to toxicity increased.

Conclusion.—This study documents ongoing survival improvements for children and adolescents with ALL. Thirty-six percent of deaths occurred among children with NCI standard-risk features emphasizing that efforts to further improve survival must be directed at both high-risk subsets and at those children predicted to have an excellent chance for cure.

▶ While it is important to learn from our own experience, the lessons may often be limited by the essence and scope (or lack thereof) of the question. This also applies to the field of oncology in which we tend to be swayed into the importance of our own experience. Thus, while the reporting of outcomes based on cooperative group trials can provide important insights, they do not necessarily reflect the outcome of all patients with a particular cancer such as those derived from population-based studies. However, the ability of group trial outcome analyses to link outcome with specific treatments is an advantage. Hunger et al report on the outcome of children and adolescents with acute lymphoblastic leukemia treated on trials from the Children's Oncology Group or precursor groups from 1990 to 2005. The article, published in 2012, interestingly does not include patients treated after 2005, even though patients who finished treatment by 2007 would still have a 5-year follow-up. Two key observations arise from these data. The first, which has been published by several previous studies, is that infants with ALL continue to have overall inferior outcomes with death related to toxicity increasing; this latter note is yet another testimony to oncologists kneeling at the altar of dose intensification. A second key point is that 36% of deaths occurred in patients with National Cancer Institute standard-risk characteristics, suggesting a subgroup that, along with infants, needs intense study of the biology of the leukemia and the host. And what about the patients who do not end up on cooperative group trials? Only national databases can approach that issue. Why population and national databases do not demand the inclusion of treatment information for such catastrophic diseases such as cancer suggests a lack of commitment and creativity on the part of governmental agencies and the groups they support.

R. J. Arceci, MD, PhD

Outcome modeling with *CRLF2, IKZF1, JAK,* and minimal residual disease in pediatric acute lymphoblastic leukemia: a Children's Oncology Group Study

Chen I-M, Harvey RC, Mullighan CG, et al (Univ of New Mexico, Albuquerque; St Jude Children's Res Hosp, Memphis, TN; et al)

Blood 119:3512-3522, 2012

As controversy exists regarding the prognostic significance of genomic rearrangements of *CRLF2* in pediatric B-precursor acute lymphoblastic leukemia (ALL) classified as standard/intermediate-risk (SR) or high-risk (HR), we assessed the prognostic significance of *CRLF2* mRNA expression, *CRLF2* genomic lesions (*IGH@-CRLF2, P2RY8-CRLF2, CRLF2* F232C), deletion/mutation in genes frequently associated with high *CRLF2* expression (*IKZF1*, *JAK*, *IL7R*), and minimal residual disease (MRD) in 1061 pediatric ALL patients (499 HR and 562 SR) on COG Trials P9905/P9906. Whereas very high *CRLF2* expression was found in 17.5% of cases, only 51.4% of high *CRLF2* expressors had *CRLF2* genomic lesions. The mechanism underlying elevated *CRLF2* expression in cases lacking known genomic lesions remains to be determined. All *CRLF2* genomic lesions and virtually all *JAK* mutations were found in high *CRLF2* expressors, whereas *IKZF1* deletions/mutations were distributed across the full cohort. In multivariate analyses, NCI risk group, MRD, high *CRLF2* expression, and *IKZF1* lesions were associated with relapse-free survival. Within HR ALL, only MRD and *CRLF2* expression predicted a poorer relapse-free survival; no difference was seen between cases with or without *CRLF2* genomic lesions. Thus, high *CRLF2* expression is associated with a very poor outcome in high-risk, but not standard-risk, ALL. This study is registered at www.clinicaltrials.gov as NCT00005596 and NCT00005603.

▶ The identification of robust prognostic factors in cancer has important implications for stratification of treatment and, ideally, reveals a pathway that can be prognostic but also therapeutically targeted. These authors report on a prognostic model built on several important, recent discoveries of aberrantly expressed or mutated genes in childhood acute lymphoblastic leukemia (ALL). One of these genes, *CRLF2*, is a surface receptor that shows increased expression and high rates of mutation in a subset of children with ALL and, interestingly, with a predilection for ALL in patients with Down syndrome (DS). However, in patients with DS, alterations in *CRLF2* do not appear to significantly influence outcomes. In patients without DS, when a combination of alterations involving *CRLF2*, *IKZF1*, *JAK* and minimal residual disease (MRD) are considered, in the National Cancer Institute risk group, presence of minimal residual disease, high *CRLF2* expression, and *IKZF1* abnormalities independently were associated with relapse-free survival. Unfortunately, it does not appear in this article that such prognostic modeling was contemporaneously validated in separate cohorts of patients. The high frequency of association of these other alterations, in conjunction with increased *CRLF2* expression, leads one to wonder whether the *CRLF2* is more like a canary in a mine. Until it can be therapeutically targeted, the targeting of the underlying gene alterations, such as *JAK* and the *BCR-ABL1*-like RNA expression pattern, may be a better investment for clinical therapeutic targeting.

R. J. Arceci, MD, PhD

Outcomes after Induction Failure in Childhood Acute Lymphoblastic Leukemia

Schrappe M, Hunger SP, Pui C-H, et al (Christian-Albrechts-Univ, Kiel, Germany; Univ of Colorado School of Medicine, Aurora; Univ of Tennessee Health Science Ctr, Memphis; et al)

N Engl J Med 366:1371-1381, 2012

Background.—Failure of remission-induction therapy is a rare but highly adverse event in children and adolescents with acute lymphoblastic leukemia (ALL).

Methods.—We identified induction failure, defined by the persistence of leukemic blasts in blood, bone marrow, or any extramedullary site after 4 to 6 weeks of remission-induction therapy, in 1041 of 44,017 patients (2.4%) 0 to 18 years of age with newly diagnosed ALL who were treated by a total of 14 cooperative study groups between 1985 and 2000. We analyzed the relationships among disease characteristics, treatments administered, and outcomes in these patients.

Results.—Patients with induction failure frequently presented with high-risk features, including older age, high leukocyte count, leukemia with a T-cell phenotype, the Philadelphia chromosome, and 11q23 rearrangement. With a median follow-up period of 8.3 years (range, 1.5 to 22.1), the 10-year survival rate (±SE) was estimated at only 32±1%. An age of 10 years or older, T-cell leukemia, the presence of an 11q23 rearrangement, and 25% or more blasts in the bone marrow at the end of induction therapy were associated with a particularly poor outcome. High hyperdiploidy (a modal chromosome number >50) and an age of 1 to 5 years were associated with a favorable outcome in patients with precursor B-cell leukemia. Allogeneic stem-cell transplantation from matched, related donors was associated with improved outcomes in T-cell leukemia. Children younger than 6 years of age with precursor B-cell leukemia and no adverse genetic features had a 10-year survival rate of 72±5% when treated with chemotherapy only.

Conclusions.—Pediatric ALL with induction failure is highly heterogeneous. Patients who have T-cell leukemia appear to have a better outcome with allogeneic stem-cell transplantation than with chemotherapy, whereas patients who have precursor B-cell leukemia without other adverse features appear to have a better outcome with chemotherapy. (Funded by Deutsche Krebshilfe and others.)

▶ Failure to respond to the most effective therapy at the time of diagnosis of cancer usually predicts a poor overall outcome. However, there are exceptions, and defining characteristics of such groups can be critical in deciding how aggressively to treat patients with primary refractory disease. In childhood acute lymphoblastic leukemia (ALL), less than 5% of all patients do not go into remission with initial induction therapy. To better understand the characteristics of this small but important cohort of patients, Schrappe et al reported on the 2.4% (1041 of 44017) of children and adolescents with ALL who did not achieve initial remission. While ALL in children and adolescents is relatively rare, the large numbers of patients studied was the result of an international collaborative effort. The results show that children younger than 6 years at the time of diagnosis and with precursor B-cell leukemia not characterized by any adverse prognostic genetic characteristics had an approximately 72% 10-year survival rate with only subsequent chemotherapy and no bone marrow transplantation. However, patients greater than 10 years of age with T-lineage ALL, with greater than or equal to 25% leukemic blasts in the bone marrow at the end of induction or with 11q23 chromosome rearrangements, had survival rates less than 50% at 10 years. Patients between 1 and 5 years with hyperdiploid B-cell precursor ALL also had a favorable outcome with chemotherapy treatment only. Of note, infants with MLL rearrangements who had primary refractory disease only had an approximately 4% to 5% 10-year survival rate, while those without mixed-lineage leukemia gene rearrangement had an approximately 65% 10-year survival rate. Of note, only those patients with T-cell ALL appeared to benefit from allogeneic bone marrow transplantation. The results of this large, retrospective study are a testimony to international cooperation and help to solidify and confirm the results of other reports with smaller numbers of patients. However, the information on the biology of the leukemia in these various groups is missing and is now a primary focus of several groups of investigators.

R. J. Arceci, MD, PhD

Neuro-Oncology

Clonal selection drives genetic divergence of metastatic medulloblastoma

Wu X, Northcott PA, Dubuc A, et al (The Hosp for Sick Children, Toronto, Ontario, Canada; et al)

Nature 482:529-533, 2012

Medulloblastoma, the most common malignant paediatric brain tumour, arises in the cerebellum and disseminates through the cerebrospinal fluid in the leptomeningeal space to coat the brain and spinal cord. Dissemination, a marker of poor prognosis, is found in up to 40% of children at diagnosis and in most children at the time of recurrence. Affected children therefore are treated with radiation to the entire developing brain and spinal cord, followed by high-dose chemotherapy, with the ensuing deleterious effects on the developing nervous system. The mechanisms of dissemination through the cerebrospinal fluid are poorly studied, and medulloblastoma metastases have been assumed to be biologically similar to the primary tumour. Here we show that in both mouse and human medulloblastoma, the metastases from an individual are extremely similar to each other but are divergent from the matched primary tumour. Clonal genetic events in the metastases can be demonstrated in a restricted subclone of the primary tumour, suggesting that only rare cells within the primary tumour have the ability to metastasize. Failure to account for the bicompartmental nature of metastatic medulloblastoma could be a major barrier to the development of effective targeted therapies.

▶ The emergence of resistance to treatment in recurrent or metastatic disease in cancer is the primary reason for treatment failures. Thus, it is not metastatic disease that kills patients but treatment-refractory metastatic disease. The distinction is important, as demonstrated in many examples, but certainly not more elegantly than in the report by Wu et al. They introduced the Sleeping Beauty mutagenesis system into a preclinical mouse model predisposed to develop medulloblastoma, a rare brain tumor of childhood. The Sleeping Beauty system introduces tractable mutations that can be identified in tumors that subsequently occur as a result of the functional alteration of potentially co-operating tumor-promoting or -modifying genes. Using this model system, they show that metastatic lesions are molecularly more similar to each other, even from different mice, than they are to the primary tumor. In some instances, the genetic mutations that characterize the metastatic lesions are found in very low frequencies in primary tumors, suggesting that selection has occurred resulting in particular clones having the ability to expand as metastatic sites. Only 1 example of a common, altered pathway in different primary tumors was observed; that pathway involved insulin-dependent signaling. Some corroboration of the results was shown in patient primary and metastatic tumors. This bicompartmental mutational patterning has potentially important implications for therapy in terms of trying to initiate therapy with agents that would eradicate those rare clones that have the capacity to generate metastases as well as how best to treat metastatic disease after it has already occurred.

R. J. Arceci, MD, PhD

Genome-Wide Analyses Identify Recurrent Amplifications of Receptor Tyrosine Kinases and Cell-Cycle Regulatory Genes in Diffuse Intrinsic Pontine Glioma

Paugh BS, Broniscer A, Qu C, et al (St Jude Children's Res Hosp, Memphis, TN; et al)

J Clin Oncol 29:3999-4006, 2011

Purpose.—Long-term survival for children with diffuse intrinsic pontine glioma (DIPG) is less than 10%, and new therapeutic targets are urgently required. We evaluated a large cohort of DIPGs to identify recurrent genomic abnormalities and gene expression signatures underlying DIPG.

Patients and Methods.—Single-nucleotide polymorphism arrays were used to compare the frequencies of genomic copy number abnormalities in 43 DIPGs and eight low-grade brainstem gliomas with data from adult and pediatric (non-DIPG) glioblastomas, and expression profiles were evaluated using gene expression arrays for 27 DIPGs, six low-grade brainstem gliomas, and 66 nonbrainstem low-grade gliomas.

Results.—Frequencies of specific large-scale and focal imbalances varied significantly between DIPGs and nonbrainstem pediatric glioblastomas.

Focal amplifications of genes within the receptor tyrosine kinase–Ras–phosphoinositide 3-kinase signaling pathway were found in 47% of DIPGs, the most common of which involved *PDGFRA* and *MET*. Thirty percent of DIPGs contained focal amplifications of cell-cycle regulatory genes controlling retinoblastoma protein (RB) phosphorylation, and 21% had concurrent amplification of genes from both pathways. Some tumors showed heterogeneity in amplification patterns. DIPGs showed distinct gene expression signatures related to developmental processes compared with nonbrainstem pediatric high-grade gliomas, whereas expression signatures of low-grade brainstem and nonbrainstem gliomas were similar.

Conclusion.—DIPGs comprise a molecularly related but distinct subgroup of pediatric gliomas. Genomic studies suggest that targeted inhibition of receptor tyrosine kinases and RB regulatory proteins may be useful therapies for DIPG.

▶ One of the primary obstacles to improving both the survival and adverse sequelae of patients with pontine gliomas has been the lack of biology. Over the last several years, the momentum and hope of personalizing treatments and improving neurosurgical methods have led to a more aggressive stance on obtaining tumor samples in patients with cancers located in anatomic sites previously considered too risky to biopsy. The issues have been even more complex when the patient is a young child who cannot provide consent. The report by Paugh et al, however, goes a long way to validate a more aggressive approach. Their work demonstrates that the childhood diffuse, intrinsic, pontine gliomas (DIPG) have significantly different molecular abnormalities compared with nonbrainstem childhood glioblastomas. In addition, 47% of DIPGs were shown to have abnormalities in the form of focal amplifications of genes encoding the important proteins, PDGFRA and MET. Of note, both of these pathways are potentially targetable with drugs already approved or currently in clinical trials. This work has thus shown that the site of the cancer in the brain results in quite different biology and that, as a Children's Oncology Group Neuro-oncology Disease Committee slogan once stated, "No brain (tumor), no gain."

R. J. Arceci, MD, PhD

Pre-Enucleation Chemotherapy for Eyes Severely Affected by Retinoblastoma Masks Risk of Tumor Extension and Increases Death From Metastasis

Zhao J, Dimaras H, Massey C, et al (Capital Med Univ, Beijing, China; The Hosp for Sick Children, Toronto, Ontario, Canada; Univ Health Network, Toronto, Ontario, Canada; et al)
J Clin Oncol 29:845-851, 2011

Purpose.—Initial response of intraocular retinoblastoma to chemotherapy has encouraged primary chemotherapy instead of primary enucleation for eyes with clinical features suggesting high risk of extraocular extension or metastasis. Upfront enucleation of such high-risk eyes allows pathologic evaluation of extraocular extension, key to management with appropriate surveillance and adjuvant therapy. Does chemotherapy before enucleation mask histologic features of extraocular extension, potentially endangering the child's life by subsequent undertreatment?

Methods.—We performed retrospective analysis of 100 eyes with advanced retinoblastoma enucleated with, or without, primary chemotherapy, in Beijing Tongren Hospital, retrospectively, from October 31, 2008. The extent of retinoblastoma invasion into optic nerve, uvea, and anterior chamber on histopathology was staged by pTNM classification. The treatment groups were compared for pathologic stage (Cochran-Armitage trend test) and disease-specific mortality (competing risks methods).

Results.—Children who received chemotherapy before enucleation had lower pTNM stage than primarily enucleated children ($P = .01$). Five patients who received pre-enucleation chemotherapy died as a result of extension into brain or metastasis. No patients who had primary enucleation died. For children with group E eyes, disease-specific survival (DSS) was lower with pre-enucleation chemotherapy ($n = 45$) than with primary enucleation ($n = 37$; $P = .01$). Enucleation longer than 3 months after diagnosis was also associated with lower DSS ($P < .001$).

Conclusion.—Chemotherapy before enucleation of group E eyes with advanced retinoblastoma downstaged pathologic evidence of extraocular extension, and increased the risk of metastatic death from reduced surveillance and inappropriate management of high-risk disease, if enucleation was performed longer than 3 months after diagnosis.

▶ Sometimes good intentions end up producing unexpectedly poor outcomes. In the case of retinoblastoma, a cancer of young children with a greater than 90% cure rate in developed countries, an important advance has been the use of upfront chemotherapy in order to shrink tumors so that enucleation-sparing local therapy can be used. In all but the most advanced stages of eye involvement, such upfront chemotherapy has successfully preserved eyes and vision. A tragic exception to this type of outcome is reported in this article. The authors present a retrospective analysis of 100 eyes with advanced retinoblastoma enucleated with or without primary chemotherapy. Although 5 patients with group E tumors who received primary chemotherapy ultimately died from extension into the brain or metastatic disease, no deaths were observed for such patients who underwent primary enucleation. Although the numbers appear low, the difference in deaths and disease-specific survival was significant between the 2 groups of patients. The authors conclude that primary chemotherapy for group E eyes downstaged actual pathologic evidence of extraocular extension; an alternative hypothesis would be that chemotherapy for group E eyes selected for a more aggressive clone. The answers to such questions are important, but the clinical lesson from the presented data is timely as well as important.

R. J. Arceci, MD, PhD

Solid Tumors

Clinical and Biologic Features Predictive of Survival After Relapse of Neuroblastoma: A Report From the International Neuroblastoma Risk Group Project

London WB, Castel V, Monclair T, et al (Children's Oncology Group Statistics and Data Ctr and Dana-Farber Children's Hosp Cancer Ctr, Boston, MA; Unidad de Oncologia Pediatrica Hospital Universitario La Fe, Valencia, Spain; Oslo Univ Hosp, Norway; et al)

J Clin Oncol 29:3286-3292, 2011

Purpose.—Survival after neuroblastoma relapse is poor. Understanding the relationship between clinical and biologic features and outcome after relapse may help in selection of optimal therapy. Our aim was to determine which factors were significantly predictive of postrelapse overall survival (OS) in patients with recurrent neuroblastoma—particularly whether time from diagnosis to first relapse (TTFR) was a significant predictor of OS.

Patients and Methods.—Patients with first relapse/progression were identified in the International Neuroblastoma Risk Group (INRG) database. Time from study enrollment until first event and OS time starting from first event were calculated. Cox regression models were used to calculate the hazard ratio of increased death risk and perform survival tree regression. TTFR was tested in a multivariable Cox model with other factors.

Results.—In the INRG database (N = 8,800), 2,266 patients experienced first progression/relapse. Median time to relapse was 13.2 months (range, 1 day to 11.4 years). Five-year OS from time of first event was 20% (SE, ± 1%). TTFR was statistically significantly associated with OS time in a nonlinear relationship; patients with TTFR of 36 months or longer had the lowest risk of death, followed by patients who relapsed in the period of 0 to less than 6 months or 18 to 36 months. Patients who relapsed between 6 and 18 months after diagnosis had the highest risk of death. TTFR, age, International Neuroblastoma Staging System stage, and *MYCN* copy number status were independently predictive of postrelapse OS in multivariable analysis.

Conclusion.—Age, stage, *MYCN* status, and TTFR are significant prognostic factors for postrelapse survival and may help in the design of clinical trials evaluating novel agents (Fig 1).

▶ While our goal in treating patients with cancer is to prevent relapse from ever occurring, in many cancers, relapse is all too common. Neuroblastoma in children is no exception, with approximately 50% of patients presenting with metastatic disease suffering relapse. Although it is clear that survival following relapse is poor overall, an important question is whether there exist subgroups of patients for whom survival is significantly better or worse. To this end, London et al examined some of the characteristics of relapse that impacted overall survival. The report that time to relapse (ie, time from initial study enrollment to first event; Fig 1), age, the International Neuroblastoma Staging System stage, and *MYCN*

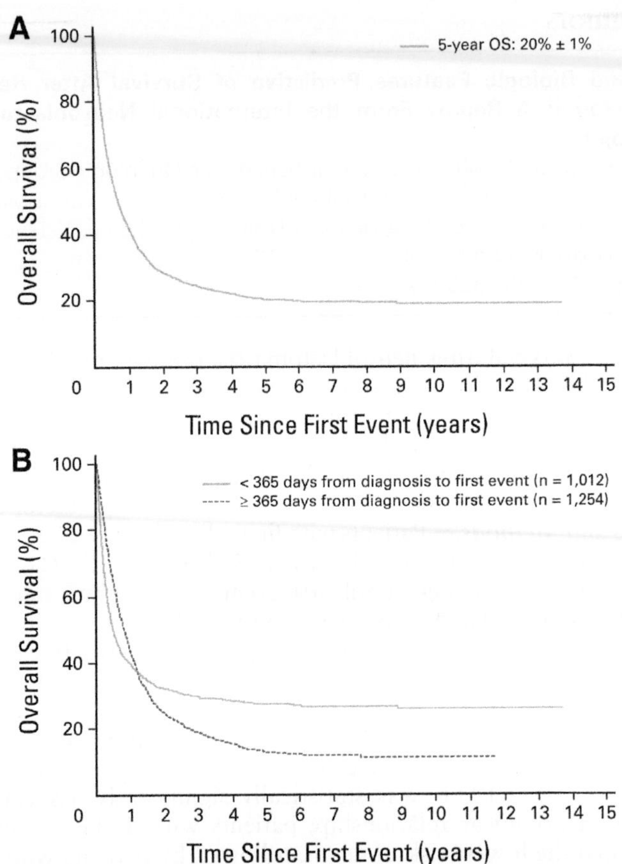

FIGURE 1.—(A) Overall survival post relapse for 2,266 patients with neuroblastoma from the International Neuroblastoma Risk Group database. Median time to first relapse (TTFR) was 13.2 months (range, 1 day to 13.1 years). (B) Overall survival post relapse. TTFR less than 365 days from diagnosis (n = 1,012) versus TTFR 365 days or more from diagnosis (n = 1,254). Log-rank test *P* value is not valid because of violation of proportional hazards assumption, which can be seen in crossing of two curves. (Reprinted from London WB, Castel V, Monclair T, et al. Clinical and Biologic Features Predictive of Survival After Relapse of Neuroblastoma: A Report From the International Neuroblastoma Risk Group Project. *J Clin Oncol.* 2011;29:3286-3292. Reprinted with permission. © 2011 American Society of Clinical Oncology. All rights reserved.)

copy number were all independent predictors of survival. Of particular note, patients who relapsed between 6 and 18 months after diagnosis had the highest risk of death. It is of potential interest that the type of treatment after relapse was not examined. It is not surprising that early relapse portends a worse prognosis, as this has been observed in multiple types of solid tumors and hematologic malignancies. Furthermore, insufficient information on the biology of early compared with late relapse tumors is mostly lacking, thus leaving open the most important question of what novel approaches to treatment could be tested in these various groups of patients.

R. J. Arceci, MD, PhD

Outcome After Surgery Alone or With Restricted Use of Chemotherapy for Patients With Low-Risk Neuroblastoma: Results of Children's Oncology Group Study P9641

Strother DR, London WB, Schmidt ML, et al (Univ of Calgary and Alberta Children's Hosp, Calgary, Canada; Children's Hosp Boston and Dana-Farber Cancer Inst, Boston, MA; Univ of Illinois at Chicago College of Medicine; et al)

J Clin Oncol 30:1842-1848, 2012

Purpose.—The primary objective of Children's Oncology Group study P9641 was to demonstrate that surgery alone would achieve 3-year overall survival (OS) ≥ 95% for patients with asymptomatic International Neuroblastoma Staging System stages 2a and 2b neuroblastoma (NBL). Secondary objectives focused on other low-risk patients with NBL and on those who required chemotherapy according to protocol-defined criteria.

Patients and Methods.—Patients underwent maximally safe resection of tumor. Chemotherapy was reserved for patients with, or at risk for, symptomatic disease, with less than 50% tumor resection at diagnosis, or with unresectable progressive disease after surgery alone.

Results.—For all 915 eligible patients, 5-year event-free survival (EFS) and OS were 89% ± 1% and 97% ± 1%, respectively. For patients with asymptomatic stage 2a or 2b disease, 5-year EFS and OS were 87% ± 2% and 96% ± 1%, respectively. Among patients with stage 2b disease, EFS and OS were significantly lower for those with unfavorable histology or diploid tumors, and OS was significantly lower for those ≥ 18 months old. For patients with stage 1 and 4s NBL, 5-year OS rates were 99% ± 1% and 91% ± 1%, respectively. Patients who required chemotherapy at diagnosis achieved 5-year OS of 98% ± 1%. Of all patients observed after surgery, 11.1% experienced recurrence or progression of disease.

Conclusion.—Excellent survival rates can be achieved in asymptomatic low-risk patients with stages 2a and 2b NBL after surgery alone. Immediate use of chemotherapy may be restricted to a minority of patients with low-risk NBL. Patients with stage 2b disease who are older or have diploid or unfavorable histology tumors fare less well. Future studies will seek to refine risk classification.

▶ It is always a challenge to reduce the amount of therapy given to patients with cancer who have an overall excellent prognosis when trying to potentially reduce the short- or long-term adverse late effects of treatment. What makes investigators and patients most uncomfortable is that the reduction of treatment may mean a higher incidence of recurrence and worse outcome. In the report by Strother et al, a reduction in therapy (ie, no chemotherapy after surgery) is examined in a large group of patients with low-stage neuroblastoma. The results nicely demonstrate that for those children with stages 2A and 2B, surgery alone resulted in event-free survival (EFS) and overall survival (OS) of about 89% and 97%, respectively. However, in the subgroup of patients with stage 2B disease characterized by unfavorable histology or diploid tumor genomes and who were older than 18 months, EFS and OS were significantly lower. Thus, in this instance, a significant subgroup of patients with neuroblastoma have been found to be able to avoid adjuvant chemotherapy if they are less than 18 months of age with low-stage tumors that have greater than 50% resection and have no unfavorable tumor characteristics.

R. J. Arceci, MD, PhD

PAX3/FOXO1 Fusion Gene Status Is the Key Prognostic Molecular Marker in Rhabdomyosarcoma and Significantly Improves Current Risk Stratification

Missiaglia E, Williamson D, Chisholm J, et al (Swiss Inst of Bioinformatics, Lausanne, Switzerland; Northern Inst for Cancer Res, Newcastle upon Tyne, UK; Royal Marsden Natl Health Service Foundation Trust, Sutton, UK; et al)
J Clin Oncol 30:1670-1677, 2012

Purpose.—To improve the risk stratification of patients with rhabdomyosarcoma (RMS) through the use of clinical and molecular biologic data.

Patients and Methods.—Two independent data sets of gene-expression profiling for 124 and 101 patients with RMS were used to derive prognostic gene signatures by using a meta-analysis. These and a previously published metagene signature were evaluated by using cross validation analyses. A combined clinical and molecular risk-stratification scheme that incorporated the *PAX3/FOXO1* fusion gene status was derived from 287 patients with RMS and evaluated.

Results.—We showed that our prognostic gene-expression signature and the one previously published performed well with reproducible and significant effects. However, their effect was reduced when cross validated or tested in independent data and did not add new prognostic information over the fusion gene status, which is simpler to assay. Among nonmetastatic patients, patients who were *PAX3/FOXO1* positive had a significantly poorer outcome compared with both alveolar-negative and *PAX7/FOXO1*-positive patients. Furthermore, a new clinicomolecular risk score that incorporated fusion gene status (negative and *PAX3/FOXO1* and *PAX7/FOXO1* positive), Intergroup Rhabdomyosarcoma Study TNM stage, and age showed a significant increase in performance over the current risk-stratification scheme.

Conclusion.—Gene signatures can improve current stratification of patients with RMS but will require complex assays to be developed and extensive validation before clinical application. A significant majority of their prognostic value was encapsulated by the fusion gene status. A continuous risk score derived from the combination of clinical parameters with the presence or absence of *PAX3/FOXO1* represents a robust approach to improving current risk-adapted therapy for RMS.

▶ The road to molecular predictors of outcome in patients with cancer is filled with obstacles and often a slippery slope to nowhere. Verification of results within the initial cohort and validation in other, matched cohorts (not always easily identified) are also major challenges. In addition, precious few RNA expression patterns as determined by microarray analysis have proven to be practically useful in defining useful risk groups for treatment stratification in prospective trials. The breast cancer–associated subset of express RNAs remains an exception. Nevertheless, investigators keep trying, journals keep publishing the results, and clinical application remains rare. Missiaglia et al attempt to ride that slippery road in their report of RNA expression patterns along with other factors to predict outcome in patients with rhabdomyosarcoma. After determining that a set of differentially expressed genes are useful in predicting outcome, they find that the presence of the *PAX3/FOXO1* fusion transcript along with TNM stage and age can basically replace the need to acquire microarray RNA expression data. However, because the model is not always 100% accurate, there must be RNA signatures that are independent of those driven by the *PAX3/FOXO1* fusion transcript. Furthermore, the data presented, although potentially useful (if prospectively validated), did not result in a pathway or altered gene expression that could be therapeutically exploited.

R. J. Arceci, MD, PhD

Pilot Induction Regimen Incorporating Pharmacokinetically Guided Topotecan for Treatment of Newly Diagnosed High-Risk Neuroblastoma: A Children's Oncology Group Study

Park JR, Scott JR, Stewart CF, et al (Seattle Children's Hosp and Univ of Washington; St Jude Children's Res Hosp, Memphis, TN; et al)

J Clin Oncol 29:4351-4357, 2011

Purpose.—To assess the feasibility of adding dose-intensive topotecan and cyclophosphamide to induction therapy for newly diagnosed high-risk neuroblastoma (HRNB).

Patients and Methods.—Enrolled patients received two cycles of topotecan (approximately 1.2 mg/m^2/d) and cyclophosphamide (400 mg/m^2/d) for 5 days followed by four cycles of multiagent chemotherapy (Memorial Sloan-Kettering Cancer Center [MSKCC] regimen). Pharmacokinetically guided topotecan dosing (target systemic exposure with area under the curve of 50 to 70 ng/mL/hr) was performed. Peripheral-blood stem cell (PBSC) harvest and surgical resection of residual primary tumor occurred after cycles 2 and 5, respectively. Patients achieving at least a partial response received myeloablative chemotherapy with PBSC rescue and radiation to the presurgical primary tumor volume. Oral 13-*cis*-retinoic acid maintenance therapy was administered twice daily for 14 days in six 28-day cycles.

Results.—Thirty-one patients were enrolled onto the study. No deaths related to toxicity or dose-limiting toxicities occurred during induction. Mucositis rarely occurred after topotecan cycles (9.7%) in contrast to 30% after MSKCC cycles. Thirty patients underwent PBSC collection with median 31.1 × 10^6 CD34+ cells/kg (range, 1.8 to 541.8 × 10^6 CD34+ cells/kg), all negative for tumor contamination by immunocytochemical analysis. Targeted topotecan systemic exposure was achieved in 26 (84%)

of 31 patients. At the end of induction, 26 patients (84%) had tumor response and one patient had progressive disease. In the overall cohort, 3-year event-free and overall survival were 37.8% ± 9.4% and 57.1% ± 9.4%, respectively.

Conclusion.—This pilot induction regimen was well tolerated with expected and reversible toxicities. These data support investigation of efficacy in a phase III clinical trial for newly diagnosed HRNB.

▶ There is a buzz on the streets and back alleys of oncology that revolves around the "era of personalized medicine." Integration of molecular profiling of tumor and patient genomes should lead to a selection of the right drugs and doses of those drugs to optimize cure rates and reduce toxicities of treatment. This approach does make more sense than giving everyone the same dose of the same drugs with the knowledge that only a percentage of those patients will experience any benefit. While there are great challenges to making all this a reality, the goal must be one that is rigorously pursued. However, despite the important impact of molecular analyses, the delivery of such treatments with predictable pharmacologic consequences is likely to be a further challenge. The report by Park et al demonstrates some of the complexities of pharmacologic targeting in pediatric patients with neuroblastoma. They focus their question on pharmacologically driven dosing of one of the drugs, topotecan, as part of an intensive induction regimen. The desired dose range was determined from xenograft mouse models, which raises immense questions as to the validity of this approach, as such studies have also shown that even within the same plasma levels, there can be great tumor drug concentration differences between animals and tumor types. In addition, only 84% of the patients in the Park et al study achieved the desired targeted exposure range. Responses appeared comparable with other nonpharmacologically dosed approaches, although a randomized trial with limited numbers of patients might have been helpful in terms of understanding differences in toxicity. Despite the many issues and questions, it is likely that more effort needs to be applied to optimally dosing chemotherapy and assessing early markers of success.

R. J. Arceci, MD, PhD

Prognostic Significance and Tumor Biology of Regional Lymph Node Disease in Patients With Rhabdomyosarcoma: A Report From the Children's Oncology Group

Rodeberg DA, Garcia-Henriquez N, Lyden ER, et al (Univ of Pittsburgh, PA; Nebraska Med Ctr, Omaha, NE; Univ of Oklahoma Health Sciences Ctr; et al)

J Clin Oncol 29:1304-1311, 2011

Purpose.—Regional lymph node disease (RLND) is a component of the risk-based treatment stratification in rhabdomyosarcoma (RMS). The purpose of this study was to determine the contribution of RLND to prognosis for patients with RMS.

Patients and Methods.—Patient characteristics and survival outcomes for patients enrolled onto Intergroup Rhabdomyosarcoma Study IV (N = 898,

1991 to 1997) were evaluated among the following three patient groups: nonmetastatic patients with clinical or pathologic negative nodes (N0, 696 patients); patients with clinical or pathologic positive nodes (N1, 125 patients); and patients with a single site of metastatic disease (77 patients).

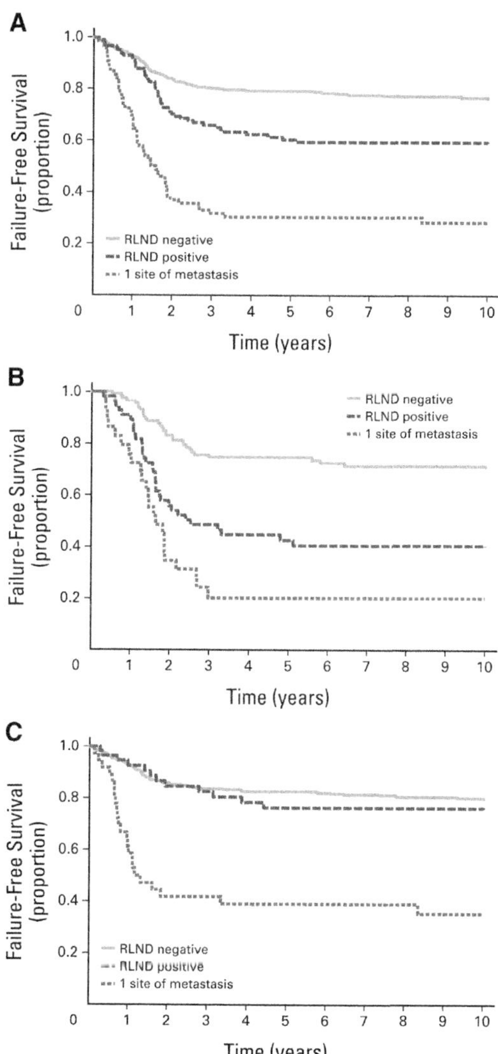

FIGURE 1.—Failure-free survival curves for patients who are regional lymph node disease (RLND) negative, patients who are RLND positive, and patients with one site of metastatic disease in (A) both embryonal and alveolar rhabdomyosarcoma (RMS), (B) alveolar RMS only, and (C) embryonal RMS only. (Reprinted from Rodeberg DA, Garcia-Henriquez N, Lyden ER, et al. Prognostic Significance and Tumor Biology of Regional Lymph Node Disease in Patients With Rhabdomyosarcoma: A Report From the Children's Oncology Group. *J Clin Oncol.* 2011;29:1304-1311. Reprinted with permission. © 2011 American Society of Clinical Oncology. All rights reserved.)

Results.—Outcomes for patients with nonmetastatic alveolar N0 RMS were significantly better than for patients with N1 RMS (5-year failure-free survival [FFS], 73% *v* 43%, respectively; 5-year overall survival [OS], 80% *v* 46%, respectively; $P < .001$). Patients with a single site of alveolar metastasis had even worse FFS and OS (23% FFS and OS, $P = .01$) when compared with patients with N1 RMS; however, the differences were not as large as the differences between patients with N0 RMS and N1 RMS. For embryonal RMS, there was no statistically significant difference in FFS or OS ($P = .41$ and $P = .77$, respectively) for patients with N1 versus N0 RMS. Gene array analysis of primary tumor specimens identified that genes associated with the immune system and antigen presentation were significantly increased in N1 versus N0 alveolar RMS.

Conclusion.—RLND alters prognosis for alveolar but not embryonal RMS. For patients with N1 disease and alveolar histology, outcomes were more similar to distant metastatic disease rather than local disease. Current data suggest that more aggressive therapy for patients with alveolar N1 RMS may be warranted (Fig 1).

▶ The outcomes for patients with advanced-stage rhabdomyosarcoma (RMS) have not substantially changed, while those with less-advanced RMS have shown significantly better outcomes. Nevertheless, a significant percentage of patients with low-stage disease have a significantly worse outcome compared with others who have the same stage disease. In order to determine what characteristics are distinctive for those patients who have poor outcomes, these authors investigated both clinical and molecular characteristics of pediatric patients with regional lymph node disease (RLND). They observed that RLND was an independent, adverse prognostic factor for patients with alveolar but not for embryonal histology (Fig 1). In addition, RNA expression analysis using microarrays showed the interesting but somewhat bewildering finding of the RLND-positive alveolar RMS having increased expression of various B-lymphocyte markers compared to those with RMS without RLND. Although the meaning of the RNA expression data remains unclear, the data clearly demonstrate both a different biology and clinical outcome for this subset of patients. Further studies like this will more than likely demonstrate further heterogeneity among different subtypes of RMS. An important consequence of such studies will be whether the findings can be used to develop more effective treatments rather than just predict outcomes with current treatment approaches.

R. J. Arceci, MD, PhD

Miscellaneous

High Risk of Symptomatic Cardiac Events in Childhood Cancer Survivors

van der Pal HJ, van Dalen EC, van Delden E, et al (Emma Children's Hosp/ Academic Med Centre, Amsterdam, the Netherlands; et al)

J Clin Oncol 30:1429-1437, 2012

Purpose.—To evaluate the long-term risk for validated symptomatic cardiac events (CEs) and associated risk factors in childhood cancer survivors (CCSs).

Patients and Methods.—We determined CEs grade 3 or higher: congestive heart failure (CHF), cardiac ischemia, valvular disease, arrhythmia and/or pericarditis (according to Common Terminology Criteria for Adverse Events [CTCAE], version 3.0) in a hospital-based cohort of 1,362 5-year CCSs diagnosed between 1966 and 1996. We calculated both marginal and cause-specific cumulative incidence of CEs and cause-specific cumulative incidence of separate events. We analyzed different risk factors in multivariable Cox regression models.

Results.—Overall, 50 CEs, including 27 cases of CHF, were observed in 42 survivors (at a median attained age of 27.1 years). The 30-year cause-specific cumulative incidence of CEs was significantly increased after treatment with both anthracyclines and cardiac irradiation (12.6%; 95% CI, 4.3% to 20.3%), after anthracyclines (7.3%; 95% CI, 3.8% to 10.7%), and after cardiac irradiation (4.0%; 95% CI, 0.5% to 7.4%) compared with other treatments. In the proportional hazards analyses, anthracycline (dose), cardiac irradiation (dose), combination of these treatments, and congenital heart disease were significantly associated with developing a CE. We demonstrated an exponential relationship between the cumulative anthracycline dose, cardiac irradiation dose, and risk of CE.

Conclusion.—CCSs have a high risk of developing symptomatic CEs at an early age. The most common CE was CHF. Survivors treated with both anthracyclines and radiotherapy have the highest risk; after 30 years, one in eight will develop severe heart disease. The use of potentially cardiotoxic treatments should be reconsidered for high-risk groups, and frequent follow-up for high-risk survivors is needed.

► The use of anthracyclines in patients with cancer has always been a double-edged sword, with both the benefits and the risks of cardiac toxicity being recognized for dozens of years. Van der Pal et al focus on the risks of cardiac events in childhood cancer survivors exposed to anthracyclines. They report 50 cardiac events, including 27 cases of congestive heart failure, in 42 survivors in a single institution study, from a cohort of 1362 patients treated between 1966 and 1996. An exponential relationship is demonstrated between the cumulative anthracycline dose, cardiac irradiation dose, and the risk of a cardiac event. Of note, 1 of 8 patients exposed to anthracyclines and cardiac radiation developed severe heart disease. Outcomes for such patients are poor. Such information has been reported previously by other studies, so why publish similar results again?

Several reasons are provided, including that this study had 90% participation compared with the Childhood Cancer Survivor Study in which only 70% of eligible survivors participated. Is this really different? Does such a difference abrogate the fact that this report is on a single institution in a single country compared with population-based study across a much larger geographical, ethnically, and racially diverse patients? Such questions are unfortunately usually not critically addressed. The report further concludes that the use of anthracyclines in patients with high-risk cancers should be re-evaluated, but no recommendation or practical advice is provided. Thus, although this report is mostly confirmatory, it again raises the key questions as to what the basic risk factors are and how can we replace or protect against the toxicity of anthracyclines.

R. J. Arceci, MD, PhD

14 Melanoma

RAS Mutations Are Associated With the Development of Cutaneous Squamous Cell Tumors in Patients Treated With RAF Inhibitors

Oberholzer PA, Kee D, Dziunycz P, et al (Broad Inst of Massachusetts Inst of Technology and Harvard, Cambridge; Peter MacCallum Cancer Centre, East Melbourne, Victoria, Australia; Univ Hosp Zürich, Switzerland; et al)

J Clin Oncol 30:316-321, 2012

Purpose.—RAF inhibitors are effective against melanomas with *BRAF* V600E mutations but may induce keratoacanthomas (KAs) and cutaneous squamous cell carcinomas (cSCCs). The potential of these agents to promote secondary malignancies is concerning. We analyzed cSCC and KA lesions for genetic mutations in an attempt to identify an underlying mechanism for their formation.

Methods.—Four international centers contributed 237 KA or cSCC tumor samples from patients receiving an RAF inhibitor (either vemurafenib or sorafenib; n = 19) or immunosuppression therapy (n = 53) or tumors that developed spontaneously (n = 165). Each sample was profiled for 396 known somatic mutations across 33 cancer-related genes by using a mass spectrometric–based genotyping platform.

Results.—Mutations were detected in 16% of tumors (38 of 237), with five tumors harboring two mutations. Mutations in *TP53, CDKN2A, HRAS, KRAS*, and *PIK3CA* were previously described in squamous cell tumors. Mutations in *MYC, FGFR3*, and *VHL* were identified for the first time. A higher frequency of activating *RAS* mutations was found in tumors from patients treated with an RAF inhibitor versus populations treated with a non–RAF inhibitor (21.1% *v* 3.2%; $P < .01$), although overall mutation rates between treatment groups were similar (RAF inhibitor, 21.1%; immunosuppression, 18.9%; and spontaneous, 17.6%; $P =$ not significant). Tumor histology (KA *v* cSCC), tumor site (head and neck *v* other), patient age (≤ 70 *v* > 70 years), and sex had no significant impact on mutation rate or type.

Conclusion.—Squamous cell tumors from patients treated with an RAF inhibitor have a distinct mutational profile that supports a mechanism of therapy-induced tumorigenesis in *RAS*-primed cells. Conceivably, cotargeting of MEK together with RAF may reduce or prevent formation of these tumors.

▶ Most experimental and especially review articles on signal transduction pathways usually present a schematic diagram that describes a sequence of interactive molecules leading to an outcome of proliferation, cell cycle progression, or both. The unfortunate truth, however, is that none of these schema reflect the truth of what is actually going on in cancer cells or, for that matter, any cell, except that which exists in the mind of the experimental scientist. This lesson has been hammered home by the observations of patients with melanoma characterized by *BRAF* V600E mutations and treated with small-molecule RAF inhibitors. An early observation was that such patients developed an extraordinarily high incidence of cutaneous cancers, particularly squamous cell carcinoma. In the study by Oberholzer et al, they perform a detailed molecular analysis of these secondary cancers. They identified already reported mutations in *TP53*, *CDKN2A*, *HRAS*, *KRAS*, and *PIK3CA* but also reported some novel mutations involved *MYC*, *FGFR3*, and *VHL*. And though overall mutation rates were approximately the same in the RAF inhibitor–treated versus the non–RAF inhibitor–treated patients, activating *RAS* mutations were found much more frequently in patients treated with RAF inhibitors (21.1% vs 3.2%). These data strongly support the ominous conclusion that RAF inhibition, which represents potentially effective treatment for such patients, results in a feedback system that predisposes to activation through alternative signal transduction pathway activation or mutation that leads to the high incidence of a secondary cancer. Thus, dual inhibition (or maybe more) may provide a more effective therapeutic strategy. These results also underline the fact that we should remain suspicious of all schematic diagrams that attempt to explain the workings of biological systems.

R. J. Arceci, MD, PhD

15 Sarcoma

Anaplastic Lymphoma Kinase Aberrations in Rhabdomyosarcoma: Clinical and Prognostic Implications

van Gaal JC, Flucke UE, Roeffen MHS, et al (Radboud Univ Nijmegen Med Centre, the Netherlands; et al)

J Clin Oncol 30:308-315, 2012

Purpose.—The aim of this study is to investigate anaplastic lymphoma kinase (ALK) protein expression and underlying genetic aberrations in rhabdomyosarcoma (RMS), with special attention to clinical and prognostic implications.

Patients and Methods.—A total of 189 paraffin-embedded RMS tumor specimens from 145 patients were collected on tissue microarray. *ALK* protein expression was evaluated by immunohistochemistry. ALK gene (2p23) copy number and translocations were determined by in situ hybridization. cDNA sequencing of the receptor tyrosine kinase domain of the *ALK* gene was assessed in 43 samples.

Results.—Strong cytoplasmic ALK protein expression was more frequently observed in alveolar RMS (ARMS) than in embryonal RMS (ERMS) (81% *v* 32%, respectively; $P < .001$). *ALK* gene copy number gain was detected in the vast majority of ARMS (88%), compared with 52% of ERMS ($P < .001$). ALK copy number correlated with protein expression in primary tumors (n = 107). We identified one point mutation (2%) and seven tumors harboring whole exon deletions (16%). In ERMS, specific *ALK* gain in the primary tumor correlated with metastatic disease (100% in metastatic disease *v* 29% in nonmetastatic disease; $P = .004$) and poor disease-specific survival (5-year disease-specific survival: 62% *v* 82% for nonspecific or no gain; $P = .046$).

Conclusion.—Because ALK aberrations on genomic and protein levels are frequently found in RMSs, in particular ARMS, and are associated with disease progression and outcome in ERMS, ALK may play a role in tumor biology and may provide a potential therapeutic target for these tumors. Future research should aim at the oncogenic role of ALK and the potential effect of ALK inhibitors in RMS.

► The molecular analysis of solid tumors, especially in children, has been difficult in part because of their rarity as well as the availability of fresh diagnostic and relapse tissue, although exceptions exist. Several molecularly based prognostic models have been published combining microarray-generated RNA expression patterns with clinical characteristics. While one of the goals of such studies is to define prognostic groups, an additional and more important goal has been to define novel factors that can be effectively targeted to improve outcomes. The identification of alterations in the anaplastic lymphoma kinase (ALK) gene have led to responses to ALK inhibitors in several disorders, such as lung cancer, neuroblastoma, lymphoma, and inflammatory myofibroblastic tumors. The report by van Gaal et al provides a descriptive pattern of expression and copy number for ALK in rhabdomyosarcoma (RMS). They demonstrated that increased ALK protein expression was more common in alveolar compared with embryonal RMS expression level and tended to correlate with ALK gene copy number. One ALK point was observed, and 7 tumors had ALK exon deletions. Of interest, only in embryonal RMS did they observe an association with metastatic disease and significant, albeit not extremely so, difference in survival rates, with specific ALK gains being associated with 5-year 62% disease-free survival compared with 82% for no gain ($P = .046$). There were several significant limitations to this study: the number of patients examined in this study was small; there was no validation cohort; immunohistochemistry controls using albumin instead of isotype control antibodies were used; and quantitation of expression was qualitative or, as is often used, *semiquantitative*. So where does such information lead us? Without more definitive data, I am afraid not much further along the road to improving treatment outcomes for such patients than where we were before.

R. J. Arceci, MD, PhD

16 Late Effects of Therapy

Anthracycline-Related Cardiomyopathy After Childhood Cancer: Role of Polymorphisms in Carbonyl Reductase Genes—A Report From the Children's Oncology Group

Blanco JG, Sun C-L, Landier W, et al (The State Univ of New York at Buffalo; Univ of California, San Diego; et al)

J Clin Oncol 30:1415-1421, 2012

Purpose.—Carbonyl reductases (CBRs) catalyze reduction of anthracyclines to cardiotoxic alcohol metabolites. Polymorphisms in *CBR1* and *CBR3* influence synthesis of these metabolites. We examined whether single nucleotide polymorphisms in *CBR1* (*CBR1* 1096G>A) and/or *CBR3* (*CBR3* V244M) modified the dose-dependent risk of anthracycline-related cardiomyopathy in childhood cancer survivors.

Patients and Methods.—One hundred seventy survivors with cardiomyopathy (patient cases) were compared with 317 survivors with no cardiomyopathy (controls; matched on cancer diagnosis, year of diagnosis, length of follow-up, and race/ethnicity) using conditional logistic regression techniques.

Results.—A dose-dependent association was observed between cumulative anthracycline exposure and cardiomyopathy risk (0 mg/m^2: reference; 1 to 100 mg/m^2: odds ratio [OR], 1.65; 101 to 150 mg/m^2: OR, 3.85; 151 to 200 mg/m^2: OR, 3.69; 201 to 250 mg/m^2: OR, 7.23; 251 to 300 mg/m^2: OR, 23.47; > 300 mg/m^2: OR, 27.59; $P_{trend} < .001$). Among individuals carrying the variant A allele (*CBR1*:GA/AA and/or *CBR3*:GA/AA), exposure to low- to moderate-dose anthracyclines (1 to 250 mg/m^2) did not increase the risk of cardiomyopathy. Among individuals with *CBR3* V244M homozygous G genotypes (*CBR3*:GG), exposure to low- to moderate-dose anthracyclines increased cardiomyopathy risk when compared with individuals with *CBR3*:GA/AA genotypes unexposed to anthracyclines (OR, 5.48; $P = .003$), as well as exposed to low- to moderate-dose anthracyclines (OR, 3.30; $P = .006$). High-dose anthracyclines (> 250 mg/m^2) were associated with increased cardiomyopathy risk, irrespective of *CBR* genotype status.

Conclusion.—This study demonstrates increased anthracycline-related cardiomyopathy risk at doses as low as 101 to 150 mg/m^2. Homozygosis for G allele in *CBR3* contributes to increased cardiomyopathy risk associated with low- to moderate-dose anthracyclines, such that there seems to be no safe dose for patients homozygous for the *CBR3* V244M G allele. These results suggest a need for targeted intervention for those at increased risk of cardiomyopathy.

▶ The reproducibility and validation of genetic studies of association with clinical outcomes has limited in many instances the practical application of such information. Predicting which cancer survivors who were exposed during their treatment to anthracyclines later develop significant cardiotoxicity remains an immense challenge. Several reports are now emerging, all of which are using somewhat different definitions of cardiotoxicity, how toxicity is measured, various groups of patients, and experimental approaches to define molecular determinants. Blanco et al report on a very focused molecular approach to identification of the potential of such molecular prognostic determinants. They hypothesize that polymorphisms in genes of the carbonyl reductases (CBRs), important in the synthesis of anthracycline-derived metabolites, would predict which patients were at highest risk for developing cardiac toxicity. Not surprisingly (or else it probably would not have been published), they identified a dose-dependent association between the cumulative anthracycline exposure, the development of cardiotoxicity, and the presence of variant alleles in the CBR1 and/or CBR3 genes. A curiosity (and not easily explained) is that the variant alleles were only predictive in patients exposed to low- or moderate-dose anthracycline and not to high-dose anthracyclines. A further caveat is that variants in these genes were not identified as risk factors in the larger screen reported by Visscher et al.[1] It is difficult to explain such discrepancies, but for such studies to have a more expeditious and practical outcome, journals and funding agencies should insist that investigators exchange materials and databases to attempt to find the truth in the matter, rather than looking for your lost keys under the lamppost because that is where the light is.

R. J. Arceci, MD, PhD

Reference

1. Visscher H, Ross CJ, Rassekh SR, et al. Pharmacogenomic prediction of anthracycline-induced cardiotoxicity in children. *J Clin Oncol.* 2012;30:1422-1428.

Congenital Anomalies in the Children of Cancer Survivors: A Report From the Childhood Cancer Survivor Study

Signorello LB, Mulvihill JJ, Green DM, et al (International Epidemiology Inst, Rockville, MD; Univ of Oklahoma; St Jude Children's Res Hosp, Memphis, TN; et al)
J Clin Oncol 30:239-245, 2012

Purpose.—Children with cancer receive mutagenic treatments, which raises concern about the potential transmissibility of germline damage to their offspring. This question has been inadequately studied to date because of a lack of detailed individual treatment exposure assessment such as gonadal radiation doses.

Methods.—Within the Childhood Cancer Survivor Study, we performed a retrospective cohort analysis of validated cases of congenital anomalies among 4,699 children of 1,128 male and 1,627 female childhood cancer survivors. We quantified chemotherapy with alkylating agents and radiotherapy doses to the testes and ovaries and related these exposures to risk of congenital anomalies using logistic regression.

Results.—One hundred twenty-nine children had at least one anomaly (prevalence = 2.7%). For children whose mothers were exposed to radiation or alkylating agents versus neither, the prevalence of anomalies was 3.0% versus 3.5% (P = .51); corresponding figures were 1.9% versus 1.7% (P = .79) for the children of male survivors. Neither ovarian radiation dose (mean, 1.19 Gy; odds ratio [OR] = 0.59; 95% CI, 0.20 to 1.75 for 2.50+ Gy) nor testicular radiation dose (mean, 0.48 Gy; OR = 1.01; 95% CI, 0.36 to 2.83 for 0.50+ Gy) was related to risk of congenital anomalies. Treatment with alkylating agents also was not significantly associated with anomalies in the children of male or female survivors.

Conclusion.—Our findings offer strong evidence that the children of cancer survivors are not at significantly increased risk for congenital anomalies stemming from their parent's exposure to mutagenic cancer treatments. This information is important for counseling cancer survivors planning to have children.

► That certain types of chemotherapies and ionizing radiation used in the treatment of patients with cancer are mutagenic is well established. However, all cells of the body may not be equally sensitive to developing sustainable mutations that lead to secondary cancers, either by their inherent resistance or as a result of their anatomic location and microenvironment. A major question in oncology has also been what the risks of exposures are to the offspring of parents who received treatment for their cancers prior to having their own children. The report by Signorello at al demonstrates that the offspring of cancer survivors do not appear to be at increased risk of congenital anomalies. While such information has been published multiple times and as early as 1979,[1] the important contribution of the Signorello et al report is that a detailed assessment of gonadal treatment exposure, especially to alkylating agents and radiation, represents a key assessment in the analysis of adverse late effects. Unfortunately, what such studies cannot assess is whether events that were not necessarily clinically evident from retrospective reviews, such as early-gestation spontaneous miscarriages, are different. Gestation is a power biological selection process for normality. In addition, another question arises as to whether such data suggest that survivors do not have germline alterations that predisposed them to developing cancer as well as influence subsequent reproductive potential. Nevertheless, the results will be helpful in counseling patients. They also should now help to contribute to international studies in which different germline genetic differences may become apparent.

R. J. Arceci, MD, PhD

Reference

1. Li FP, Fine W, Jaffe N, Holmes GE, Holmes FF. Offspring of patients treated for cancer in childhood. *J Natl Cancer Inst.* 1979;62:1193-1197.

Nonmalignant Late Effects and Compromised Functional Status in Survivors of Hematopoietic Cell Transplantation

Khera N, Storer B, Flowers MED, et al (Fred Hutchinson Cancer Res Ctr, Seattle, WA)

J Clin Oncol 30:71-77, 2012

Purpose.—Our objective was to describe the incidence of nonmalignant late complications and their association with health and functional status in a recent cohort of hematopoietic cell transplantation (HCT) survivors.

Patients and Methods.—We determined the incidence of 14 nonmalignant late effects in adults who underwent transplantation from January 2004 through June 2009 at Fred Hutchinson Cancer Research Center who survived at least 1 year after HCT. Data were derived from review of medical records and annual self-reported questionnaires.

Results.—The 1,087 survivors in the study had a median age at HCT of 53 years (range, 21 to 78 years) and were followed for a median of 37 months (range, 12 to 77 months) after HCT. The prevalence of preexisting conditions ranged from 0% to 9.8%. The cumulative incidence of any nonmalignant late effect at 5 years after HCT was 44.8% among autologous and 79% among allogeneic recipients; 2.5% of autologous and 25.5% of allogeneic recipients had three or more late effects. Survivors with three or more late effects had lower physical functioning and Karnofsky score, lower likelihood of full-time work or study, and a higher likelihood of having limitations in usual activities. Predictors of at least one late effect were age ≥50 years, female sex, and unrelated donor, but not the intensity of the conditioning regimen.

Conclusion.—The burden of nonmalignant late effects after HCT is high, even with modern treatments and relatively short follow-up. These late effects are associated with poor health and functional status, underscoring the need for close follow-up of this group and additional research to address these complications.

▶ Most people would agree that going through a bone marrow transplant is not easy. The immediate, short-, and long-term toxicities are significant and often considered the tradeoff for a potentially life-saving treatment. Several studies in pediatric and adult patients who have undergone transplant have reported significant late effects that have major impact on quality-of-life measures. The report by Khera et al helps further define the adverse consequences of having undergone a bone marrow transplant. They examined 1087 survivors of either autologous or allogeneic bone marrow transplant at a single institution. The age range was 21 to 78 years with an entire study cohort median of 53. The majority of the allogeneic transplants received myeloablative preparatory regimens. Fourteen nonmalignant adverse late effects were examined, which revealed that approximately 45% and 79%, respectively, of survivors of autologous and allogeneic transplants had significant late toxicities. Those with 3 or more adverse late effects had lower physical functional and Karnofsky score and lower likelihood of full-time work. Age greater than 50 years, being female, or receiving an unrelated donor transplant all correlated with worse outcomes. Interestingly, the intensity of the conditioning regimen did not appear to impact the frequency of adverse late effects. It is postulated that this may be because those who underwent nonablative regimens were older. While such studies may be biased because of reporting differences of various groups of survivors, the results do pose important challenges and future questions, especially as to how such complications can be reduced and whether nonablative preparatory regimens will be able to contribute to this reduction in younger patients. The report also stresses the need for a carefully articulated and concise medical survivorship document to be part of each patient's medical record.

R. J. Arceci, MD, PhD

Pharmacogenomic Prediction of Anthracycline-Induced Cardiotoxicity in Children

Visscher H, Canadian Pharmacogenomics Network for Drug Safety Consortium (Univ of British Columbia, Vancouver; et al)

J Clin Oncol 30:1422-1428, 2012

Purpose.—Anthracycline-induced cardiotoxicity (ACT) is a serious adverse drug reaction limiting anthracycline use and causing substantial morbidity and mortality. Our aim was to identify genetic variants associated with ACT in patients treated for childhood cancer.

Patients and Methods.—We carried out a study of 2,977 single-nucleotide polymorphisms (SNPs) in 220 key drug biotransformation genes in a discovery cohort of 156 anthracycline-treated children from British Columbia, with replication in a second cohort of 188 children from across Canada and further replication of the top SNP in a third cohort of 96 patients from Amsterdam, the Netherlands.

Results.—We identified a highly significant association of a synonymous coding variant rs7853758 (L461L) within the *SLC28A3* gene with ACT (odds ratio, 0.35; $P = 1.8 \times 10^{-5}$ for all cohorts combined). Additional associations ($P < .01$) with risk and protective variants in other genes including *SLC28A1* and several adenosine triphosphate–binding cassette transporters (*ABCB1*, *ABCB4*, and *ABCC1*) were present. We further explored combining multiple variants into a single-prediction model together with clinical risk factors and classification of patients into three risk groups. In the high-risk group, 75% of patients were accurately predicted to develop ACT, with 36% developing this within the first year alone, whereas in the low-risk group, 96% of patients were accurately predicted not to develop ACT.

Conclusion.—We have identified multiple genetic variants in SLC28A3 and other genes associated with ACT. Combined with clinical risk factors, genetic risk profiling might be used to identify high-risk patients who can then be provided with safer treatment options.

▶ While the risk of cardiotoxicity following exposure to anthracyclines has been known for decades, there has been little information except for some general dose and clinical exposures that could predict which patient would develop such toxicities. To this end, Visscher et al have applied a relatively large-scale molecular association study examining 2977 single-nucleotide polymorphisms (SNPs) in 220 drug biotransformation genes in 3 separate cohorts of childhood survivors following anthracycline exposures of different degrees. They report that a synonymous coding variant of the *SLC28A3* gene was significantly associated with an increased risk of cardiotoxicity development. When combined with specific clinical risk factors, a model was constructed that had a 75% accuracy of predicting in a high-risk group the development of significant cardiotoxicity, while in a lower-risk group, 96% of patients were accurately predicted (Fig 2 in the original article). While not perfect (and biological predictions rarely are), these data represent a potentially important contribution. Furthermore, a significant strength of the report is the use of 3 independent cohorts for validation. Unfortunately, this study only examined a subset of SNPs within a preselected group of genes, leaving open whether the genes in question were key or associated with other genomic predispositions. Nevertheless, this is more than a beginning. The real question is whether such information can be translated into preemptive practice to modify therapies while maintaining cure rates.

R. J. Arceci, MD, PhD

Secondary solid cancers after allogeneic hematopoietic cell transplantation using busulfan-cyclophosphamide conditioning

Majhail NS, Brazauskas R, Rizzo JD, et al (Ctr for International Blood and Marrow Transplant Res, Minneapolis, MN; et al)

Blood 117:316-322, 2011

Risks of secondary solid cancers among allogeneic hematopoietic cell transplant (HCT) recipients who receive conditioning without total body irradiation are not well known. We evaluated the incidence and risk factors for solid cancers after HCT using high-dose busulfan-cyclophosphamide conditioning in 4318 recipients of first allogeneic HCT for acute myeloid leukemia in first complete remission (N = 1742) and chronic myeloid leukemia in first chronic phase (N = 2576). Our cohort represented 22 041 person-years at risk. Sixty-six solid cancers were reported at a median of 6 years after HCT. The cumulative-incidence of solid cancers at 5 and 10 years after HCT was 0.6% and 1.2% among acute myeloid leukemia and 0.9% and 2.4% among chronic myeloid leukemia patients. In comparison to general population incidence rates, HCT recipients had

1.4× higher than expected rate of invasive solid cancers (95% confidence interval, 1.08-1.79, $P = .01$). Significantly elevated risks were observed for tumors of the oral cavity, esophagus, lung, soft tissue, and brain. Chronic graft-versus-host disease was an independent risk factor for all solid cancers, and especially cancers of the oral cavity. Recipients of allogeneic HCT using busulfan-cyclophosphamide conditioning are at risk for developing solid cancers. Their incidence continues to increase with time, and lifelong cancer surveillance is warranted in this population.

► The risk of secondary malignancies following treatment of patients with a new diagnosis of cancer remains one of the primary adverse risks. Most of these secondary malignancies are also likely to be treatment related. In the bone marrow transplant setting, the use of total body irradiation (TBI) as part of preparative regimens has been shown to be associated with an increased risk of secondary malignancies, particularly breast, thyroid, lung, and brain tumors. Less is known about non-TBI-based conditioning regimens. The report by Majhail et al focuses on the incidence and type of secondary cancers in survivors of non-TBI-containing preparative transplant regimen (busulfan/cyclophosphamide) with allogeneic donors in patients with acute myeloid leukemia (AML) or chronic myeloid leukemia (CML). Close to 6000 patients met criteria for their study. The cumulative incidence of solid cancers at 10 years following transplant was 1.2% and 2.4% for patients with AML and CML, respectively. Of note, the highest incidence was for lung cancer and with a suggestion that this increased frequency was more associated with patients with a history of smoking. There was also no plateau in the occurrence of secondary cancers over time (Fig 1 in the original article). The report raises important issues. Clearly, non-TBI-based transplant regimens are associated with an increased incidence of posttransplant solid secondary malignancies. Furthermore, prior life exposures may be an important consideration in determining which preparative regimen might reduce the incidence of specific secondary cancers. In addition, such patients need to be carefully followed for the rest of their lives. Early detection of secondary cancers, such as breast, thyroid, lung, and others, is far more curable than when the diagnosis made is at an advanced cancer stage.

R. J. Arceci, MD, PhD

17 Novel Targets

Paraneoplastic Thrombocytosis in Ovarian Cancer

Stone RL, Nick AM, McNeish IA, et al (Univ of Texas M.D. Anderson Cancer Ctr, Houston, TX; Univ of London, UK; et al)

N Engl J Med 366:610-618, 2012

Background.—The mechanisms of paraneoplastic thrombocytosis in ovarian cancer and the role that platelets play in abetting cancer growth are unclear.

Methods.—We analyzed clinical data on 619 patients with epithelial ovarian cancer to test associations between platelet counts and disease outcome. Human samples and mouse models of epithelial ovarian cancer were used to explore the underlying mechanisms of paraneoplastic thrombocytosis. The effects of platelets on tumor growth and angiogenesis were ascertained.

Results.—Thrombocytosis was significantly associated with advanced disease and shortened survival. Plasma levels of thrombopoietin and interleukin-6 were significantly elevated in patients who had thrombocytosis as compared with those who did not. In mouse models, increased hepatic thrombopoietin synthesis in response to tumor-derived interleukin-6 was an underlying mechanism of paraneoplastic thrombocytosis. Tumor-derived interleukin-6 and hepatic thrombopoietin were also linked to thrombocytosis in patients. Silencing thrombopoietin and interleukin-6 abrogated thrombocytosis in tumor-bearing mice. Anti-interleukin-6 antibody treatment significantly reduced platelet counts in tumor-bearing mice and in patients with epithelial ovarian cancer. In addition, neutralizing interleukin-6 significantly enhanced the therapeutic efficacy of paclitaxel in mouse models of epithelial ovarian cancer. The use of an antiplatelet antibody to halve platelet counts in tumor-bearing mice significantly reduced tumor growth and angiogenesis.

Conclusions.—These findings support the existence of a paracrine circuit wherein increased production of thrombopoietic cytokines in tumor and host tissue leads to paraneoplastic thrombocytosis, which fuels tumor growth. We speculate that countering paraneoplastic thrombocytosis either directly or indirectly by targeting these cytokines may have therapeutic potential. (Funded by the National Cancer Institute and others.)

► Thrombocytosis as a paraneoplastic manifestation (defined as a platelet count of greater than 450 000) has been well-described and known for more than a century. The mechanism is thought to be mediated through interleukin-6, which stimulates the production of hepatic thrombopoietin, which in turn causes the thrombocytosis. Cancers associated most frequently with thrombocytosis include those of the gastrointestinal tract, breast, lung, and ovaries. The phenomenon is associated with a poor prognosis. According to the literature, nearly 40% of patients with thrombocytosis in the absence of inflammation or iron deficiency turn out to have an occult malignancy. Further evidence suggests that platelets can contribute to the progression of the disease process by a number of mechanisms. This study evaluated the impact of neutralizing the interleukin-6 with an antibody and reducing the platelet count with an antiplatelet antibody and found that the former enhanced the therapeutic efficacy of paclitaxel at least in mice and that the latter reduced tumor growth and angiogenesis in both mice and patients with ovarian cancer. These observations support further investigation of therapy directed at thrombocytosis and its underlying mechanism as another approach to treatment of these patients with a poor prognosis.

J. T. Thigpen, MD

18 Supportive Care

Impact of Awareness of Terminal Illness and Use of Palliative Care or Intensive Care Unit on the Survival of Terminally Ill Patients With Cancer: Prospective Cohort Study

Yun YH, Lee MK, Kim SY, et al (Natl Cancer Ctr, Gyeonggi-do, Korea)

J Clin Oncol 29:2474-2480, 2011

Purpose.—We conducted this study to evaluate the validity of the perception that awareness of their terminal prognosis and use of palliative care or nonuse of an intensive care unit (ICU) causes patients to die sooner than they would otherwise.

Patients and Methods.—In this prospective cohort study at 11 university hospitals and the National Cancer Center in Korea, we administered questionnaires to 619 consecutive patients immediately after they were determined by physicians to be terminally ill. We followed patients during 6 months after enrollment and assessed how their survival was affected by the disclosure of terminal illness and administration of palliative care or nonuse of the ICU.

Results.—In a follow-up of 481 patients and 163.8 person-years, we identified 466 deceased patients. Nineteen percent of the patients died within 1 month, while 41.3% lived for 3 months, and 17.7% lived for 6 months. Once the cancer was judged terminal, the median survival time was 69 days. On multivariate analysis, neither patient awareness of terminal status at baseline (adjusted hazard ratio [aHR], 1.20; 95% CI, 0.96 to 1.51), use of a palliative care facility (aHR, 0.96; 95% CI, 0.76 to 1.21), nor general prostration (aHR, 1.23; 95% CI, 0.96 to 1.57) was associated with reduced survival. Use of the ICU (aHR, 1.47; 95% CI, 1.06 to 2.05) and poor Eastern Cooperative Oncology Group performance status (aHR, 1.37; 95% CI, 1.10 to 1.71) were significantly associated with poor survival.

Conclusion.—Patients' being aware that they are dying and entering a palliative care facility or ICU does not seem to influence patients' survival.

► Oncologists are routinely presented with patients whose prognosis is poor and there are few if any reasonable treatment options left. Yet we struggle in our ability to verbalize this to patients, thinking that if we say "you are terminal; we have no other treatments to offer," it will hasten their demise. Slowly but surely more data are emerging to support this frank communication with our patients and the use of the palliative care option.

The data presented in this prospective cohort study are another example of the appropriate use of this ever-emerging field of medicine. Patients who are told they are terminal and have access to palliative care personnel do not die sooner, as shown in this study. In fact these and other data looking at the role of palliative care services show that not only do patients not die sooner, their quality of life can improve given appropriate palliative care. We as oncologists need to access this option sooner rather than later for our terminal patients and their families.

C. Lawton, MD

Semuloparin for Thromboprophylaxis in Patients Receiving Chemotherapy for Cancer

Agnelli G, for the SAVE-ONCO Investigators (Univ of Perugia, Italy; et al)
N Engl J Med 366:601-609, 2012

Background.—Patients receiving chemotherapy for cancer are at increased risk for venous thromboembolism. Limited data support the clinical benefit of antithrombotic prophylaxis.

Methods.—In this double-blind, multicenter trial, we evaluated the efficacy and safety of the ultra-low-molecular-weight heparin semuloparin for prevention of venous thromboembolism in patients receiving chemotherapy for cancer. Patients with metastatic or locally advanced solid tumors who were beginning to receive a course of chemotherapy were randomly assigned to receive subcutaneous semuloparin, 20 mg once daily, or placebo until there was a change of chemotherapy regimen. The primary efficacy outcome was the composite of any symptomatic deep-vein thrombosis, any nonfatal pulmonary embolism, and death related to venous thromboembolism. Clinically relevant bleeding (major and nonmajor) was the main safety outcome.

Results.—The median treatment duration was 3.5 months. Venous thromboembolism occurred in 20 of 1608 patients (1.2%) receiving semuloparin, as compared with 55 of 1604 (3.4%) receiving placebo (hazard ratio, 0.36; 95% confidence interval [CI], 0.21 to 0.60; $P < 0.001$), with consistent efficacy among subgroups defined according to the origin and stage of cancer and the baseline risk of venous thromboembolism. The incidence of clinically relevant bleeding was 2.8% and 2.0% in the semuloparin and placebo groups, respectively (hazard ratio, 1.40; 95% CI, 0.89 to 2.21). Major bleeding occurred in 19 of 1589 patients (1.2%) receiving semuloparin and 18 of 1583 (1.1%) receiving placebo (hazard ratio, 1.05; 95% CI, 0.55 to 1.99). Incidences of all other adverse events were similar in the two study groups.

Conclusions.—Semuloparin reduces the incidence of thromboembolic events in patients receiving chemotherapy for cancer, with no apparent increase in major bleeding. (Funded by Sanofi; ClinicalTrials.gov number, NCT00694382.)

▶ Patients with advanced cancer, particularly those with lung cancer and cancers of the gastrointestinal tract, incur an increased frequency of venous thrombosis. This increased risk is enhanced further in patients receiving chemotherapy for their cancer diagnosis. Anecdotal observations have suggested that low-dose anticoagulation may prevent some episodes of venous thrombosis. This study proposed to evaluate the premise that anticoagulation could reduce the likelihood of venous thrombosis in patients with lung, pancreatic, colorectal, stomach, bladder, and ovary cancers. Patients were randomized to placebo or once daily semuloparin, an ultra–low-molecular-weight heparin, at the start of a chemotherapy regimen and continued on treatment until a change in chemotherapy regimen became necessary. The results demonstrated a lowering of the incidence of venous thrombosis from 3.4% to 1.2% without an increase in significant bleeding and without a compromise in the outcome of the patient's disease process. The authors do not speculate on whether they feel this should become a standard treatment approach, and they do point out that National Comprehensive Cancer Network guidelines suggest that further study is needed.

J. T. Thigpen, MD

19 Miscellaneous

What Oncologists Believe They Said and What Patients Believe They Heard: An Analysis of Phase I Trial Discussions

Jenkins V, Solis-Trapala I, Langridge C, et al (Univ of Sussex, Falmer, Brighton, UK; Lancaster Univ, UK; Churchill Hosp, Oxford, UK)
J Clin Oncol 29:61-68, 2011

Purpose.—Evaluation of the communication and informed consent process in phase I clinical trial interviews to provide authentic, practice-based content for inclusion in a communication skills training intervention for health care professionals.

Patients and Methods.—Seventeen oncologists and 52 patients from five United Kingdom cancer centers consented to recording of phase I trial discussions. Following each consultation, clinicians completed questionnaires indicating areas they felt they had discussed, and researchers conducted semistructured interviews with patients examining their recall and understanding. Patients and oncologists also completed the Life Orientation Test-Revised questionnaire, measuring predisposition toward optimism. Independent researchers coded the consultations identifying discussion of key information areas and how well this was done. Observed levels of agreement were analyzed for each consultation between oncologist-coder, oncologist-patient, and patient-coder pairs.

Results.—In several key areas, information was either missing or had been explained but was interpreted incorrectly by patients. Discussion of prognosis was a frequent omission, with patients and coders significantly more likely to agree that oncologists had not discussed it (odds, 4.8; $P < .001$). In contrast, coders and oncologists were more likely to agree that alternate care plans to phase I trial entry had been explained (odds, 2.5; $P = .023$).

Conclusion.—These data indicate that fundamental components of communication and information sharing about phase I trial participation are often missing from interviews. Important omissions included discussion of prognosis and ensuring patient understanding about supportive care. These findings will inform educational initiatives to assist communication about phase I trials.

► As oncologists we are constantly discussing treatment options with patients and their families. We are taught as residents/fellows the importance of open, clear, and honest communication with patients regarding risks and benefits of the treatment options available. This expression of open, honest, and clear communication becomes even more critical when we discuss participation in clinical trials. Of all the clinical trials available to patients, in phase I trials, in which toxicity is the endpoint, the discussions need to be even more explicit, as supportive care is often the obvious alternative.

It is very clear from this dataset that what we as oncologists feel that we have communicated is not in fact what the patients feel they have heard. Lack of discussion of prognosis, as the patients documented in this report, is of significant concern.

These data behoove all oncologists to rethink their approach to discussions of participations in clinical trials in general and particularly in discussion of phase I trial participation. Consideration of multiple meetings with patients potentially enrolling in clinical trials and consideration of patients meeting with clinical trial nurses as a separate visit are both important to enhance the overall understanding of a patient who ponders clinical trial participation.

C. Lawton, MD

Article Index

Chapter 1: Cancer Biology

Clinically Relevant Changes in Family History of Cancer Over Time 1

Intratumor Heterogeneity and Branched Evolution Revealed by Multiregion Sequencing 2

Chapter 2: Cancer Prevention

Effect of daily aspirin on risk of cancer metastasis: a study of incident cancers during randomised controlled trials 5

Chapter 3: Cancer Therapies

American society for radiation oncology (ASTRO) and american college of radiology (ACR) practice guideline for the performance of high-dose-rate brachytherapy 7

Chapter 4: Chemotherapy: Mechanisms and Side Effects

Appropriate Chemotherapy Dosing for Obese Adult Patients With Cancer: American Society of Clinical Oncology Clinical Practice Guideline 9

Chapter 5: Breast Cancer

Characteristics and Outcomes of Breast Cancer in Women With and Without a History of Radiation for Hodgkin's Lymphoma: A Multi-Institutional, Matched Cohort Study 11

Quality-of-Life Measurement in Randomized Clinical Trials in Breast Cancer: An Updated Systematic Review (2001–2009) 13

Dietary fiber intake and risk of breast cancer: a meta-analysis of prospective cohort studies 16

Tumor-Infiltrating $CD8^+$ Lymphocytes Predict Clinical Outcome in Breast Cancer 18

Adjuvant Therapy in Stage I Carcinoma of the Breast: The Influence of Multigene Analyses and Molecular Phenotyping 20

Association of Occult Metastases in Sentinel Lymph Nodes and Bone Marrow With Survival Among Women With Early-Stage Invasive Breast Cancer 21

Bevacizumab Added to Neoadjuvant Chemotherapy for Breast Cancer 22

Comparisons between different polychemotherapy regimens for early breast cancer: meta-analyses of long-term outcome among 100 000 women in 123 randomised trials 23

Disease-Related Outcomes With Long-Term Follow-Up: An Updated Analysis of the Intergroup Exemestane Study 25

Preoperative Chemotherapy Plus Trastuzumab, Lapatinib, or Both in Human Epidermal Growth Factor Receptor 2–Positive Operable Breast Cancer: Results of the Randomized Phase II CHER-LOB Study 26

Effect of Obesity on Prognosis After Early-Stage Breast Cancer 27

Effect of Occult Metastases on Survival in Node-Negative Breast Cancer 28

Lapatinib with trastuzumab for HER2-positive early breast cancer (NeoALTTO): a randomised, open-label, multicentre, phase 3 trial 30

Ductal Carcinoma In Situ Treated With Breast-Conserving Surgery and Accelerated Partial Breast Irradiation: Comparison of the Mammosite Registry Trial With Intergroup Study E5194 31

Comparison of treatment outcome between breast-conservation surgery with radiation and total mastectomy without radiation in patients with one to three positive axillary lymph nodes 32

Breast Imaging Training and Attitudes: Update Survey of Senior Radiology Residents 34

Screening Breast MR Imaging in Women with a History of Chest Irradiation 36

Effect of HER2 status on risk of recurrence in women with small, node-negative breast tumours 38

Factors influencing survival in patients with breast cancer and single or solitary brain metastasis 40

Accelerated partial breast irradiation with interstitial implants: risk factors associated with increased local recurrence 42

Accelerated partial breast irradiation: 5-year results of the German-Austrian multicenter phase II trial using interstitial multicatheter brachytherapy alone after breast-conserving surgery 44

Age, Comorbidity, and Breast Cancer Severity: Impact on Receipt of Definitive Local Therapy and Rate of Recurrence among Older Women with Early-Stage Breast Cancer 46

Early-stage young breast cancer patients: Impact of local treatment on survival 47

Fractionation for whole breast irradiation: An American Society for Radiation Oncology (ASTRO) evidence-based guideline 50

Irradiation effect after mastectomy on breast cancer recurrence in patients presenting with locally advanced disease 53

Liver resection and local ablation of breast cancer liver metastases – A systematic review 55

Phase III randomized equivalence trial of early breast cancer treatments with or without axillary clearance in post-menopausal patients results after 5 years of follow-up 57

Subsets of women with close or positive margins after breast-conserving surgery with high local recurrence risk despite breast plus boost radiotherapy 61

Effect of Very Small Tumor Size on Cancer-Specific Mortality in Node-Positive Breast Cancer 65

Axillary Dissection vs No Axillary Dissection in Women With Invasive Breast Cancer and Sentinel Node Metastasis: A Randomized Clinical Trial 66

Timing of radiotherapy and outcome in patients receiving adjuvant endocrine therapy 68

Adjuvant Tamoxifen Reduces Subsequent Breast Cancer in Women With Estrogen Receptor–Positive Ductal Carcinoma in Situ: A Study Based on NSABP Protocol B-24 71

Ductal Carcinoma In Situ Treated With Breast-Conserving Surgery and Radiotherapy: A Comparison With ECOG Study 5194 72

Everolimus in Postmenopausal Hormone-Receptor–Positive Advanced Breast Cancer 74

Loss of Human Epidermal Growth Factor Receptor 2 (HER2) Expression in Metastatic Sites of HER2-Overexpressing Primary Breast Tumors 75

Pertuzumab plus Trastuzumab plus Docetaxel for Metastatic Breast Cancer 76

Management of hot flashes in patients who have breast cancer with venlafaxine and clonidine: a randomized, double-blind, placebo-controlled trial 77

Nodal status and clinical outcomes in a large cohort of patients with triple-negative breast cancer 78

Chapter 6: Genitourinary

10-year experience with I-125 prostate brachytherapy at the Princess Margaret Hospital: results for 1,100 patients 81

American Society for Radiation Oncology (ASTRO) and American College of Radiology (ACR) practice guideline for the transperineal permanent brachytherapy of prostate cancer 82

Behavioral Therapy With or Without Biofeedback and Pelvic Floor Electrical Stimulation for Persistent Postprostatectomy Incontinence: A Randomized Controlled Trial 83

Comparison of Health-Related Quality of Life 5 Years After SPIRIT: Surgical Prostatectomy Versus Interstitial Radiation Intervention Trial 85

Cost-Effectiveness of Prostate Specific Antigen Screening in the United States: Extrapolating From the European Study of Screening for Prostate Cancer 86

Definition of medical event is to be based on the total source strength for evaluation of permanent prostate brachytherapy: A report from the American Society for Radiation Oncology 87

Does hormone therapy reduce disease recurrence in prostate cancer patients receiving dose-escalated radiation therapy? An analysis of Radiation Therapy Oncology Group 94-06 89

Dose escalation and quality of life in patients with localized prostate cancer treated with radiotherapy: long-term results of the Dutch randomized dose-escalation trial (CKTO 96-10 Trial) 90

Fifteen-year biochemical relapse-free survival, cause-specific survival, and overall survival following I^{125} prostate brachytherapy in clinically localized prostate cancers: Seattle experience 91

Phase I dose-escalation study of stereotactic body radiation therapy for low and intermediate-risk prostate cancer 92

Progression From High-Grade Prostatic Intraepithelial Neoplasia to Cancer: A Randomized Trial of Combination Vitamin-E, Soy, and Selenium 93

Radiotherapy and Short-Term Androgen Deprivation for Localized Prostate Cancer 95

Radical Prostatectomy versus Watchful Waiting in Early Prostate Cancer 96

Vitamin E and the Risk of Prostate Cancer: The Selenium and Vitamin E Cancer Prevention Trial (SELECT) 97

Association of diagnostic radiation exposure and second abdominal-pelvic malignancies after testicular cancer 99

Management of Seminomatous Testicular Cancer: A Binational Prospective Population-Based Study From the Swedish Norwegian Testicular Cancer Study Group 100

Randomized Trial of Carboplatin Versus Radiotherapy for Stage I Seminoma: Mature Results on Relapse and Contralateral Testis Cancer Rates in MRC TE19/EORTC 30982 Study (ISRCTN27163214) 101

Chapter 7: Gynecology

A Multicenter, Randomized, Phase 2 Clinical Trial to Evaluate the Efficacy and Safety of Combination Docetaxel and Carboplatin and Sequential Therapy With Docetaxel Then Carboplatin in Patients With Recurrent Platinum-Sensitive Ovarian Cancer 103

A Phase 3 Trial of Bevacizumab in Ovarian Cancer 104

A systematic review evaluating the relationship between progression free survival and post progression survival in advanced ovarian cancer 106

CA-125 can be part of the tumour evaluation criteria in ovarian cancer trials: experience of the GCIG CALYPSO trial 107

Evolution of surgical treatment paradigms for advanced-stage ovarian cancer: Redefining 'optimal' residual disease 108

Final overall survival results of phase III GCIG CALYPSO trial of pegylated liposomal doxorubicin and carboplatin *vs* paclitaxel and carboplatin in platinum-sensitive ovarian cancer patients 109

Incorporation of Bevacizumab in the Primary Treatment of Ovarian Cancer 110

Is comprehensive surgical staging needed for thorough evaluation of early-stage ovarian carcinoma? 112

OCEANS: A Randomized, Double-Blind, Placebo-Controlled Phase III Trial of Chemotherapy With or Without Bevacizumab in Patients With Platinum-Sensitive Recurrent Epithelial Ovarian, Primary Peritoneal, or Fallopian Tube Cancer 113

Olaparib Maintenance Therapy in Platinum-Sensitive Relapsed Ovarian Cancer 114

Ovarian low-grade serous carcinoma: A comprehensive update 115

Phase II, Open-Label, Randomized, Multicenter Study Comparing the Efficacy and Safety of Olaparib, a Poly (ADP-Ribose) Polymerase Inhibitor, and Pegylated Liposomal Doxorubicin in Patients With *BRCA1* or *BRCA2* Mutations and Recurrent Ovarian Cancer 116

Randomized, Double-Blind, Placebo-Controlled Phase II Study of AMG 386 Combined With Weekly Paclitaxel in Patients With Recurrent Ovarian Cancer 118

Reclassification of Serous Ovarian Carcinoma by a 2-Tier System: A Gynecologic Oncology Group Study 119

Vignette-Based Study of Ovarian Cancer Screening: Do U.S. Physicians Report Adhering to Evidence-Based Recommendations? 120

A multi-institutional phase II trial of paclitaxel and carboplatin in the treatment of advanced or recurrent cervical cancer 122

Chemoradiation and adjuvant chemotherapy in advanced cervical adenocarcinoma 123

Comparison of treatment outcomes between squamous cell carcinoma and adenocarcinoma in locally advanced cervical cancer 124

Consensus guidelines for delineation of clinical target volume for intensity-modulated pelvic radiotherapy for the definitive treatment of cervix cancer 125

Management of recurrent cervical cancer: A review of the literature 126

Association of number of positive nodes and cervical stroma invasion with outcome of advanced endometrial cancer treated with chemotherapy or whole abdominal irradiation: A Gynecologic Oncology Group study 127

Metformin potentiates the effects of paclitaxel in endometrial cancer cells through inhibition of cell proliferation and modulation of the mTOR pathway 128

Recurrence and Survival After Random Assignment to Laparoscopy Versus Laparotomy for Comprehensive Surgical Staging of Uterine Cancer: Gynecologic Oncology Group LAP2 Study 130

The role of lymphadenectomy in endometrial cancer: Was the ASTEC trial doomed by design and are we destined to repeat that mistake? 131

A phase II trial of radiation therapy and weekly cisplatin chemotherapy for the treatment of locally-advanced squamous cell carcinoma of the vulva: A gynecologic oncology group study 132

Chapter 8: Gastrointestinal

Association Between Lymph Node Evaluation for Colon Cancer and Node Positivity Over the Past 20 Years 135

Adjuvant capecitabine and oxaliplatin for gastric cancer after D2 gastrectomy (CLASSIC): a phase 3 open-label, randomised controlled trial 136

Bevacizumab in Combination With Chemotherapy As First-Line Therapy in Advanced Gastric Cancer: A Randomized, Double-Blind, Placebo-Controlled Phase III Study 138

Salvage Chemotherapy for Pretreated Gastric Cancer: A Randomized Phase III Trial Comparing Chemotherapy Plus Best Supportive Care With Best Supportive Care Alone 140

Gemcitabine Alone Versus Gemcitabine Plus Radiotherapy in Patients With Locally Advanced Pancreatic Cancer: An Eastern Cooperative Oncology Group trial 141

A Phase II Trial of Neoadjuvant Chemoradiation and Local Excision for T2N0 Rectal Cancer: Preliminary Results of the ACOSOG Z6041 Trial 142

Primary Tumor Response to Preoperative Chemoradiation With or Without Oxaliplatin in Locally Advanced Rectal Cancer: Pathologic Results of the STAR-01 Randomized Phase III Trial 144

Long-term risk of colorectal cancer after negative colonoscopy 145

Chapter 9: Hematologic Malignancies

Clonal origins of relapse in *ETV6-RUNX1* acute lymphoblastic leukemia 147

Radiation therapy for leukemia cutis 148

The genetic basis of early T–cell precursor acute lymphoblastic leukaemia 149

TP53 alterations in acute myeloid leukemia with complex karyotype correlate with specific copy number alterations, monosomal karyotype, and dismal outcome 150

A phase 1/2 study of chemosensitization with the CXCR4 antagonist plerixafor in relapsed or refractory acute myeloid leukemia 151

Acute leukemia incidence and patient survival among children and adults in the United States, 2001-2007 152

Age-Related Prognostic Impact of Different Types of *DNMT3A* Mutations in Adults With Primary Cytogenetically Normal Acute Myeloid Leukemia 154

Assessment of *BCR-ABL1* Transcript Levels at 3 Months Is the Only Requirement for Predicting Outcome for Patients With Chronic Myeloid Leukemia Treated With Tyrosine Kinase Inhibitors 155

Chronic myeloid leukemia stem cells are not dependent on Bcr-Abl kinase activity for their survival 156

DNMT3A mutations in acute myeloid leukemia: stability during disease evolution and clinical implications 157

Frequency and prognostic impact of mutations in *SRSF2*, *U2AF1*, and *ZRSR2* in patients with myelodysplastic syndromes 158

Increased BMI correlates with higher risk of disease relapse and differentiation syndrome in patients with acute promyelocytic leukemia treated with the AIDA protocols 159

Outcomes after matched unrelated donor versus identical sibling hematopoietic cell transplantation in adults with acute myelogenous leukemia 160

Pediatric-inspired intensified therapy of adult T-ALL reveals the favorable outcome of *NOTCH1/FBXW7* mutations, but not of low *ERG/BAALC* expression: a GRAALL study 162

Poor response to second-line kinase inhibitors in chronic myeloid leukemia patients with multiple low-level mutations, irrespective of their resistance profile 163

Prediction of Early Death After Induction Therapy for Newly Diagnosed Acute Myeloid Leukemia With Pretreatment Risk Scores: A Novel Paradigm for Treatment Assignment 164

Prognostic and therapeutic implications of minimal residual disease detection in acute myeloid leukemia 165

Prognostic Relevance of Integrated Genetic Profiling in Acute Myeloid Leukemia 166

Minimal Disseminated Disease in High-Risk Burkitt's Lymphoma Identifies Patients With Different Prognosis 167

Chapter 10: Thoracic Cancer

DNA Repair Capacity in Peripheral Lymphocytes Predicts Survival of Patients With Non–Small-Cell Lung Cancer Treated With First-Line Platinum-Based Chemotherapy 169

Genetic Variations and Patient-Reported Quality of Life Among Patients With Lung Cancer 170

Occult metastases in lymph nodes predict survival in resectable non–small-cell lung cancer: report of the ACOSOG Z0040 trial 171

Phase III Comparison of Prophylactic Cranial Irradiation Versus Observation in Patients With Locally Advanced Non–Small-Cell Lung Cancer: Primary Analysis of Radiation Therapy Oncology Group Study RTOG 0214 173

Randomized Phase III Study of Surgery Alone or Surgery Plus Preoperative Cisplatin and Gemcitabine in Stages IB to IIIA Non–Small-Cell Lung Cancer 174

Randomized Phase III Study of Thoracic Radiation in Combination With Paclitaxel and Carboplatin With or Without Thalidomide in Patients With Stage III Non–Small-Cell Lung Cancer: The ECOG 3598 Study 175

Reduced Lung-Cancer Mortality with Low-Dose Computed Tomographic Screening 176

First-SIGNAL: First-Line Single-Agent Iressa Versus Gemcitabine and Cisplatin Trial in Never-Smokers With Adenocarcinoma of the Lung 178

Impact on disease-free survival of adjuvant erlotinib or gefitinib in patients with resected lung adenocarcinomas that harbor EGFR mutations 179

Ipilimumab in Combination With Paclitaxel and Carboplatin As First-Line Treatment in Stage IIIB/IV Non–Small-Cell Lung Cancer: Results From a Randomized, Double-Blind, Multicenter Phase II Study 180

Prospective Molecular Marker Analyses of *EGFR* and *KRAS* From a Randomized, Placebo-Controlled Study of Erlotinib Maintenance Therapy in Advanced Non–Small-Cell Lung Cancer 182

Randomized Phase II Trial of Erlotinib Alone or With Carboplatin and Paclitaxel in Patients Who Were Never or Light Former Smokers With Advanced Lung Adenocarcinoma: CALGB 30406 Trial 183

Randomized, Double-Blind, Placebo-Controlled Phase II Study of Single-Agent Oral Talactoferrin in Patients With Locally Advanced or Metastatic Non–Small-Cell Lung Cancer That Progressed After Chemotherapy 185

Weekly *nab*-Paclitaxel in Combination With Carboplatin Versus Solvent-Based Paclitaxel Plus Carboplatin as First-Line Therapy in Patients With Advanced Non–Small-Cell Lung Cancer: Final Results of a Phase III Trial 186

Sunitinib Plus Erlotinib Versus Placebo Plus Erlotinib in Patients With Previously Treated Advanced Non–Small-Cell Lung Cancer: A Phase III Trial 187

Vandetanib Versus Placebo in Patients With Advanced Non–Small-Cell Lung Cancer After Prior Therapy With an Epidermal Growth Factor Receptor Tyrosine Kinase Inhibitor: A Randomized, Double-Blind Phase III Trial (ZEPHYR) 188

Carboplatin- or Cisplatin-Based Chemotherapy in First-Line Treatment of Small-Cell Lung Cancer: The COCIS Meta-Analysis of Individual Patient Data 189

Cisplatin, Irinotecan, and Bevacizumab for Untreated Extensive-Stage Small-Cell Lung Cancer: CALGB 30306, a Phase II Study 191

Randomized Phase II Study of Dulanermin in Combination With Paclitaxel, Carboplatin, and Bevacizumab in Advanced Non–Small-Cell Lung Cancer 192

Randomized Phase II Study of Erlotinib in Combination With Placebo or R1507, a Monoclonal Antibody to Insulin-Like Growth Factor-1 Receptor, for Advanced-Stage Non–Small-Cell Lung Cancer 193

Randomized, Placebo-Controlled Phase III Study of Docetaxel Plus Carboplatin With Celecoxib and Cyclooxygenase-2 Expression as a Biomarker for Patients With Advanced Non–Small-Cell Lung Cancer: the NVALT-4 Study 194

Longitudinal Perceptions of Prognosis and Goals of Therapy in Patients With Metastatic Non–Small-Cell Lung Cancer: Results of a Randomized Study of Early Palliative Care 196

ROS1 Rearrangements Define a Unique Molecular Class of Lung Cancers 197

Chapter 11: Endocrine

Combination Chemotherapy in Advanced Adrenocortical Carcinoma 199

Chapter 12: Head and Neck

A Phase 2 Trial of Bortezomib Followed by the Addition of Doxorubicin at Progression in Patients With Recurrent or Metastatic Adenoid Cystic Carcinoma of the Head and Neck: A trial of the Eastern Cooperative Oncology Group (E1303) 201

A prospective, comparative study on the early effects of local and remote radiation therapy on carotid intima–media thickness and vascular cellular adhesion molecule-1 in patients with head and neck and prostate tumors 202

Chapter 13: Pediatric Cancer

Anti–*Escherichia coli* asparaginase antibody levels determine the activity of second-line treatment with pegylated *E coli* asparaginase: a retrospective analysis within the ALL-BFM trials 205

Developmental origins and impact of *BCR-ABL1* fusion and *IKZF1* deletions in monozygotic twins with Ph$^+$ acute lymphoblastic leukemia 206

Improved Survival for Children and Adolescents With Acute Lymphoblastic Leukemia Between 1990 and 2005: A Report From the Children's Oncology Group 207

Outcome modeling with *CRLF2, IKZF1, JAK*, and minimal residual disease in pediatric acute lymphoblastic leukemia: a Children's Oncology Group Study 208

Outcomes after Induction Failure in Childhood Acute Lymphoblastic Leukemia 210

Clonal selection drives genetic divergence of metastatic medulloblastoma 211

Genome-Wide Analyses Identify Recurrent Amplifications of Receptor Tyrosine Kinases and Cell-Cycle Regulatory Genes in Diffuse Intrinsic Pontine Glioma 212

Pre-Enucleation Chemotherapy for Eyes Severely Affected by Retinoblastoma Masks Risk of Tumor Extension and Increases Death From Metastasis 213

Clinical and Biologic Features Predictive of Survival After Relapse of Neuroblastoma: A Report From the International Neuroblastoma Risk Group Project 215

Outcome After Surgery Alone or With Restricted Use of Chemotherapy for Patients With Low-Risk Neuroblastoma: Results of Children's Oncology Group Study P9641 217

PAX3/FOXO1 Fusion Gene Status Is the Key Prognostic Molecular Marker in Rhabdomyosarcoma and Significantly Improves Current Risk Stratification 218

Pilot Induction Regimen Incorporating Pharmacokinetically Guided Topotecan for Treatment of Newly Diagnosed High-Risk Neuroblastoma: A Children's Oncology Group Study 219

Prognostic Significance and Tumor Biology of Regional Lymph Node Disease in Patients With Rhabdomyosarcoma: A Report From the Children's Oncology Group 220

High Risk of Symptomatic Cardiac Events in Childhood Cancer Survivors 223

Chapter 14: Melanoma

RAS Mutations Are Associated With the Development of Cutaneous Squamous Cell Tumors in Patients Treated With RAF Inhibitors 225

Chapter 15: Sarcoma

Anaplastic Lymphoma Kinase Aberrations in Rhabdomyosarcoma: Clinical and Prognostic Implications 227

Chapter 16: Late Effects of Therapy

Anthracycline-Related Cardiomyopathy After Childhood Cancer: Role of Polymorphisms in Carbonyl Reductase Genes—A Report From the Children's Oncology Group 229

Congenital Anomalies in the Children of Cancer Survivors: A Report From the Childhood Cancer Survivor Study 230

Nonmalignant Late Effects and Compromised Functional Status in Survivors of Hematopoietic Cell Transplantation 232

Pharmacogenomic Prediction of Anthracycline-Induced Cardiotoxicity in Children 233

Secondary solid cancers after allogeneic hematopoietic cell transplantation using busulfan-cyclophosphamide conditioning 234

Chapter 17: Novel Targets

Paraneoplastic Thrombocytosis in Ovarian Cancer 237

Chapter 18: Supportive Care

Impact of Awareness of Terminal Illness and Use of Palliative Care or Intensive Care Unit on the Survival of Terminally Ill Patients With Cancer: Prospective Cohort Study 239

Semuloparin for Thromboprophylaxis in Patients Receiving Chemotherapy for Cancer 240

Chapter 19: Miscellaneous

What Oncologists Believe They Said and What Patients Believe They Heard: An Analysis of Phase I Trial Discussions 243

Author Index

A

Admane S, 196
Advani SH, 185
Aghajanian C, 113
Agnelli G, 240
Al-Mamgani A, 90
Alexander C, 61
Alexandre J, 107
Ali S, 132
Allred DC, 71
Anderson H, 9
Anderson SJ, 71
Ando M, 122
Andriole GL, 86
Argiris A, 201
Aschele C, 144
Ashikaga T, 28
Avril A, 57

B

Bae K, 89, 173
Bagnardi V, 159
Bakst R, 148
Baldwin L-M, 120
Ballman KV, 21, 66
Bang Y-J, 136
Bantema-Joppe EJ, 47
Bartelink H, 20
Baselga J, 30, 74, 76
Bassett LW, 34
Bear HD, 22
Beitsch PD, 31
Ben Abdelali R, 162
Bent C, 34
Bentzen SM, 50
Berchuck A, 103
Bergenfeldt M, 55
Bergethon K, 197
Beyer DC, 82
Bill-Axelson A, 96
Biolo A, 202
Bittner NH, 82
Blanco JG, 229
Blank SV, 113
Blasinska-Morawiec M, 182
Bliss JM, 25
Bodurka DC, 119
Boekhout AH, 77
Boike TP, 92
Bondarenko I, 180, 186
Bordeleau LJ, 13
Boren T, 112
Borg J, 81
Borthakur G, 164
Bosco JLF, 46
Bottini A, 26
Brazauskas R, 234
Breccia M, 159
Brenner H, 145
Bristow RE, 108
Broniscer A, 212
Brown C, 107
Brugger W, 182
Buccisano F, 165
Bullinger L, 150
Burger RA, 110
Burgio KL, 83
Burstein HJ, 20
Burtness B, 201

C

Campone M, 74
Cardenes H, 141
Castel V, 215
Cazzaniga G, 206
Chang S-J, 108
Chang-Claude J, 145
Chavez-Macgregor M, 78
Chen D, 193
Chen I-M, 208
Chen K, 65
Chiodini P, 189
Chisholm J, 218
Cho LC, 92
Cionini L, 144
Coeffic D, 107
Coleman RE, 25
Colman S, 147
Correa CR, 50
Crook J, 81
Crook JM, 85
Curtis RE, 152

D

Dahlberg SE, 175
Dalesio OB, 77
d'Amore ES, 167
de Andrade M, 170
De Munck L, 47
Deavers MT, 119
Decker P, 170
Decker PA, 171
Del Principe MI, 165
Demanes DJ, 7, 87
Devesa SS, 152
Devidas M, 207
Di Maio M, 189
Diaz-Padilla I, 115
Dimaras H, 213
Ding L, 149
Dong J-Y, 16
Dong Q, 169
Donnelly B, 93
Dores GM, 152
Dubuc A, 211
Dudek AZ, 191
Dziunycz P, 225

E

Earle C, 99
Elkin EB, 11
Erickson BA, 7
Evans A, 81
Ewertz M, 27

F

Fassnacht M, 199
Feng Y, 141
Fergusson D, 99
Field TS, 46
Figueroa ME, 166
Filiaci VL, 127
Fleshner NE, 93
Flowers MED, 232
Flucke UE, 227
Foppa M, 202
Frassoldati A, 26

G

Garcia-Aguilar J, 142
Garcia-Henriquez N, 220
Garcia-Soto AE, 112
Gerlinger M, 2
Gerß J, 205
Ghebremichael M, 201
Giuliano AE, 21, 66
Goff BA, 113
Gomez-Iturriaga A, 85
Gönen M, 166
Gonzales AM, 11
Goode PS, 83
Goodwin PJ, 13

Gore EM, 173
Gourley C, 114
Goyal S, 31, 72
Green DM, 230
Greer JA, 196
Griggs JJ, 9
Grimm PD, 91
Groen HJ, 194
Guarneri V, 26
Gunnarsdóttir KÁ, 27

H

Hagan M, 87
Hamilton A, 156
Han J-Y, 178
Hanna RK, 128
Harter P, 114
Harvey RC, 208
Hawes D, 21, 171
Hayashi N, 75
He K, 16
Helgason GV, 156
Hernandez-Aya LF, 78
Higgins RV, 103
Hildebrandt G, 42, 44
Hillaby K, 106
Hirsh V, 188
Ho M, 163
Hoang T, 175
Holmfeldt L, 149
Horick NK, 1
Horsley S, 147
Horswell S, 2
Hou H-A, 157
Hunger SP, 207, 210
Hunt D, 95
Hunt KK, 66

I

Ibbott GS, 7
Ibrahim AR, 155

J

Janjigian YY, 179
Jänne PA, 183
Jenkins V, 243
Jensen BV, 55
Jensen M-B, 27
Johnson TM II, 83
Jones CU, 95

K

Kade S, 158
Kang JH, 140
Kapusta L, 93
Karaseva NA, 186
Karlan BY, 118
Karlsson P, 68
Katanyoo K, 124
Katsumata N, 122
Kawaguchi H, 38
Kaye SB, 116
Kee D, 225
Khera N, 232
Kilburn LS, 25
Kim S-W, 178
Kim SI, 32
Kim SY, 239
Kinney AY, 1
Kitagawa R, 122
Klein EA, 97
Klem ML, 11
Koh W-J, 132
König T, 205
Krag DN, 28
Krzakowski M, 187
Kuntz KM, 135
Kuo Y-Y, 157

L

Landier W, 229
Langridge C, 243
Largillier R, 109
Ledermann J, 114
Lee CH, 36
Lee JS, 188
Lee MK, 239
Lee SI, 140
Lei X, 78
Lemieux J, 13
Lim DH, 140
Lim K, 125
Liu C-Y, 157
Liu J, 75
Lo Nigro L, 206
Loehrer PJ Sr, 141
Lonardi S, 144
London WB, 215, 217
Lotan Y, 92
Lu X, 207
Lubinski J, 116
Lucas C, 155
Luft A, 180
Lupe K, 61
Lyden ER, 220
Lynch TJ, 180

M

Mahmoud SMA, 18
Majhail NS, 234
Malloy KM, 128
Malpica AL, 115
Mangu PB, 9
Manusirivithaya S, 124
Marcucci G, 154
Marin D, 155
Màrk Z, 192
Marth C, 109
Massey C, 213
Matthews B, 120
Matulonis U, 116
Maurillo L, 165
Mazzarella L, 159
McGowan DG, 95
McNeish IA, 237
Mead GM, 101
Metzeler KH, 154
Michalski J, 89
Minig L, 115
Missiaglia E, 218
Monclair T, 215
Moore DH, 132
Moran MS, 72
Morris AD, 53
Morris EA, 36
Motabi IH, 151
Motwani SB, 72
Mullighan CG, 208
Mulvihill JJ, 230
Murawska M, 40
Mussolin L, 167

N

Nag S, 87
Nakamura Y, 38
Naumann RW, 131
Neville BA, 65
Nick AM, 237
Niikura N, 75
Niwińska A, 40
Northcott PA, 211

O

Oberholzer PA, 225
Ohtsu A, 138

Oliver RTD, 101
Opie S, 160
Othus M, 164
Ott OJ, 42
Ou SH, 197
Oza AM, 118

P

Paik S, 71
Paish EC, 18
Pang HH, 191
Parikh PM, 185
Park BJ, 179
Park HS, 32
Park JR, 219
Park K, 178, 188
Park S, 32
Parker WT, 163
Parsons HM, 135
Pastorino U, 174
Patel JP, 166
Paugh BS, 212
Peiretti M, 126
Pereira Lima MN, 202
Perren TJ, 104
Piccart M, 74
Piedmonte MR, 130
Pillon M, 167
Pogoda K, 40
Pötter R, 42, 44
Powe DG, 18
Price JF, 5
Prout MN, 46
Pui C-H, 210

Q

Qu C, 212

R

Ramalingam SS, 193
Rastogi P, 22
Ready NE, 191
Rettig MP, 151
Richardson GE, 118
Rizzo JD, 160, 234
Rodeberg DA, 220
Roeffen MHS, 227
Rosenthal SA, 82
Rossi A, 189
Rothwell PM, 5
Rowan AJ, 2
Rücker FG, 150
Rusch VW, 171
Rustin GJS, 101

S

Saber W, 160
Sanguanrungsirikul S, 124
Sayre JW, 34
Scagliotti GV, 174, 187
Schemionek M, 156
Schiller JH, 175
Schlarmann C, 158
Schlenk RF, 150
Schmidt ML, 217
Schrappe M, 210
Schwartz GF, 20
Schwind S, 154
Scott HS, 163
Scott JR, 219
Secord AA, 103
Seiler CM, 145
Shah MA, 138
Shaw AT, 197
Shi Q, 142
Shteynshlyuger A, 86
Sietsma H, 194
Signorello LB, 230
Skjoldbye B, 55
Sloan JA, 170
Smaaland R, 100
Smith BD, 50
Socinski MA, 183, 186
Solberg A, 100
Solis-Trapala I, 243
Soria JC, 192
Spigel DR, 193
Spirtos NM, 127, 130
Stewart CF, 219
Stone RL, 237
Storer B, 232
Strnad V, 41
Strother DR, 217
Sun C-L, 229
Sundar S, 106
Sung JS, 36
Sylvester JE, 91
Szczesna A, 187

T

Tanaka K, 38
Tandstad T, 100
Tang G, 22
Tang J, 123
Tang Y, 123
Tangen CM, 97
Taras AR, 53
Temel JS, 196
Tewari KS, 127
Thol F, 158
Thomas CR Jr, 142
Thompson IM Jr, 97
Thorpe JD, 53
Tian C, 119
Triller N, 182
Trivers KF, 120
Truong PT, 61
Tuttle TM, 135

U

Uy GL, 151

V

Vaid A, 185
Valicenti RK, 89
Van Cutsem E, 138
van Dalen EC, 223
van Delden E, 223
van Delft FW, 147, 206
van der Pal HJ, 223
van der Wielen GJ, 90
van Gaal JC, 227
van Putten WLJ, 90
van Walraven C, 99
Vansteenkiste JF, 174
Vicini F, 31
Vincent A, 194
Vincent AD, 77
Visscher H, 233
Visser O, 47

W

Wagner U, 109
Walker JL, 130
Wallace K, 85

Walter RB, 164
Wang L-E, 169
Wang P, 16
Wang X, 183
Weaver DL, 28
Willer A, 205
Williamson D, 218
Wilson M, 5
Wingo SN, 112
Wo JY, 65
Wong J, 91
Wong SJ, 173
Wu J, 106
Wu X, 211

Y

Yahalom J, 148
Yang J, 123
Yin M, 169
Yun YH, 239

Z

Zakowski MF, 179
Zanagnolo V, 126
Zapardiel I, 126
Zatloukal P, 192
Zhang J, 149
Zhao J, 213
Zhou C, 128
Ziogas A, 1

Printed and bound by CPI Group (UK) Ltd, Croydon, CR0 4YY
08/05/2025
01864678-0002